1993

Germany: One Nation United, With Health Care for All

Germany: One Nation With Health Care for All

by Richard A. Knox

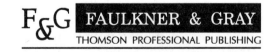

F&G FAULKNER & GRAY
THOMSON PROFESSIONAL PUBLISHING

Faulkner & Gray, Inc., New York
Healthcare Information Center, Washington DC

ISBN 1-881393-11-9

The sponsoring editor was Luci S. Koizumi; production
director was Susan Namovicz-Peat; project editor was
Amy Kilgallon Lee; indexed by L. Pilar Wyman.

Published by Faulkner & Gray's
Healthcare Information Center

1133 Fifteenth Street, NW
Washington DC 20005

PRINTED IN THE UNITED STATES OF AMERICA

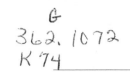
DEDICATION

To the memory of
A.L. Knox (1911-1989)
who believed in honest public debate.

ACKNOWLEDGEMENTS

This project was a perilous undertaking, especially for someone whose German language instruction was a long time ago and mostly useful these days only for singing Bach. I have tried to guard against errors of fact and interpretation, but I know some must lurk herein. Accept my apologies, and please don't blame my sources. From my German friends and readers, I ask special indulgence; I beg them to consider that an outsider's perspective may sometimes be valid even when it departs from conventional German wisdom.

This book owes everything to the generosity, patience, and support of a large number of people on both sides of the Atlantic, and to a few institutions. The *Boston Globe*'s willingness to let me have time off during an inconvenient period was a *sine qua non*, and I thank Jack Driscoll, Al Larkin, Ben Bradlee, and my reporting colleagues who had to take up the slack. Special thanks are due Kathy Everly and Alice Dembner, who shepherd the health and science specialists, for their faith and support. Also indispensable was the Commonwealth Fund, which provided a travel grant that took me to Germany twice. I am grateful to Thomas Moloney and Penny Duckham for their support, interest, faith, and flexibility. Robert Blendon, Karen Donelan, and their colleagues at the Harvard School of Public Health provided wonderful encouragement and advice. Bonnie Blanchfield shared information and insights from her investigation of German hospital finance.

On this side of the Atlantic are several impressive scholars who have long recognized the need for more information and analysis about German health care, and who were invaluable, both in their written work and in generously offering personal advice and insights. Among these are Deborah Stone, Donald W. Light, William A. Glaser, and Christa Altenstetter. Meg Murray, an American currently in Berlin studying the German health system, appeared by fax just when I needed her. Douglas Webber in Paris generously responded to my queries for information on the politics of German health care.

Special thanks go to my friend and colleague Joe Neel, Washington bureau chief of *Physician's Weekly*, who contributed the chapter on the German pharmaceutical industry. He was especially well equipped for this assignment, having studied and worked in Germany. More important, he has a keen analytical mind and a sure instinct for what is important. He contributed to this book in many other ways, material and spiritual.

Of course this kind of project depends critically on the assistance of the real experts on the German system — who often happen to be German. I am especially fortunate to have met Michael Arnold when he gave a fascinating talk at Harvard in the fall of 1990 that first inspired my interest. Professor Arnold, who established a center for health services research at the University of Tübingen, served for six years as chairman of the expert advisory panel of the national Council on Concerted Action in Health Care. He makes it his business to know everybody in German health care, and, equally important, he is unfailingly generous in arranging introductions, interviews, and itineraries for importunate Americans with unending questions. He will not agree with everything I have written as a result, but since he loves a good argument, I trust he will not consider me ungrateful.

Other Tübingen colleagues were also indispensable. Dr. Christoph Straub was a conscientious and hard-working coauthor of the chapter on the German hospital system despite other pressing priorities. Dominik von Stillfried provided valuable translation and research assistance, and was especially helpful on the history of the German system and on the pharmaceutical sector. Dr. Walburga Armann cheerfully answered a slew of data questions, and offered hospitality as well. Dr. Karl Lauterbach, who commutes these days between Tübingen and Boston, was always available for questions. Dr. Hans-Konrad Selbmann is an honest and generous investigator of data on the German health system. Frau Nixdorf and Frau Kukal efficiently did Prof. Arnold's bidding on my behalf, arranging and rearranging *Reisepläne* and appointments. Special thanks go to Jürgen in der Schmitten, who was an especially sensitive and indefatigable translator, has become a lifelong friend, and will make a wonderful doctor.

Claudia Himmelreich of the *Boston Globe*'s Berlin bureau was a super scout for up-to-the-minute health care reform and reunification news, and efficiently helped locate academic papers and data otherwise out of reach for a stateside reporter.

There are dozens of others in Germany who deserve thanks for their time and patience in helping me through the maze of their health system (and their language). Many, though regrettably by no means all of them, are named in the following pages. I need to make special mention of Dr. Hartmut Reichwage, a gentle man and dedicated physician who opened his home to me and spoke movingly about what it was like to emerge from 40 years behind the Iron Curtain. Dr. Peter Helmich offered insights about West German medical practice along with gracious hospitality.

Luci Koizumi and Amy Kilgallon Lee at Faulkner & Gray have been patient and understanding under terrific deadline pressure.

Finally, the fullest measure of gratitude belongs to my wife, Jean McBee Knox, whose support was crucial. To her, and to our wonderful daughters Elizabeth and Sarah ("Is your book finished yet, Dad?"), go undying thanks and love.

Dorchester, Massachusetts
April 11, 1993

PROLOGUE

For anyone who cares about health policy, this is a suspenseful time. Will the United States finally join the company of developed nations providing decent and secure health care to all their citizens as a matter of right? Or will a once-in-a-generation opportunity collapse, as it has so often, in a confused storm of partisan bickering, interest group-induced paralysis, and recrimination?

The stakes are incalculable, not only for President Clinton, Hillary Rodham Clinton, and the Democratic Party, but for every child, woman, and man in the nation, and for millions of unborn Americans. The number of people pushed outside the tattered tent of U.S. health insurance coverage seems certain to grow, absent some bold action. Those remaining inside will continue to find themselves sliding backwards, not only in terms of health coverage but in terms of the discretionary income they can devote to raising and educating their children, paying the mortgage, and saving for retirement. The relationship between U.S. employees and their employers will grow more embittered as companies slice coverage, shift costs, or drop health insurance altogether. Inequities will widen. Feelings will harden. Defensive maneuvers by health care providers will increase, further draining the depleted reservoir of moral authority and good will that U.S. hospitals and doctors used to take for granted. What remains of Americans' faith in government's ability to address *any* problem will evaporate. And, although this will be the least of America's problems in the event of such a failure, other nations will justifiably conclude that U.S. democracy is indeed in terminal decline.

Yet success — even a good solid start on the road to U.S. health care reform — is by no means assured. No other domestic problem could harder to solve. The fact that other nations are grappling successfully with the Hydra-headed health care monster offers needed encouragement to jaded Americans. It is heartening to know that the world's oldest health care financing scheme, the one that most closely resembles America's public-private approach, is confronting many of the same challenges as we are and managing to cope. Germany has not compromised yet on its long commitment to universal coverage, fairness, comprehensiveness, and high-quality health care. Germany's health care system is troubled, for many of the same reasons as America's. But the Germans are far from immobilized. They are meeting the challenge of extending the West's high standard of health care to 16 million new citizens in the East — a task proportionately greater than the mainstreaming of America's 37 million uninsured citizens. Moreover, reunification is not deflecting Germans from their effort to reform their health care system so it might withstand the buffeting of cost-increasing new technology, a rapidly aging population, and an uncertain economic future.

Clearly, American policymakers need to know more about how Germany's well-tested health care system works. Too many reject the notion that the U.S. has something useful to learn from Germany's (or any other nation's) health care system. The often-repeated reasons — Americans are too individualistic, our standards are unequalled, our social burdens would overwhelm any system of universal health care entitlement, and so forth — are shallow truisms. Their subtext is: Accept the *status quo*, or some minor reworkings of it at best.

Faulkner & Gray's Luci Koizumi would tell you that I vacillated a good deal when she approached me in late 1992 to ask if I would write this book. At the time it looked like Bill Clinton was really going to win. As a medicine and health reporter for the *Boston Globe* who covered President Nixon's ill-fated health reform proposal, it seemed unwise to take myself out of the loop for even a few months as the Clinton Administration prepared to take its shot at the Hydra. A health reporter's chance to cover presidential-level health care reform can't be counted on to come around more than twice in a career span. But I allowed myself to be tempted. A trip to Germany during a Harvard sabbatical in 1991 had whetted my appetite to know more about the German health care system — and what better way to learn more than to write a book?

Now that the task is done, I *still* want to know more about how the Germans do it. But I trust that the increasing number of Americans who seem open-minded and curious about the question will find in the following pages the beginning of an answer. My hope is that this effort will open a few more minds, encourage a positivist attitude toward U.S. health care reform, and stimulate health service researchers to help all of us understand better the tradeoffs Germans have made so that we — and they — might proceed more wisely.

TABLE OF CONTENTS

CHAPTER 1

The Relevance of Germany's Achievement for U.S. Health Policy

G ermany's system of universal national health insurance, which is 110 years old in 1993, ranks as the world's oldest and, by many measures, the world's most successful. "The German health care system," notes J.-Matthias Graf von der Schulenburg, director of the Institute for Insurance Economics at the University of Hannover, "has managed to achieve a number of partly conflicting goals at the same time: comprehensive coverage and equal access for everyone, freedom of choice, high-quality medicine, and cost containment."[1]

The overriding lesson of the German experience is simply that it is feasible to provide high-quality health care through a universal, affordable, and equitable financing mechanism with impressive durability.

At the same time, Germany is struggling with major health care problems. These issues have recently prompted enactment of some of the most sweeping reforms in the history of its system, and German authorities expect more to come. The difficulties that prompted the 1993 reforms are familiar to all industrialized nations, though some are peculiar to the German way of organizing and financing medical services. But it is important to remember that Germany's latest health care problems would not loom so large or require such urgent action were it not for the unique burdens of German reunification coinciding with economic stagnation.

Making It Work in the U.S.

Is the success of this system achievable only under the particular historical and cultural circumstances that have shaped Germany's health system and strongly undergird it today? Can major aspects of Germany's achievement be adapted to America's very different ethos, world view, and political constraints?

Ultimately, these questions are unanswerable without real world, trial-and-error experimentation (which is, in fact, precisely the way Germany's system evolved). An assessment of whether such an experiment would be wise or foolish requires thoughtful consideration of how Germany's system actually works, and how it got to its present stage of evolution.

Given the documented record, it is not surprising that Germany's health system has recently been cited as a possible model, at least in part, for reform of the U.S. health care system. In fact, Germany and Canada have become the most frequently mentioned models in the current U.S. debate. This marks the first time in decades American policymakers and analysts have looked to other industrialized nations for "elements...that might prove useful in the restructuring of a system troubled by problems of spiraling costs and limited access to care for an increasing proportion of the population," says Harvard University professor Robert J. Blendon.[2] Keen interest in the German model spans a broad portion of America's ideological spectrum. Germany's federal structure for negotiating health expenditures and controling costs shaped major aspects of the "HealthAmerica" reform proposal drafted by Democratic leaders of the U.S. Senate.[3] "The German system," James S. Todd, MD, executive vice president of the American Medical Association, has said, "has more relevance to the need for reform in this country than any other nation we've looked at yet....We don't see the deficiencies in the German system that we see in the Canadian system."[4] A recent report issued by the Health Insurance Association of America, noting that Germany "now seems to be the focus of particular attention," ascribed the interest to the fact that the German system "bears more resemblance to the U.S. system" than Canada's does, is "decidedly pluralistic," and "has been more successful at limiting the rate of increase of costs."[5]

During his successful 1992 campaign for the U.S. Presidency, Bill Clinton—who speaks and reads German himself[6]—often cited Germany as an example of a health care system that works. "For the last five years, Germany's health care costs have gone up slightly less than the rate of inflation," Clinton noted in the most extended health policy speech of his campaign. "That may be one reason why the average German factory worker makes 20 percent more than the average American for working a shorter work week, gets four weeks paid vacation, family leave, and has comprehensive health care."[7]

"No wonder President-elect Clinton and his health care advisers sing the praises of Germany's insurance system," wrote Marc Fisher, the *Washington Post's* Bonn correspondent. "Unlike other much-ballyhooed national health programs, Germany's approach to health care boasts much of what Americans say they want: private physicians, job-based insurance, and no bloated federal bureaucracy."[8]

Snapshot of a Health System

Despite this recent enthusiasm, detailed knowledge of how the German health care system works is largely lacking among many otherwise sophisticated U.S. policymakers and academic authorities. The English-language literature on the German system is relatively sparse, and what exists is the health services equivalent of "anatomy" rather than "physiology." In other words, it summarizes the system's principal features rather than detailing how it actually works and why it has been, relatively speaking, so successful. Even in Germany, health services research is an infant field and in-depth analyses are surprisingly rare, according to both foreign and native scholars. Quality assurance is likewise underdeveloped by American standards. Even basic epidemiological data to judge the performance of the system in terms of the public's health "is very sketchy."[9]

Keeping the Costs Down

The most enviable aspect of Germany's health care system, from an American vantage point, is its success so far in constraining costs. "Among industrialized countries, West Germany's health insurance system came closest during the 1980s to limiting increases in spending to a rate that equaled the growth of its national income," observes John K. Iglehart, national correspondent of the *New England Journal of Medicine*. "The disparity between the two measures was greatest in the United States."[10]

As a proportion of national wealth, the measure most often used in international comparisons of health expenditures, Germany spent 8.1 percent of its gross domestic product (GDP) on health care in 1990, ranking ninth-highest among 24 member nations of the Organization for Economic Cooperation and Development (OECD). Germany's 1990 expenditure was 38 percent lower than the United States'.[11] (Table 1.1)

This is all the more striking when one considers that Germany is not as wealthy as the U.S.; thus, its significantly lower share of health spending was in relation to an economic base substantially smaller than America's. On a per capita basis, German GDP was $18,317 in 1990, 20 percent lower than the Americans' per capita GDP of $21,933.

Another way to capture the priority a society places on health care is to compare per capita health spending. Germans spent $1,486 per person on health care in 1990, while the U.S. spent $2,566—73 percent more. Canada, with a per capita GDP about the same as Germany's, spent 20 percent more per person in 1990 on health care.[12]

Such a snapshot still fails to convey Germany's most notable achievement: its ability in recent years to keep health costs relatively stable compared to other modern societies. George Schieber of the U.S. Health Care Financing Administration and his colleagues recently analyzed health expenditure trends in six developed nations—the United States, Canada, United Kingdom, Germany, France, and Japan—and found Germany was the only one to have experienced a decline in health spending as a percentage of GDP between 1980 and 1990. Among all 24 OECD countries, Germany is one of only four, including Sweden, Denmark, and Japan, that experienced a decline in health's share of national spending during the 1980s. Of the six countries, Germany also had the lowest growth rate in per capita health spending on an inflation-adjusted basis, only 1.1 percent per year in the 1980s.[13]

A graph of per capita health spending shows a steady upward trend since 1960 for many developed nations. However, Germany and the United States stand out—Germany because its health expenditures appeared to level off and even decline in the late 1980s, and the United States because its per capita health spending steadily accelerated at a rate that diverges from the OECD norm in the past 15 years.[14] (Figure 1.1) During the 1980s, U.S. health

Table 1.1

Ranking of OECD Nations in Total Health Expenditures as a Percent of Gross Domestic Product, 1990

Country	Health spending as percent of GDP	Compound annual growth rate 1980-90
United States	**12.1%**	**2.7%**
Canada	9.3%	2.3%
France	8.8%	1.6%
Iceland	8.6%	2.9%
Sweden	8.6%	-0.9%
Austria	8.4%	0.6%
Australia	8.2%	1.1%
Netherlands	8.2%	0.2%
Germany	**8.1%**	**-0.4%**
Finland	7.8%	1.9%
Italy	7.7%	1.2%
Switzerland	7.7%	0.5%
Belgium	7.5%	1.2%
New Zealand	7.4%	0.2%
Norway	7.4%	1.1%
Luxembourg	7.2%	0.5%
Ireland	7.0%	-2.6%
Portugal	6.7%	1.2%
Spain	6.6%	1.7%
Japan	6.5%	0.1%
Denmark	6.3%	-0.8%
United Kingdom	6.2%	0.7%
Greece	5.5%	2.4%
Turkey	4.0%	0.0%

Source: George J. Schieber et. al., Health Care Financing Review, *Summer 1992.*

Figure 1.1

Per Capita Health Spending in U.S. Dollars, Selected OECD Countries, 1960–91

Listed using purchasing power parities instead of exchange rates

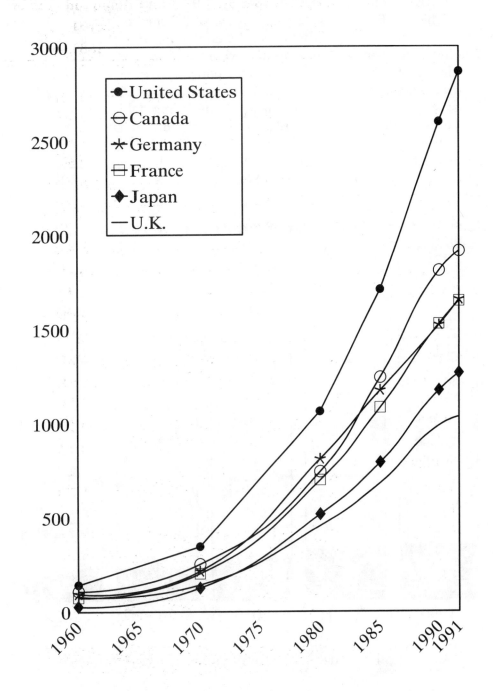

Source: Health OECD, Facts and Trends *(Paris: OECD, Forthcoming).*

expenditures outpaced economic growth by 33 percent per year, on average. This is 10 times higher than excess health care inflation in Germany during that period.[15]

Germany has achieved relative control of health care costs in the face of an aging population that is exerting a strong upward push in medical spending. In 1988 (the most recent figure available), 15.4 percent of Germany's population was older than 65 years. This surpasses the average in all OECD nations except the United Kingdom (with 15.6 percent in 1988) and Denmark (with 15.4 percent). The over-65 population in the U.S. was 12.3 percent in 1988, 20 percent lower than Germany's. This is not a recent trend in Germany; the cost pressures of an aging population have operated for years. As long ago as 1975, the over-65 population of West Germany was 14.3 percent, a level which will not be reached in Japan until the year 2000 and not until 2005 in France.[16] (Figure 1.2) At the same time, the overall population is declining, which means that the medical bills of Germany's aged will be borne by a dwindling number of actively

Figure 1.2

Projection of German Population, by Age, 1990 to 2030 (in millions)

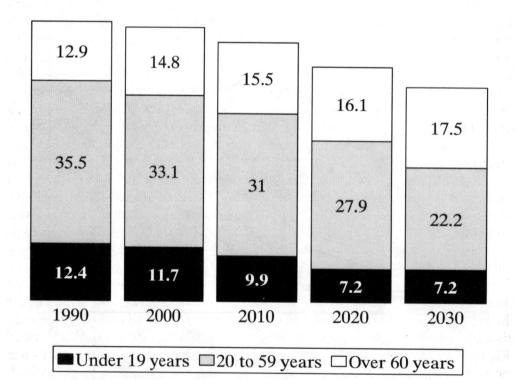

Source: Federal Minister for Youth, Family Affairs, Women and Health, The Health Care System in the Federal Republic of Germany (Bonn-Bad Godesberg, February 1988).

employed citizens. While the burden is still tolerable, the demographic trend will pose a serious challenge to the system in the future, as German policymakers are well aware.

What Do the Germans Think?

Given the success of the German health care system up to now, one might wonder if Germany has purchased cost control by stinting on the quality or quantity of medical services, or by oppressing its health care providers. The available evidence—supplemented by interviews with a wide variety of German health care providers, administrators, government officials, and analysts—does not support this contention. On the contrary, West Germans are among the most satisfied citizens surveyed in major industrialized nations about their health care arrangements. Available data indicate that most German patients and providers are satisfied with most aspects of their system.

For instance, a 1990 Louis Harris survey of citizens in six nations commissioned by the Harvard Community Health Plan found that 8 percent of (West) Germans expressed dissatisfaction with their health care—slightly less than the 10 percent registered by U.S. patients. Among Germans, 92 percent said they were "somewhat" or "very" satisfied, compared to 88 percent of Americans. In that survey, Germans' overall satisfaction with their health services trailed that of Canadians (who spent 60 percent more per capita on health care in 1990 than Germans), but was higher than the British, Swedes, or Japanese.[17]

Germans were less likely to be satisfied than Americans with particular aspects of their health care system, such as waiting times for a doctor's appointment, personal control, access to technology, and access to elective surgery. However, citizens of both nations were fairly comparable in their satisfaction with health care quality, the availability of top-quality care for everyone, and out-of-pocket expenses—despite the fact that Germans' out-of-pocket medical expenses are much lower than Americans'. Germans are much less likely than Americans to say that spending on such items as medical technology, patient care, physicians, or hospitalization is "too high."[18] (Figure 1.3)

A 1992 German poll also found that two-thirds of respondents supported the existing government-guaranteed system of social security, which includes health coverage. More than half said their financial contributions to health insurance were appropriate, and one-third said the burden was too high (1.1 percent said contributions were too low and 10 percent said they didn't know).[19]

A recent 10-nation public opinion survey, conducted by researchers at the Harvard School of Public Health, Louis Harris Associates, and the Institute for the Future, found that significant minorities of citizens in all the countries were dissatisfied with health care in some degree, and Germany was no exception.[20] (Figure 1.4) The Harvard analysts concluded that Americans' dissatisfaction is rooted in a widespread feeling of insecurity about their health coverage, which can disappear entirely with loss of employment or changing job status and is being sharply eroded even for those who have insurance. Whatever their complaints, this is a worry that does not concern Germans. "People would not accept that they wouldn't have insurance, or if they lose their job they lose their insurance," comments Ulrich Bopp, director of the Bosch Foundation in Stuttgart, a leading German philanthropy. "It's part of our political culture."[21]

Even the Doctors Approve

Health care providers in Germany are also happier with their system than their U.S. counterparts, judging from a recent Harvard School of Public Health survey of doctors in the United States, (West) Germany, and Canada.[22]

A majority of doctors in all three nations said major changes are needed to make their respective health systems work better—a reflection of the fact that

Figure 1.3

Percentage of Respondents Indicating "Very Satisfied" or "Somewhat Satisfied" with All Aspects of Health Care System: Germany and the United States

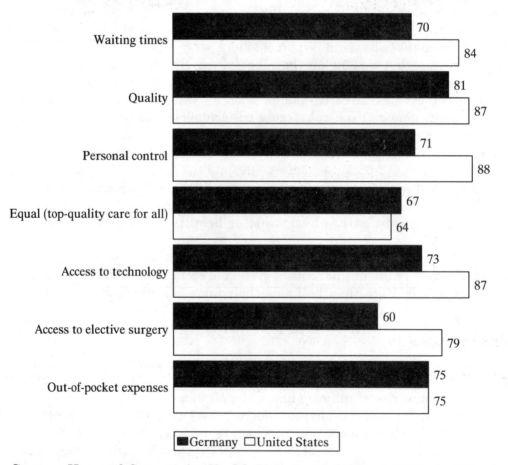

Source: Harvard Community Health Plan, Annual Report 1990: An International Comparison of Health Care Systems, *(Brookline, MA: Harvard Community Health Plan, 1990).*

Figure 1.4

Citizens' View of Their Health Care Systems in the United States and Germany, 1990

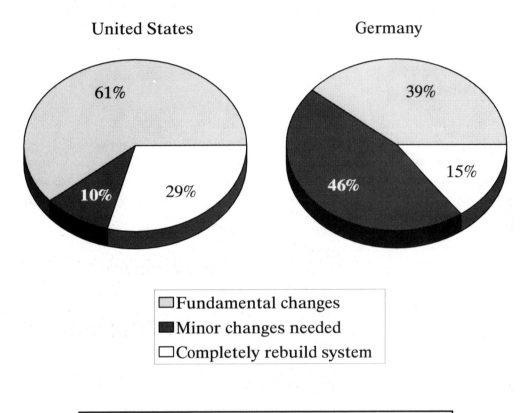

Per Capita Health Expenditures (in U.S. dollars)	
U.S.	$2,051
Germany	$1,486

Source: Health Affairs, *Summer 1990.*

no nation has yet found the magic formula that balances cost, access, and quality considerations well enough to keep patients and providers fully content. But 48 percent of German physicians thought their system "works pretty well and only minor changes are necessary to make it work better," whereas only 23 percent of American doctors agreed with that statement. Only one in five German physicians complained about lack of access to well-equipped facilities, compared to one in seven U.S. doctors. And German doctors were less likely to advise a student against a career in medicine (33 percent said they would do so) than U.S. doctors (37 percent).

Like America's, a Pluralistic System

Germany's achievement in stabilizing health costs while retaining broad popular and provider support for the health financing system is not the only feature attractive to American reformers. The German system is not government-run, in either its financing or its delivery. This also has appeal for Americans ideologically opposed to government sponsorship and for others convinced that a tax-financed, government-administered health system is unlikely to gain political favor in the U.S. Objections voiced by pragmatists include
- American distrust of government,
- the political clout of the health insurance industry and other interests opposed to a British- or Canadian-style system, and
- U.S. budget deficits that would preclude any major new on-budget social program.

The German approach suggests another path. It presents an alternate role for government—a limited and collaborative one, but sovereign and effective nonetheless. Under this role, which is still evolving to meet new circumstances after 11 decades, the government
- mandates financing of health care by employers and employees;
- sets the rules by which those parties must pay contributions to health plans, called *Krankenkassen* or "sickness funds" (but does not set each plan's premiums);
- requires and defines coverage and payment mechanisms for pensioners;
- subsidizes or pays outright the health insurance premiums of the unemployed and destitute;
- specifies which payer and provider organizations may participate in the mandatory health insurance system;
- defines and regulates the market for private health insurance;
- requires explicit cross-subsidization among insured groups in order to equalize risks, and forbids hidden, involuntary cross-subsidies;
- authorizes specific organizations of payers and providers to bargain over the flow of payments at the federal, state, and regional levels;
- sets limits to providers' claims on health care funds;
- monitors the operation of the system in collaboration with major stake-holders;
- tries to anticipate problems and takes corrective action to modify any of the above parameters when the affected parties cannot resolve difficulties or meet societal goals.

These powers are formidable, but they are fundamentally different from the part in health care financing played by Britain's National Health Service, Canada's provincial governments, Sweden's County Councils—or, indeed, the U.S. Government's Medicare and Medicaid programs, the first- and second-largest U.S. third-party payers. Whatever the differences in these systems, they are alike in that government acts directly to collect taxes and pay providers, with all the powers this implies. It determines benefits, sets fees and prices, processes and pays bills, reviews utilization, and otherwise polices providers and intermediaries.

Generally, the German government does not directly finance or pay for health care services. The only exceptions to this are
   □ direct payments that local governments sometimes make for the care of the chronically unemployed—what Americans would call "welfare" clients;
   □ direct contributions government makes to the medical bills of higher-level civil servants, such as teachers and professors; and
   □ direct coverage government provides to police and members of the military.

Public expenditures for health care account for only 13 percent of the federal budget, compared to 42 percent in the U.S. The government's role in Germany is to mandate, specify, authorize, referee, consult, collaborate, regulate, monitor, and supervise. To help the federal government "steer" the system, the German Parliament in 1977 created an advisory panel called "Concerted Action in Health Care" chaired by the Minister of Health. This panel is and made up of representatives of all the interested parties, including payers, physicians, hospitals, pharmaceutical companies, medical equipment manufacturers, and others—but, significantly, no consumer representatives. (Table 1.2) The Concerted Action panel has no statutory powers and seems to work mainly through moral suasion "and the incentive the participants have to avoid further cost-containment laws."[23] Its twice-yearly pronouncements influence negotiations of providers and payers as well as the shape of remedial legislation.

Cooperation and Consensus

As a number of commentators have observed, the success of the German system depends upon a disposition on the part of all players—indeed, of the political culture—to achieve consensus. There is "a cultural preference that favors reaching compromises before deadlock occurs—a preference that is quite evident throughout German life," John L. Iglehart observed in a two-part 1991 series on German health care in the *New England Journal of Medicine*.

This is a very different orientation from the American temper, which is adversarial rather than collaborative. It is easy to overplay this consensual impulse, however. Germany's health care stage is also crowded with fierce adversaries. Politics, after all, is politics. The difference is that opposing interests in the U.S. are not given official roles and responsibilities. Germany has developed a framework of countervailing forces in which the considerable power of the medical and dental professions, insurance funds, pharmaceutical companies, hospital interests, and other players is carefully checked. In addition, government waits in the wings to impose a resolution if negotiations break

Table 1.2

Concerted Action in Health Care

Composition of Germany's "Concerted Action in Health Care Panel" members are named by the Federal Minister of Health from the following groups:

National Association of Local Sickness Funds

National Association of Factory-Based Sickness Funds

National Association of Craftsmen's Funds

National Association of Farmers' Sickness Funds

Miners' Sickness Fund

National Association of Substitute Sickness Funds

National Association of Private Health Insurers

National Association of Statutory Health Insurance Physicians

National Association of Statutory Health Insurance Dentists

National Physicians Chamber (deals with licensure and ethics)

National Dentists Chamber (deals with licensure and ethics)

German Hospital Association

National Association of German Pharmacists

National Association of Pharmaceutical Manufacturers

National Association of Trade Unions (blue-collar workers)

German Association of Salaried Employees (white-collar workers)

German Civil Servants Union

National Association of Employers' Associations

National Association of Communities

State Ministers of Labor

State Conference of Health Ministers

State Conference of Social Affairs

Federal Health Ministry

Federal Economics Ministry

Federal Ministry of Labor

Source: Klaus-Dirk Henke (1988). "Funktionsweise und Steuerwirksamkeit der Konzertierten Aktion im Gesundheitswesen (KAiG)." In Gerard Gafgen (ed.), Neokorporatismus und Gesundheitswesen. *Baden-Baden: Nomos Verlagsgesellschaft, pp. 113-158.*

down or the system is not performing the way it is supposed to. This process will be discussed in detail in later chapters.

Financing the Care

The difference is expressed most visibly in the structure of the German health system, often characterized as corporatism. That is, discrete private health care interests are organized into powerful groups and given official standing by statute to represent their interests in the bargaining process that determines the flow of funds as well as in the daily operation of the system. The governing principle is that socially undesirable concentrations of power in one or another vested interest can be prevented by giving these organizations powers over one another. Corporatism "is a form of managed conflict," observes political scientist Donald W. Light.[24] In a sense, this is similar to the U.S. division of government powers, within the federal and state governments and between these levels. But in the U.S. such checks and balances are never officially extended to the private sector, nor is economic power ever formally delegated, by statute, to private groups.

"American solutions," observes Deborah Stone, a Brandeis University political scientist who has written extensively on the German health care system, "have typically been based on the idea of structuring authority so as to *fragment* strong groups." U.S. antitrust law is one prominent example. Germany, Stone notes, has taken a very different approach, deliberately *consolidating* the power of private economic interests in order to define it, set countervailing groups against one another, and manage the system.[25]

Because of this multiplicity of formal roles, the German health care system seems forbiddingly complex to an outsider (as the pluralistic but less structured U.S. system undoubtedly appears to non-Americans). Germany has more than 1,100 separate statutory health insurance funds of seven different types for a population of 83 million.[26] These are publicly chartered nonprofit corporations which alone have legal authority to receive federally mandated payroll contributions from workers and their employers. In addition, there are 50 private for-profit health insurers. By comparison, the U.S. has only about 1,250 health insurers for a population three times larger.[27]

Private Insurance—Public Rules

Health care financing in Germany operates through largely private channels, but according to strict and rather detailed federal laws. Contributions to sickness funds are mandatory for most of the population. Every citizen earning up to 58,500 deutschmarks ($36,270 in terms of 1991 currency exchange rates, $24,570 in terms of purchasing power parity conversion) must enroll in a statutory sickness fund. For practical purposes, this is a payroll tax, but technically it is not. Contributions are not collected by any government entity but are paid directly to the sickness funds, which are self-governing, private corporations operating under public charter.

Federal statute in Germany requires that contributions to sickness funds (what Americans call "premiums") and to private insurers (called "tariffs" by Germans) must be split evenly by employers and employees. By law sickness funds must offer a standard package of benefits that is quite generous by U.S. standards. They encompass

- unlimited ambulatory physician care, generally without copayment, including home visits;
- unlimited hospital care, with minor copayments, limited to 10 days;
- maternity care (including household help);
- prescription drugs, with limited copayments;
- medical supplies and devices;
- preventive care;
- family planning services;
- rehabilitative services, including attendants;
- periodic "rest cures" at certified health spas;
- dental care, with copayments for dentures;
- optical services and eyeglasses; and
- ambulance transport.

However, Germany's liberal benefits do not include much long term care coverage, though recently sickness funds have been paying for some respite care and home care for elders. Private insurers may depart from statutory benefits, but usually match them. Private policies often impose deductibles and copayment requirements on their subscribers, at least for ambulatory services.[28]

Who Is Covered By Which Fund?

About two-thirds of the German population must obtain health care coverage through a sickness fund. These are workers and their dependents whose annual income falls below approximately the same income ceiling that is the basis for sickness fund contributions. Many of the mandatory sickness fund members have no choice of which fund to join, either because they work for a company with its own sickness fund (12 percent of sickness fund members and dependents) or because they are not eligible for any fund other than one of the 268 geographically based local funds, which enroll 42 percent of the 55 million people[29] who belong to sickness funds.

The local sickness funds, company-based funds, and others dedicated to craftsmen, agricultural workers, seamen, and miners are called **primary funds**, or *RVO* funds (for *Reichsversicherungsordnung* or "state insurance regulation," referring to the 1911 law that is the statutory basis for the social insurance system). The other major category of sickness funds is called **substitute funds**, or *Ersatzkassen*. These seven funds, open primarily to white-collar workers, enroll about 35 percent of all sickness fund members. Substitute funds provide almost identical benefits as the primary funds, but they carry a degree of social cache because membership is an emblem of higher employment status and because they pay doctors about twice as much as RVO funds do. Thus, substitute funds are seen as buying their members better service.

Other Kinds of Coverage

Though the sickness funds cover 88 percent of the German population, they account for only about half the nation's total health care expenditures. The rest comes from pension funds, private insurers, accident insurers, and government programs of various kinds.[30]

Retired people generally have coverage through the sickness fund or private insurer they belonged to as active workers. Premiums are set at the national average for active workers and, like workers, the contributions are evenly split between retirees (withheld from monthly pension checks) and a government pension fund.[31] But these contributions cover only about half the cost of pensioners' care. The difference comes from surcharges on active workers' premiums, adjusted for each sickness fund's number of retirees to equalize the burden nationally.[32,33]

Because their incomes are above the statutory income threshold, 20 to 30 percent of all Germans can opt out of the statutory sickness funds and insure themselves privately. Only one-third of them, or fewer, do.[34] The economic incentives of private insurance in Germany strongly favor those who are single or childless couples. Premiums are calculated on an individual-insured basis; that is, a separate, risk-rated premium is charged for each member of a family, while sickness fund members pay a flat premium regardless of family size. Those who are self-employed, including many professionals, also buy private insurance because they cannot gain access to sickness funds. Certain civil servants whose medical bills are partially paid by their respective government employers buy supplemental private coverage to pay the unpaid balance. Still, only about 10 percent of the population is privately insured. While this market has shown some growth in recent years, some analysts do not expect substantial increases among the privately insured in future years.[35]

The Delivery System: Similar Yet Different

If the financing side of German health care seems complex, the delivery side is no less so. Outwardly, Germany's delivery system bears strong resemblance to America's. Ambulatory doctors are private entrepreneurs, their offices are well-equipped, and they are paid by the fee-for-service method that still dominates U.S. medical practice. The hospital community is a mixture of private nonprofit institutions, publicly owned facilities, some for-profit private hospitals, and university teaching hospitals. Outwardly German hospitals resemble their U.S. counterparts; the flagship institutions compare favorably in terms of physical plant and equipment.

The internal organization of German medical providers differs in significant ways from those in the U.S., however, and their relationships with payers is quite different. Within the medical profession, the most striking difference is the wall that separates hospital-based physicians from ambulatory doctors. With few exceptions, doctors who practice in hospitals may not treat outpatients and, until very recently, they could not even perform preadmission tests on patients.[36] Office-based physicians may not treat their patients once they have entered a hospital. Payment methods are different on either side of the wall too. Hospital-based doctors are salaried, and only department chiefs may collect extra fees above the salary, while office-based doctors are paid a fee for each service they provide. The multispecialty group practices and salaried staff-model health maintenance organizations common in the U.S. have no counterparts in German medicine. (The German states of former East Germany retain some multispecialty clinics where physicians are salaried. As will be discussed in a Chapter Seven, these clinics are remnants of the East German health care system, and their future is in doubt.)

German hospitals, in addition to having full-time salaried medical staff, differ in other important ways from their U.S. counterparts. A bare majority of them are publicly owned (by states, as is the case of all teaching hospitals, and by municipalities), while only 29 percent of U.S. hospitals are public institutions. Consequently, a much higher proportion of U.S. hospitals are not-for-profit voluntary institutions (60 percent) compared to Germany (35 percent). Many more voluntary institutions in Germany are church-sponsored (either Roman Catholic or Protestant). The proportion of investor-owned hospitals is similar—14 percent in Germany versus 11 percent in the U.S.

A Different Style of Care

The statistics also suggest that German hospitals provide a very different style of care. There are almost twice as many acute-care beds per 1,000 population as in the U.S. Occupancy rates are 30 percent higher, and the number of patient-days per 1,000 people is two-and-one-half times higher. Germans are admitted to the hospital 46 percent more often and, once admitted, spend 72 percent longer there than Americans. Inpatient care is less intensive, as reflected by a staffing ratio 56 percent lower than in U.S. hospitals.[37]

These "anatomical" differences owe a great deal to the very different relationship that German hospitals have with those who pay the bills. Most strikingly, there is a sharp division in hospital financing between operating costs (which come from the various third-party payers) and capital funds (which since 1972 have come from government—even for private, for-profit institutions). Between 1982 and 1986, capital funds came from the federal and state governments. Since 1986, they have come exclusively from state governments, called *Länder*. Capital funds are allotted through a health planning process similar to state Certificate-of-Need programs in the U.S.

This absolute state control over inpatient infrastructure is a relatively recent phenomenon that has only begun to reverse a widely recognized overcapacity problem. Excess hospital capacity has been fueled by a per diem reimbursement mechanism which rewards high admission rates and long lengths-of-stay.

Paying the Providers

This brings us to the key difference between the German and U.S. health systems: the relationship between providers and payers. This is where the corporatist structure of the German system really makes a difference—for better and for worse—in terms of function and cost.

Major providers of health services are organized, for the purpose of reimbursement, into layered arrays of associations at the federal, state, and regional levels. At the federal level, provider and payer groups bargain over annual expenditure constraints and how they should apply to various sectors. They also argue over changes in policy designed to correct failures in cost control and equity in financing. State associations of providers and payers translate these goals to their realms and oversee their regional constituents as they implement the policies. Regional negotiations are "where the rubber meets the road." This is where most sickness funds negotiate actual annual budgets with local provider groups. (The seven substitute funds are organized on a national, not a regional, basis.)

Physicians. Office-based doctors are obliged to belong to a regional **Association of Sickness Fund Physicians** if they wish to treat the 88 percent of the population insured through the statutory sickness funds. They also must belong to their respective state **Physician Chambers**, which have authority over licensing, specialty certification, and physician discipline. Of course, they may—and usually do—belong to voluntary associations, such as one that represents physicians in ambulatory practice, another that represents hospital-based doctors, groups of hospital department chiefs, specialty societies, and so forth. The compulsory associations, which have no close U.S. counterparts, have statutorily delegated powers and responsibilities, whereas the others are similar to U.S. interest groups such as the American Medical Association or the American College of Surgeons.

The Associations of Sickness Fund Physicians, called *kassenärztliche Vereinigungen* or *KVs*, who represent only office-based doctors, have two main functions.

1. They negotiate annually with sickness funds over the total amount of payment they will receive from the funds, based on the projected number of insurees and anticipated expenditure per enrollee. Since 1977, these negotiations have been constrained by a federal law that does not allow ambulatory physician expenditures to grow faster than the average German wage.
2. They are reimbursement intermediaries between sickness funds and their member physicians. They receive quarterly lump-sum payments from the funds based on the negotiated budgets, and they pay member physicians.

Physician payment is based on quarterly vouchers, called *Krankenscheine* or **sickness certificates**. Sickness funds provide these vouchers to their members, who hand them over to physicians in exchange for treatment. Technically, patients are supposed to get one *Krankenschein* per quarter, but Germans say it is easy to obtain more, thus enabling them to see more than one primary physician at a time, or to self-refer to specialists. Ambulatory doctors itemize the services they have provided to each sickness fund's members on each voucher then submit the collected *Krankenscheine* to the respective sickness funds. Services are enumerated in point values set at the federal level and based on the relative time, skill, and resources involved; for example, a telephone consultation may be worth 80 points, a home visit 360 points, and an x-ray between 360 and 900 points. Doctors may not "balance-bill," or charge sickness fund members extra beyond fund reimbursement. Private insurers pay doctors approximately twice as much as statutory sickness funds, leading to the widespread belief that private patients enjoy such amenities as fixed appointment times and greater attention.

Because of the federally determined annual expenditure cap on ambulatory physician services, doctors are financially at risk. If they bill for more services (i.e., more points) than was allowed for in the annual budget negotiations, the value of each point will be reduced so the overall expenditure cap for that region will not be exceeded. Certain services deemed socially desirable, such as cancer screenings, well-child visits, and other preventive care, are exempt from the cap. The threat of reduced reimbursement is an incentive not to provide unnecessary services, but it works imperfectly. Doctors complain bitterly that much additional utilization is beyond their control because the physician supply is rising much faster than population growth.

Because expenditure caps alone have not controlled physician costs, the Associations of Sickness Fund Physicians also perform utilization review in conjunction with associations of sickness funds. The mechanisms and scope of these activities will be discussed in Chapter Five.

Dentists. Dentists' reimbursement works along much the same lines as physician payment, except that there is no expenditure cap. Dental care is a more important component of health insurance in Germany than it is in the U.S.

Hospitals. The relationship between hospitals and third-party payers is also regional, but hospital associations do not play a direct role in determining reimbursement levels, budgets, or actual payment. Instead, annual global budgets are set through direct annual negotiations between individual hospitals and sickness funds. The local sickness funds, called the *Allgemeine Ortskrankenkasse*, normally take the lead in these negotiations because they claim the most members and thus contribute the largest share of hospitals' operating revenues.

The key budget-setting calculation is an historically projected number of patient days. Once a global budget is agreed upon, the allowed revenue is simply divided by the expected number of patient-days to derive the *Pflegesatz*, or per diem rate, that each sickness fund will pay the hospital. Private insurers reimburse more generously than sickness fund, but their payments are also based on an average daily rate. In negotiating the budget, sickness funds conduct a detailed review of hospitals' operating costs, including

☐ staffing ratios and compensation (including physicians),
☐ routine depreciation,[38]
☐ occupancy,
☐ utilization trends, and
☐ other inputs.

Sickness funds have the advantage of considerable data from all hospitals in their area, and they use this—as they are authorized by law to do—to bargain down the budgetary demands of less-efficient hospitals. Agreement is almost always reached, since the alternative is considered unpalatable by both sides: binding arbitration by a state government panel. Teaching hospitals have special status in these regional negotiations, since they are part state governments and also answerable to a powerful federal science advisory council when they wish to expand services. But they still must justify their budgets to the sickness funds that pay their per diem rates.

Hospital budget discipline is enforced through **reimbursement corridors**, to use the American term. That is, if hospitals generate more patient-days than anticipated, their marginal reimbursement will be 25 percent of the established per diem rate. If they have underestimated their volume, they will be penalized by a per diem rate 75 percent of the negotiated level. Certain high-tech services, such as organ transplants, are exempted from the general per diem reimbursement scheme and paid for on a fee-for-service basis. The rationale is that these services attract referrals from a wide area and should not be solely the responsibility of the sickness funds in the hospitals' locality.

Drug Makers and Sellers. The relationship between pharmaceutical manufacturers, pharmacies, and third-party payers is characterized recently by increasingly stringent federal price-setting. This is a reflection of mounting discontent among policymakers and politicians over the utilization and cost of prescription drugs—both of which are among the world's highest. Historically, the lack of significant cost-sharing by patients has made for very weak price competition, and doctors have had no incentive not to prescribe liberally.

A major feature of a German health reform law of 1989 was a scheme to set fixed prices on certain drugs. This step was intended initially to encompass up to two-thirds of the prescription drug market, but in practice it has fallen considerably short of that target. In the first phase, sickness funds were to pay no more than a "reference price" for drugs with generic equivalents—about a third of the market. The reference price was pegged to the generic price. Doctors were free to prescribe more expensive drugs, but the patient would have to pay the difference. Eventually, the plan was to set reference prices for "therapeutically equivalent" drugs, those with the same active ingredients and those which operate in pharmacologically similar ways. However, this effort has reportedly bogged down. Still, the practical effect of the 1989 law was a dramatic reduction in drug prices for pharmaceuticals that came under the fixed-price plan, with a consequent savings of DM 1.2 billion a year (about $720 million in currency-exchange terms, or $504 million in purchasing power parities).[39]

One recent reform law, effective in 1993, takes pharmaceutical cost control one big step further by making physicians financially responsible if they prescribe drugs that cost, in the aggregate, more than a fixed annual budget for prescription drugs established by Parliament on the basis of 1991 expenditures. Legislators decided that rising drug prices were a smaller component of the nation's 10-plus percent inflation rate in pharmaceuticals than rising prescription volume.[40]

Summary

To understand how the German system works, why it is more successful, or why the Germans are engaged in major tinkering with it, one must study how it evolved. In particular, one must understand something about the controlling idea behind it—**social solidarity**.

Solidarity is a term unfamiliar to Americans outside its use in labor union rhetoric, where it connotes workers standing together against management. In Germany, the term means something quite different: The collective agreement to share the risks and costs of a necessary good—in this case, health care—so that the rich subsidize the poor, the healthy support the sick, the young pay for the old, workers help the unemployed, and single and childless couples subsidize families and children. As insurance theorist William A. Glaser points out, social solidarity is inherently redistributive. "A large number of people are taxed in order to cover the costs of those who use health care services, even though the high payers are often low users and the high users are often low payers."[41] However, health care is different from what Americans call "welfare" programs designed solely to redistribute from rich to poor. Instead, health care programs redistribute very broadly, in such a way that everyone who pays into the system understands that he or she may someday benefit. "Social solidarity and redistributive financing began on a small scale among friends," Glaser has written, "but became universal and nationwide."[42] The closest example that exists in the U.S. is a monumental one, and telling in its popularity—Social Security and Medicare.

In the next chapter, we will explore the roots of this idea, how it has shaped the German health care system, and how it operates today. This discussion should serve as a foundation for more detailed exploration of the workings of Germany's system, what it may have to teach American reformers, and what Germany might learn from the U.S. experience.

References and Notes

1. Schulenburg J-M (1989). International Symposium on Health Care Systems. Taipei, Taiwan.

2. Blendon, RJ, et.al. (1992). Physician Perspectives on Caring for Patients in Three Different Health Systems, *New England Journal of Medicine,*Vol. 328, No 14, pp. 1011-1016.

3. Sen. Edward M. Kennedy, personal communication, June 28, 1991.

4. Knox, RA (1992). "Lessons from a Medical System that Works," *The Boston Globe,* page 1, and personal communication, May 12.

5. Wicks, EK (1992). *German Health Care: Financing, Administration and Coverage*, Health Insurance Association of America, Washington, D.C., pp. v, 1.

6. Honan, WH (1992). *The New York Times*, December 10, p. C15.

7. Gov. Bill Clinton (1992). speech at Merck Pharmaceuticals, Rahway, NJ, September 24.

8. Fisher, M (1992). *The Washington Post*, December 28, p.A1.

9. Arnold M. *Health Care in the Federal Republic of Germany* Deutscher Ärzte-Verlag, Cologne, *1191, p. 14.*

10. Iglehart, JK (1991). "Germany's Health Care System (First of Two Parts)," *New England Journal of Medicine*, Vol. 324, No. 7, Feb. 14, p. 503.

11. Schieber GJ et. al. (1992). *Health Care Financing Review*, Summer.

12. These figures are given in U.S. dollars as measured in gross domestic product purchasing power parities (PPPs), as calculated by George J. Schieber and Leslie M. Greenwald of the U.S. Department of Health and Human Services and Jean-Pierre Poullier of the Organization for Economic Cooperation and Development (OECD). PPPs are based on comparisons of a weighted "market basket" of goods and services and are often considered more stable and meaningful for international comparisons than simple currency exchange rates. PPPs will be used in this text whenever possible; when currency exchange rate-based figures are used, this will be noted.

13. Schieber GJ 1992.

14. Schieber GJ and Poullier (1991). *Health Affairs*, Spring, pp. 106-116.

15. Iglehart (1991). *NEJM*, February 14, p. 503.

16. Arnold M (1991), p. 13.

17. Harvard Community Health Plan, (1990). *Annual Report 1990: An International Comparison of Health Care Systems,* Brookline, MA; Harvard Community Health Plan.

18. Ibid.

19. Dehlinger, E and Brennecke, R (1992). Die Akzeptanz der sozialen Sicherung in der Bevölkerun der Bundesrepublik Deutschland (Acceptance of social security by the population of the Federal Republic of Germany), *Gesundheitswesen*, 54, 229-243, Stuttgart-New York.

20. Blendon, RJ et.al., (1990) "Satisfaction with Health Systems in Ten Nations," *Health Affairs* Vol.9, No. 2 (Summer), 186-192. Sample size in the United States and West Germany exceeded 1,000 respondents, and sampling error was +\- 3-4 percent.

21. Bopp, U (1991). Personal interview in Stuttgart, March.

22. Blendon, RJ, et.al., (1992).

23. Hurst, J (1992). *The Reform of Health Care: A Comparative Analysis of Seven OECD Countries*, OECD, Paris, p. 62.

24. Light, DW and Schuller, A (1986). *Political Values and Health Care: The German Experience*. Cambridge, MA and Oxford: The MIT Press, p. 5.

25. Stone, DA (1980). *The Limits of Professional Power: National Health Care in the Federal Republic of Germany*, Chicago: University of Chicago Press, pp. 17-18.

26. Based on 1987 census figures. The total includes 61.2 million in former West Germany and 16 million in former East Germany.

27. Health Insurance Association of America, personal communication, (1993). The number of third-party payers in the United States may be much larger; for instance, the Mayo Clinic estimates that it deals with 2,400 separate insurers. (*New York Times*, January 24, p. 1.)

28. Wicks, EK (1992) p. 31.

29. These figures are for former West Germany only in 1989. The source is Der Bundesminister für Arbeit und Sozialordnung (Ministry of Labor and Social Welfare), *Die gesetzliche Krankenversicherung in der Bundesrepublik Deutschland im Jahre 1989: Statistischer und finanzieller Bericht* (Bonn, 1990).

30. Schulenburg, J-M. "The German Health Care System: A Close-Up View," *The Internist*, May, 1991, p.11.

31. Wicks, EK (1992), p. 25.

32. Hurst, J (1992) ,p. 60.

33. Wicks, EK (1992), p. 25-26.

34. Ibid.

35. Ibid.

36. Stone, DA (1990), p. 57.

37. Wicks EK (1992), p. 18.

38. There is no amortization of large-scale hospital debt incurred to purchase new equipment or bricks and mortar, since these expenses are met through outright grants from state governments, which are written off as soon as the investments are made.

39. Schulte, G, German Federal Ministry of Health, at a conference on "German and American Health Care Systems: A Comparison," Goethe Institute of Boston, October 16-18, 1992.

40. Ibid.

41. Glaser, *Health Insurance in Practice: International Variations in Financing, Benefits and Problems,* 1991, p. 14.

42. Ibid.

CHAPTER 2

The Roots of the German Health System: Evolution of an Idea

T he birth date of Germany's health care system is customarily given as 1883, when Otto von Bismarck, who unified the disparate German states into a nation, persuaded the 12-year-old Parliament to enact a national system of health insurance in a statute running to only 87 paragraphs.[1] In fact, the roots of Bismarck's system reach back centuries, to cooperative medieval organizations called then, as now, **sickness funds**. They were important fixtures of German life well before Bismarck's landmark legislation. The "iron chancellor," as Bismarck was known for his autocratic style, preferred discarding the sickness fund model for a tax-supported system with a more direct administrative role for government, but even he could not prevail against the funds' powerful and well-entrenched sponsors. The resulting compromise—the government prescribes policy but autonomous private parties finance and deliver services—persists to the present day.

The Origins of Social Solidarity

Sickness funds, like the craft guilds that gave them birth, embody a notion of enlightened self-interest and voluntarism. In feudal society, economic security depended on the protection of kings and local nobility and guilds provided an economic niche founded on self-regulation among kindred craftsmen. The founding idea, of course, was protectionism against renegade competitors. **Guilds** defined the qualifications a craftsman needed to call himself a goldsmith, a baker, a carpenter, a blacksmith. They specified training requirements and created hierarchies of novices, journeymen, and masters that not only controlled quality but also limited entry into their respective fields. The protectionism was reinforced with initiation fees and dues. Guilds also provided meeting places where members could discuss common interests. Imposing guild halls, which still stand in the market squares of many German towns, testify to the power and prominence these organizations forged for themselves in medieval society.

Getting Sick in the Middle Ages

Not surprisingly, these economic affinity groups developed a response to something that threatened every member's livelihood: illness and injury. In exchange for initiation fees and annual fixed amounts, capitation fees, usually payable in installments two or three times a year on feast days of patron saints, sickness fund members could count on cash benefits—sick pay—when they were injured or fell ill, sparing them and their families from destitution. These contributions did not vary by family size, so the funds inherently redistributed money from unmarried members and those with small families to those with large families. In some guilds, the contributions were based upon the number of goods a member sold or jobs performed, so there was some link between the size of the contribution and the member's income.[2] Upon a member's death, his widow was assured funeral expenses (a benefit that only recently has been curtailed, much to the consternation of undertakers). In the Middle Ages, cash grants were by far the most important benefits, since the medicine of the day had little to offer; gradually, sickness funds began to cover the services of physicians.

Social Solidarity vs Insurance

The reciprocal relationship among sickness fund members benefited the funds' sponsoring guilds, which depended on group cohesion. "This cohesion was fostered wherever their members could count on help in times of need based on a solidarity related to their specific profession," notes Michael Arnold, M.D., director of the Institute of Health Systems Research at the University of Tübingen.[3] The idea that individuals' interests "can best be served by a set of stable, occupationally based membership groups is a profound tradition in German politics which has significantly influenced the structure of social welfare programs," writes Deborah Stone, a Brandeis University analyst of the German health system.[4]

The European idea of social solidarity as the basis for financing health care is quite distinct from the Anglo-Saxon tradition that shaped America's approach in this area. As social policy analyst William A. Glaser noted,

> The Americans were heirs of Anglo-Saxon self-interested individualism, and the European philosophy and methods of social solidarity were less influential. The Anglo-Saxons have defined social programs as charity, a fallback because of failures of private enterprise, to be paid for temporarily by government and phased out eventually.[5]

There is also an important distinction to be made between a solidarity-based health system and the notion of health *insurance* as it has developed in the United States. Glaser explains:

> "Insurance" implies a person's self-centered calculations to protect himself against loss. A self-centered insurance company creates pools to spread risks, so it can market policies, bear the risks, and earn profits. But "insurance" in this form is designed to avoid exceptionally risky persons, not to protect them at a loss for a social good.[6]

Expansion of the Sickness Fund Model

The sickness fund system that developed in middle Europe half a millennium ago clearly served a perceived need for individuals and communities. By the 16th century, sickness funds had been extended from craftsmen to miners, initially as a self-help effort, since early mines were owned by the miners as shareholders and later as a cooperative effort between labor and management. As long ago as 1784, the Kingdom of Prussia gave legal protection and standing to existing sickness funds. In 1854 a Prussian law obligated all mines and foundries to have sickness funds, and required sickness funds to offer sick pay, medication, and rehabilitation—marking the first compulsory, regulated health insurance system. The 1854 law also authorized communities to require, at their option, both employer and employees in artisan shops to join the sickness fund of their respective guild. The statute signified the social and political value that had accrued to sickness funds by the mid-19th century and it also prefigured the decentralized structure that would characterize the sickness fund movement for more than a century to come.[7]

Sickness Funds Meet the Industrial Revolution

The 19th century in Europe was a time of enormous economic and social transition—from feudal to industrial society and from an agrarian to an urban landscape. In the lands that were to become united as Germany in 1871, these monumental changes shaped the politics and the policy debates that led to Bismarck's social legislation, including compulsory health insurance. As Peter Rosenberg, a policy analyst at the Federal Ministry of Labor, notes,

> Until the end of the 19th century, half of the population was engaged in agriculture, the rest primarily in trade and commerce. At the beginning of the 19th century there were approximately 300,000 factory workers in the area of the future German Reich. Their numbers grew to 2,000,000 by 1867 and then rapidly to 12,000,000 by 1900. Thus, a new social class developed which included almost half the population by the turn of the century.[8]

By drawing so many people into cities, industrialization broke the familial and community bonds that supported laborers and their dependents when illness or accident struck. Church-sponsored charity was not up to the burgeoning task—though the Roman Catholic Church and Catholics' influential *Zentrum* (Center) Party (until the 1890s) strongly resisted state intervention on philosophical grounds. The Church said intervention was against the "natural law" that required individuals to be responsible to themselves and dependent only on God, but it also knew state-sponsored social relief would undercut the Church's power. Due to the vacuum created by this resistance, the deteriorating state of workers' living conditions loomed in 1871 as one of the most urgent priorities of the newly unified nation. One reflection of this was the emigration of an annual average of 62,500 Germans to the U.S. between 1871 and 1880.[9] Bismarck and his ministers were even worried about the military implications of poor health due to alarming reports that recruits from industrial areas were unfit for service. "Welfare socialism," they concluded, "was essential if the fatherland was to survive in a hostile world."[10]

In 1876, the new Parliament enacted regulations over sickness funds setting national standards for minimum contributions and management; but the law stopped short of requiring workers to join or employers to contribute. "Since the benefits were often insufficient, the workers did not always utilize the sickness funds; they preferred to depend upon charity in case of illness."[11]

Bismarck's Strategy: A Carrot, Not a Stick

The young German state, its monarchy and its conservative ruling faction found themselves threatened by unrest within the new laboring class--encouraged by the followers of Karl Marx. Organization among the workers sparked political countermeasures in 1878: laws against socialism, trade unions, and the Social Democratic Party. Though a conservative, Bismarck realized that repressive laws would not work in the long term since they did nothing about the underlying social problems. The opening sentence of Emperor Wilhelm I's Imperial message of 1881 introduced Bismarck's social welfare legislation to the Parliament, or *Reichstag*, tellingly: "The healing of social damages cannot be found merely through repression of Social Democratic transgressions."[12,13]

It is an abiding irony that Bismarck conceived the 1880s succession of German social welfare measures—beginning with health insurance and extending to accident insurance for factory workers (1884), agriculture workers (1886), and old-age and disability pensions (1889)[14]—in order to coopt the socialists and blunt socialism's appeal for restive laborers. But Arnold points out that Prince Bismarck's own background also inclined him toward an attitude of *noblesse oblige*. There has been, he notes,

> a reluctance to appreciate Bismarck's conviction and motivation as a big landowner and member of the feudal class, a class also committed to Christian principles, that he had the lord of the manor's obligation to take care of "his people." He also recognized very clearly that statutory coverage against the risks of sickness would serve to secure social contentment and increase loyalty to the state.[15]

Also influential in setting the young nation's course was the philosophy of German idealism, exemplified by Johann Gottlieb Fichte and Georg Wilhelm Friedrich Hegel. They argued that the individual's identity sprang from association with social groups, from the family to the State, and taught that "the welfare of each goes together with the welfare of all."[16] This moral philosophy legitimized the familiar model of the sickness fund, helping to make it the natural basis for Bismarck's social reform. The timing of Germany's emerging identity as a nation-state also played a role. "Partly because Germany industrialized later and faster," sociologist Paul Starr has noted, "its traditional forms of social protection had partly survived when it faced the challenge of socialism. Perhaps as a result, it made a more direct transition to the social protection of the welfare state."[17]

A Government-Run System Averted

If Bismarck had his way, Germany's health care system would have resembled the model enacted 68 years later in postwar Britain—a government-run, centrally administered health service. "Bismarck and his associates thought this strategy would induce the working class to favor the new national government," Glaser writes. "But the business and agricultural interests in the *Reichstag* opposed the financing provisions; and the provincial governments and conservatives opposed the expanded role of the national government."[18] After several attempts to set up an Imperial Insurance Institute to administer both health and accident insurance, Bismarck finally scrapped the plan. The sickness fund model, marrying federal government superintendency with private financing and administration by autonomous institutions, became a complex but durable compromise.

The social welfare system Germany enacted in the 1880s was Europe's first, but one should not overestimate its initial reach. Estimates vary on the number of Germans initially covered by the 1883 health insurance statute, from about 3 million workers and their families[19] to 4.3 million workers, not including dependents[20]. In any event, it was a small fraction of an estimated German-speaking population approaching 60 million.[21] The law did not at first require universal coverage—nor does it today, though compulsory insurance now embraces about 78 percent of the German population and another 7 percent voluntarily participate in the statutory sickness funds.[22]

Occupational Coverage: The Roots of Complexity

Bismarck realized from Prussia's earlier efforts that entirely voluntary health insurance would not do the job, so the 1883 law made coverage compulsory—for all laborers. Blue-collar workers paid hourly wages were compelled to join regardless of their income. Sickness fund participation for salaried, or white-collar, workers was mandatory only if they were lower-income; the income ceiling for mandatory coverage was set at a point that initially excluded most salaried workers.[23] Obviously, the statutory scheme left out many Germans within and outside the workforce—farmers and farm workers, self-employed people outside of guilds, pensioners, civil servants, and many others. Partly through adding categories of people and partly by raising the income ceiling for salaried workers, more Germans were brought within the embrace of statutory health insurance. Stone estimated that statutory health insurance covered 11 percent of the German population in 1888, 17 percent in 1900, and about 20 percent in 1910.[24] The system was not complete until 1975. (Table 2.1)

Sickness fund members originally paid two-thirds of the contribution necessary for their respective sickness fund to cover benefit costs, and their employers paid one-third. However, the amount that workers could be assessed was initially capped at 1.5 to 3 percent of the workers' daily wages (depending on the type of worker). Benefits, both in sickness pay and in medical service, were accordingly limited, to a combined total of 13 weeks.[25] The sickness funds were governed by elected boards representing workers and management initially proportionate to the 2:1 contributions; they still are self-governed today, though the ratio of contributions and worker-employer representation now is 1:1.

The 1883 law preserved the historical link between employment category and sickness funds, retaining the **guild- or craft-based funds** (called *Innungskassen, Innung* meaning "guild") and **miners' funds** (called *Kappschaftskasssen, Knappschaft* meaning "body of miners"). The statute also added new categories: **local sickness funds** (*Allgemeine Ortskrankenkassen,* or *AOK* for short, *Allgemeine* meaning "general," and *Ort* meaning "place" or "locality") and **company sickness funds** (*Betriebskrankenkassen, Betrieb* meaning "factory"), which were optional for firms of sufficient size (450 workers in recent years). Outside the definition of "statutory" sickness funds, but a component of health insurance that would become increasingly important in the mid- to late-20th century, were mutual-aid societies for salaried employees, called **substitute funds** or *Ersatzkassen.* Substitute funds were not originally included in the official scheme, though they were allowed to exist and to benefit from the same government policies that fostered the statutory funds. Bismarck chose to focus on lower-income, hourly wage workers rather than salaried office employees. This distinction would later come back to haunt Germany in its efforts to create and maintain a single-class system of health care and it causes troublesome political disputes even now.

When statutory health insurance was enacted, Germany already had a formidable preexisting sickness fund infrastructure: approximately 20,000 sickness funds existed in 1885, averaging 215 compulsory members each, not including family members.[26] The number of sickness fund members grew steadily over the ensuing decades, while the number of funds shrank as a result of consolidation into ever-larger organizations—a trend that continues today. (Figure 2.1)

Growing Popularity— Except Among Doctors

By the end of its third decade, the statutory insurance system had grown tremendously, reaching 15 million members. It also grew in popularity, even among the Social Democrats who fought it bitterly at the outset as insufficient response to workers' misery, and as the creature of their enemy Bismarck. The system's obvious benefits won over such opponents as the leaders of the Roman Catholic Church and many employers, who had staunchly opposed state involvement in the lives of individuals and businesses. But one group was increasingly unhappy: physicians.

The tumultuous early relationship between sickness funds and doctors, which took five decades to stabilize, is important to understand. Obviously, physicians are not the only providers of health care, and other payer-provider relationships are important in their own way. But the politics of the sickness fund-physician dyad shaped Germany's current health care system more than any other factor. It continues to dominate momentous policy decisions, such as the shape of the medical care system in the *Neue Bundesländer*—the five new states that formerly made up East Germany. In Germany, notes health economist J.-Matthias Graf von der Schulenburg, "office-based physicians play the dominant role in the health care sector as a whole."[27]

Table 2.1

Categorical Expansion of Statutory Insurance in Germany

1983   Blue-collar workers

1901   Transport and commercial (office) workers

1911   Agricultural and forestry workers, domestic servants

1914   Civil service employees

1918   Unemployed people

1927   Seamen

1930   Dependents of fund members

1941   Voluntary participants (workers no longer eligible for compulsory insurance due to wage increases that put their income over the ceiling could now continue coverage with the same fund on a voluntary basis)

1941   Pensioners

1966   Farmworkers and salesmen

1972   Self-employed agricultural workers and dependents

1975   Students and disabled persons

Source: Stone, DA (1980). The Limits of Professional Power: National Health Care in the Federal Republic of Germany. *Cambridge, MA: The MIT Press, P.78.*

Figure 2.1

Growth in Sickness Fund Members and Consolidation of Funds

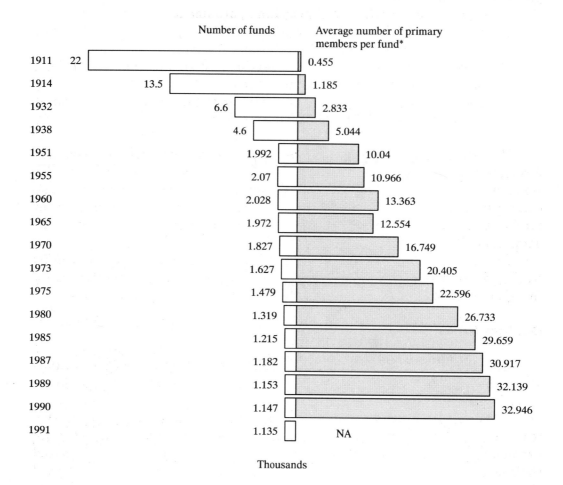

Number of funds — Average number of primary members per fund*

Year	Number of funds	Avg members per fund
1911	22	0.455
1914	13.5	1.185
1932	6.6	2.833
1938	4.6	5.044
1951	1.992	10.04
1955	2.07	10.966
1960	2.028	13.363
1965	1.972	12.554
1970	1.827	16.749
1973	1.627	20.405
1975	1.479	22.596
1980	1.319	26.733
1985	1.215	29.659
1987	1.182	30.917
1989	1.153	32.139
1990	1.147	32.946
1991	1.135	NA

Thousands

*Primary members = without dependents.

Sources: *Bundesministerium für Arbveit und Sozialordnug, Ürbersicht die Siziale Sicherung, 1975 (1911-1973 data) and Bundesministeriums für Gesundheit,* Daten des Gesundheitswesens, *1991 (1975-1991 data).*

The medical profession had not been involved in—or even particularly exercised about—the passage of the *Health Insurance Act of 1883.*[28] In fact, doctors were not even mentioned in the law. In its early years, statutory insurance posed no great threat to physicians, since enrollment was not a large share of any doctor's potential market. But three factors conspired to engender physicians' concern, then alarm:

- exponential growth in sickness fund enrollment;
- an increase in the number of physicians, from a ratio of 3,000 people per doctor in 1883 to 2,000 in 1913;[29]
- sickness funds' practice of contracting with individual doctors on a salaried basis to care for a defined number of fund members, effectively freezing out private physicians who wanted access to the burgeoning market of sickness fund patients.

"In effect, social insurance created two patient pools where there had formerly been one," Stone says. "The creation of two separate markets for health services had a strong influence on the development of medical politics. Physicians were in the ironic position of trying to restrict the size of the public sector (and thus preserve the private sector) and to increase their access to it at the same time."[30]

In addition, many doctors chafed at being employed and supervised by worker-dominated organizations. Their irritation grew along with physicians' increasing sense of professional, privileged status.

Doctors Strike Back

The 1883 law had not addressed what relationship the sickness funds should have with physicians nor what the qualifications of doctors should be, leaving both up to the funds. Since medical practice was not itself legally defined, sickness fund were free to hire anyone to provide any type of care. Due to the increasing competition among physicians, sickness funds "could negotiate extremely low fees, especially in contracts with physicians who had not passed their board exams."[31] "Panel doctors" with sickness fund contracts complained they were exploited and overworked while outside doctors demanded access to sickness fund patients. Both groups formed unions and began to call strikes that attracted wide attention, within Germany and among medical colleagues in other countries. The most successful effort was launched by a group of 21 doctors who called themselves the *Leipziger Vorband* (after the founding city of Leipzig) and later the *Hartmannbund,* after the Leipzig physician who was its founding father. The *Hartmannbund,* which exists today as the voice of office-based physicians, organized hundreds of successful strikes and boycotts against sickness funds in the first decade of the new century; its membership swelled from the founding 21 physicians to include nearly three-quarters of all German doctors by the decade's end. Its principal goal was to guarantee all doctors the right to treat sickness fund patients.[32]

The long-brewing conflict came to a head in 1911, as the government prepared a codification of the health insurance program through an **Imperial Insurance Decree** (*Reichsversicherungsordnung,* often referred to as the *RVO*). The decree regulated the details of sickness fund contribution levels, benefits, and other components neglected in Bismarck's legislation. It also exacerbated the physicians' problem by expanding the population covered by compulsory insurance from 20 to nearly 30 percent of all Germans. Furthermore, it authorized funds for the first time to reimburse patients for medical services (an indemnity benefit) rather than only to contract directly with physicians. This step undercut the leverage physicians had wielded against the sickness funds by striking or refusing to sign contracts.

To meet the threat of the *RVO*, the physicians demanded that:

☐ only credentialed physicians be allowed to treat sickness-fund patients, undercutting the funds' ability to contract more cheaply with uncertified physicians;

☐ sickness fund patients be guaranteed free choice of physician; and

☐ sickness fund membership be restricted, lest it expand among higher-income white-collar employees who constituted the private market for medical care.

The government responded to the physicians' demand. The 1911 insurance decree required sickness funds to give their members a choice between at least two physicians (but did not guarantee totally free choice) and ordained that doctors must be paid by fee-for-service rather than by salary or capitation. The *RVO* also required funds to pay only physicians with full credentials.[33,34]

Berlin Treaty of 1913: A Temporary Peace

However, the doctors were not satisfied. Within two years, the national umbrella group of medical associations, the *Deutsche Ärztevereinsbund* or *DÄV*, which had refrained from militancy in favor of the feistier *Hartmannbund,* called for a general physicians' strike. The government was forced to mediate, resulting in the landmark *Berlin Treaty of 1913,* narrowly averting the strike. The agreement did not guarantee physicians full access to sickness fund practice, but did set up joint committees for doctors and statutory health insurers to negotiate their differences and set standards on crucial issues such as the required ratio of physicians to fund members (though *not* how much doctors should be paid). This new machinery, an alternative to the confrontational, ad hoc mode of labor disputes, strikes, and physician boycotts, was the foundation on which the lasting payer-provider relationships characteristic of the German system would be built.

The *Berlin Treaty* bought relative peace between sickness funds and physicians for a decade or so, but the 1920s saw renewed strife. The underlying cause was the overwhelming economic crisis brought on by Germany's defeat in World War I — the burden of reparations and territorial losses dictated by the *Treaty of Versailles,* combined with enormous internal debt and astronomical inflation (in 1923 the dollar was worth 4 billion marks[35]). Postwar industrial production declined to one-third of pre-war levels. The late 1920s saw striking economic recovery, but it was interrupted by depression following the 1929 Wall Street crash; by 1932 German unemployment reached 30 percent. Not surprisingly, the deteriorating economy threatened the very existence of the health insurance system. "Inflationary price increases and corresponding pay raises made it necessary to increase the income limits for mandatory members," Rosenberg writes. "At the same time benefits were being reduced, members were required to pay for various services individually, and the administrative control of the physicians as well as of the members was intensified."[36] Unhappy with burgeoning sickness fund contributions, business leaders joined with doctors in attacking the dominance of workers in the funds' governing structure, which was closely identified with the Social Democratic leaders of the shaky Weimar Republic government of 1919-33.

Doctors Win a Collective Victory

Faced with doctors' strikes and fast-eroding sickness fund finances, the government issued a series of emergency decrees in 1923, 1930, and 1931 to save the system. The orders "dramatically changed the character of sickness fund-physician relationships and shaped the countervailing power model on which today's system is based," Stone notes.[37]

The most far-reaching of these decrees was the 1931 *Weimar Settlement*, which more than doubled the number of doctors sickness funds were obliged to admit into their panels (the required ratio of doctors to fund members was changed from 1:1,350 to 1:600) and, more importantly, established associations of sickness fund doctors to negotiate collectively with the funds over reimbursement.[38] Physicians were legally obligated to belong to one of these regional **sickness fund physicians' associations**, called *kassenärztliche Vereinigungen*, or *KVs*, in order to receive sickness fund payments.

The establishment of *KVs*, long sought by doctors' lobbies, was a watershed in the development of the German system. It created a counterforce to the sickness funds in annual negotiations over fees and in all dealings between the two parties. Henceforth all funds for ambulatory physician payment would flow from sickness fund coffers to *KVs*, which would distribute payment to member physicians; doctors would submit bills to their organization rather than directly to the funds. The advent of *KVs* also meant that funds could no longer pit doctors against each other by negotiating with individual physicians on a take-it-or-leave-it basis. The innovation gave the doctors' groups statutory standing; in the German phrase, they are "bodies of public law," not merely private associations. The sickness funds had no choice but to deal with the authorized physician associations.

"One of the advantages of the *Weimar Settlement* for the doctors was that they were organized as a bargaining monopoly, whereas their negotiating partners were divided into several different kinds of funds," notes Douglass Webber of the European Institute of Business Administration.[39] This advantage has never been mitigated, despite later attempts by local funds (the *Allgemeine Ortskrankenkassen* or *AOKs*), unions, and Social Democrats to even the score by establishing a single large sickness fund (or at least a single fund type in each region).

The *Weimar Settlement* also marked the arrival of the medical profession as a nationally recognized profession instead of merely a business. Individual German states had earlier recognized medicine as a profession, but before 1931, the national government had not.[40]

The sickness funds were not entirely on the losing side of the *Weimar Settlement*. They won the ability to impose an overall ceiling on annual payments for ambulatory care, based on a capitated amount for each fund member and the financial condition of the fund. This put sickness fund doctors at financial risk if they overspent the budget, a precedent that would be important in the 1970s, when expenditure caps would be reestablished for office-based physicians. In addition, sickness funds were given statutory authority to set standards of "necessary and economical" care, monitor doctors' practices, and recover the costs of physician services deemed excessive.

The *Berlin Treaty* and the *Weimar Settlement* exemplified and extended a larger pattern characteristic of the German system: government's limited scope in the regulation of health care. As Webber points out, health sector regulation in Germany has been a story of

- ☐ "procedural regulation" by the state, which has set the rules and blessed the processes of financing, dispute resolution, administrative machinery, and cost-control; and
- ☐ "substantive regulation" by the joint self-administration of sickness funds and organized groups of health care providers.

"The combined impact of these two processes has been to narrow the scope for the operation of market mechanisms in health care regulation," Webber writes.[41]

Stone sees in this pattern a deliberate German strategy of setting up countervailing powers. "The government's solution to the problem of controlling a group with a monopoly on valued technical expertise," she writes, "was to make the group more powerful, but to confront it with an equally powerful opponent."[42]

The *Weimar Settlement* altered the balance of power between sickness funds and doctors in the physicians' favor. But the ensuing 12-year period of National Socialism tipped that balance decisively in favor of organized medicine by destroying the funds' governing structure and by stifling funds' experiments with alternative forms of medical care delivery such as ambulatory clinics and salaried group practices resembling contemporary "closed panel" health maintenance organizations. At the same time, Adolph Hitler strengthened the associations of sickness fund physicians, by giving them the status of "bodies of public law" with quasi-public responsibilities, a legal standing that does not exist in the United States. Hitler also formally declared medicine a special profession, exempt from trade regulations.[43] Organized medicine's fortunes (at least for "Aryan" physicians) were no doubt enhanced by the close contacts Hitler had with physician leaders. It has been reported, for instance, that the leader of the Nazi doctors' association, a physician named Wagner, had lunch with Hitler three times a week.[44]

Hitler's Health Care Agenda

The Nazis were initially hostile to the sickness funds, partly because they had become leading vehicles of power and influence for the rival Social Democrats and, thus, identified with the Weimar governments. More fundamentally, sickness funds were often governed and staffed by Jews active in the labor movement.

Hitler and his advisers saw social policy as an instrument to promote the Third Reich's goal of a healthy, productive, fit and racially pure German state.[45] Those who were not "perfect human material" were not to be beneficiaries of health insurance and other forms of social welfare, and they were certainly not to administer the agencies for funding and delivering medical care.

One of the first decrees after Hitler's accession to the chancellorship in 1933 was designed to purge the civil service—including managers of sickness funds since they were independent "public bodies"—of "nationally unreliable" elements and "non-Aryan" persons. Yet another early Nazi decree abolished the sickness funds' self-government. In 1934, the Hitler government transferred all decision-making power within sickness funds from an elected council of members and employers to a single *führer,* or chief.

Sickness fund staff were also "purified" of elements deemed undesirable. Relying on archival material of the Nazi Ministry of Labor, Stephan Leibfried of the University of Bremen and Florian Tennstedt of the University of Kassel have estimated that up to 4,000 sickness fund employees were purged throughout the Third Reich—as many as one-quarter of the total.[46] The chief of a local sickness fund in Nuremberg, in a 1938 memoir, explained Hitler's purpose: "The issue was to win back the sickness funds and devote them to the original purpose, that is, to insure all working Germans, and thus to free them from domination by Marxists and Jews."[47]

A parallel effort barred "non-Aryan" doctors from sickness fund practice. Jewish physicians represented approximately 15 percent of practicing physicians in Prussia (roughly the northern half of what is now Germany) at this time, but in Berlin the proportion of "non-Aryan" physicians approached 60 percent. In other major cities they comprised 25 to 30 percent of practicing doctors.[48]

"The Nazis rolled out the red carpet for 'Aryan' physicians," said a 45-year-old Hamburg physician whose father was a Nazi doctor. "Jewish doctors were kicked out of the sickness funds."[49] Aryan physicians were indoctrinated in eugenics and had to pass exams in "racial hygiene." The medical profession had the highest proportion of Nazi party members of any, followed by teachers.[50]

Purging of the Sickness Funds

Some believe it would be a mistake to assume that the Nazi animus against Jewish doctors and sickness fund managers was motivated solely by racism. Instead, or rather in addition to the racist motive, Leibfried and Tennstedt assert that Nazi officials wanted to crush the sickness funds' union-dominated governing structure, which represented an independent power base for the Social Democrats that was threatening to the Nazi Party. In this they had common cause with leaders of private-practice medicine, who had for decades opposed union-inspired innovations in medical-care delivery, such as fund-owned ambulatory clinics with salaried doctors, a drug formulary commission, and prevention-oriented public health programs. The sickness funds' governing councils and the reformist doctors often tended to be Jewish.

> Jewish doctors in the main industrial cities, especially Berlin, had consistently supported health reform initiatives of diverse sorts. As providers of social services, they opposed or at least transcended the private-practice outlook of the medical profession's association, and they believed that the self-government of the sickness funds, with their strong union base, made progress in social service delivery possible.[51]

The net effect of all the Nazi-era changes was to change the culture and decimate the power of sickness funds, while strengthening the dominant role of ambulatory physicians and their associations. The main point is that the fundamentals of the German health system survived the brutalities and tumult of the Nazi years relatively intact; the mechanisms of health care financing and delivery were one set of German institutions that Allied occupation forces did not have to worry much about. But the system's internal dynamics were altered in ways that resonate today; for instance, in the controlling influence that western physicians wielded in the transformation of East Germany's health care after the Berlin Wall fell in 1989, as examined in Chapter Seven.

Health Care in a Divided Germany

After the Third Reich fell on May 8, 1945, health care (and virtually everything else) in Germany bifurcated into systems that became virtually diametrical:

1. the three Allied sectors that were to become the Federal Republic of Germany (FRG), a continuation of the decentralized, largely private system of finance and delivery launched two generations earlier; and
2. the Soviet sector, the future German Democratic Republic (GDR), a strongly centralized, state-operated, command-and-control health system loosely modelled on the USSR's.

The GDR system, however, had some important differences from the Soviets. For instance, a system of financing based on the traditional German system was retained, with workers and employers sharing premium costs but with administration concentrated in two large "sickness funds," one for workers and another for business managers, professionals, farmers, and artisans.[52]

Naturally, ideology played a controlling role in postwar health care policy—on both sides of the Allied divide. The Soviets quickly dispatched an elite group of 60 health specialists to Berlin to design the new system, reporting directly to the Health Ministry in Moscow. As Stefan Kirchberger points out, health care offered the Soviets:

> the possibility of creating a model situation in an area of social life affecting the entire population, especially the workers...thereby demonstrating the achievements a socialist society can realize.[53]

There was no such attention given to health care in the Allied sectors. Insofar as it was addressed at all, Kirchberger reports, the Americans considered the issue "a matter for private initiative...not to be guided by the state," and were interested only in immediate issues such as the threat of epidemics and the distribution of scarce drugs. The British administered health affairs in a more centralized fashion reflecting their governmental structure, while the French tried to restrict Germans' authority in a decentralized, state-by-state model to prevent the development of a strong central authority.

While the Allies' respective ideologies determined their approach to Germany's postwar health care, the physical state of affairs that confronted them required emergency solutions. In the Soviet sector, these top-down measures became institutionalized—and seemed to justify the ideology. Living conditions throughout Germany were at or below subsistence levels, but conditions were worse in the east. Food shortages and resulting malnutrition were dire and the threat of epidemic disease was greater. Soviet authorities launched drastic measures against infectious disease, mandating registration of all cases of typhoid, malaria, tuberculosis, and other contagions, vaccinating against typhoid, and sometimes requiring hospitalization.

The Ideology of Venereal Disease Control

The way western and Soviet occupation authorities dealt with postwar epidemics of venereal disease offers an interesting case study of the two Germanies at the earliest stage of the split. The Soviets ordered the establishment of ambulatory VD clinics for every 50,000 to 70,000 people in their sector, staffed by specialists, to provide both counseling and treatment. This ended the monopoly of private, office-based practitioners to provide outpatient treatment. "War was openly declared on private practice," according to Renata Baum, a fellow of the East Europe Institute at the Free University of Berlin.[54] Private doctors protested, but the Soviet authorities directed supplies of scarce penicillin and Salvarsan, then the only effective drugs against venereal diseases, toward the state-run clinics. The VD clinics represented the first step toward the system of ambulatory clinics, factory-based clinics and multispecialty "polyclinics" that were to characterize the East German health system for the next 45 years.

In the western sectors, occupation authorities also tried to establish VD clinics but were blocked by German medical practitioners, who "saw in this measure a threat to their existence, the first step toward 'socialization of medicine.'"[55] Doctors also raised the question of who would pay them if the VD patient did not belong to a sickness fund and could not afford expensive penicillin. The payment issue sometimes produced "insufficient interest" among physicians in attacking rampant venereal disease, according to a contemporary account.[56] There were disputes, as well, over the role of VD specialists in consultation with general practitioners. The generalists complained about the interference of VD specialists and blocked any direct contact between consultant and patient as undue intrusion on their turf.

Western Doctors Consolidate Their Gains

While doctors in the Soviet sector ultimately had no choice but to give up the cherished notion of private practice, the *laissez-faire* policy of Allied authorities in the west permitted doctors there to maintain the gains they had made in the Weimar and Nazi periods. Dealing from strength, they fought fiercely against even marginal intrusions upon their independent, solo-practice, office-based turf. For instance, western physicians were able to enact bans against
- a physician employing (or working for) another physician;
- group practice, unless the participating doctors were relatives (a proscription not lifted until 1968);
- physician advertising, competition, or criticism of colleagues; and
- public-health and occupational-health physicians engaging in patient care.

Through such rigorous barriers German physicians have preserved a solo-practice, fee-for-service mode of medical practice far more successfully than their American colleagues have managed to do.

Due to mostly hands-off attitudes on the part of occupation forces, the structure of health care in West Germany continued as an unbroken thread from Bismarck's time. Interestingly, American occupation authorities did attempt, with temporary success, to break up German doctors' economic power, partly on the grounds that the physicians' associations violated U.S. principles of anti-trust law—a *non sequitur* as far as German law is concerned, then or now. The Allies abolished the Physicians' Chamber (responsible for licensure and ethics) and the association of sickness fund physicians, or *KVs*, at the national level, though not at the regional level. Doctors in some states seized the opportunity to abolish the regional *KVs* and consolidate all their power in state Physicians' Chambers, but sickness funds objected to this maneuver because it was too great a concentration of physicians' power, and it was reversed. The old structure of regional groups of sickness fund physicians designated to act as bargaining agents was restored, though the Americans' antitrust qualms blocked a return to the *status quo ante* in their sector until the early 1950s.

The reason this is worth noting is more than merely historical. As Americans debate how to create the mechanisms necessary to impose economic bargaining and "global budgeting" on physicians and other health providers, citing the German system as a model, U.S. antitrust law looms as one of the major obstacles. One of the fundamental legal differences between the German and U.S. health systems, which surfaced briefly in the late 1940s, seems likely to emerge again on this side of the Atlantic.

Despite Skirmishes, a Return to Normalcy in West Germany

After the Federal Republic of Germany was established in the western sectors on May 23, 1949, the local sickness funds, labor unions, and the Social Democratic Party campaigned for creation of a single insurance fund for health care, unemployment benefits, and pensions to replace the fragmented system of *Krankenkassen* and other funds. (At this point, there were approximately 2,000 sickness funds in West Germany with an average membership of about 10,000 each.) A unitary insurance fund would have had enormous bargaining leverage over the monopoly that ambulatory physicians enjoyed; its advocates argued that the step would merely even the score that had been unbalanced in favor of the doctors for more than a dozen years. Ultimately the leftists' aim during the 1950s and 1960s, in Germany and other European countries, was a tax-supported, governmentally administered health system.

However, the new German republic's first parliamentary elections in August 1949, resulted in a coalition led by the more conservative Christian Democratic Party. That thwarted the single-fund plan, which was strongly opposed by doctors, sickness fund managers, hospital associations, and businessmen.[57,58] Instead, the government, in 1955, acted to confirm the Weimar Settlement provisions that gave the associations of sickness fund doctors a statutory monopoly over ambulatory care; in return, the doctors promised not to strike.[59]

Outwardly, the health care system of the new FRG was remarkably consistent with what existed before and during the Nazi dictatorship. The same structure persists today. There are

☐ six types of statutory (*RVO*) sickness funds, governed by equal representation from members (labor unions) and employers;

- ☐ "substitute" funds for white-collar workers, governed by members exclusively;
- ☐ private insurance purchased by about 10 percent of the population who have higher incomes and by the self-employed;
- ☐ coverage for pensioners (added to the statutory sickness fund system in 1941) through continuing membership in the sickness funds they belonged to as workers; and
- ☐ government-sponsored insurance (with contributions from the insureds) for civil servants, police, members of the armed services, and the unemployed.

Annual bargaining over total reimbursement takes place between sickness funds and regional associations of ambulatory physicians, and between the funds and individual hospitals. Contribution rates, shared equally between employers and employees, flow to the sickness funds, substitute funds and private insurers. These agencies pay ambulatory doctors through their associations; reimburse hospitals (and hospital-based doctors) directly; and remit the cost of prescription drugs through regional associations of pharmacies.

Seeds of Trouble in Modern Germany

Behind this outwardly unchanged flow chart, however, forces were at work in the 1950s, '60s, and '70s that would have powerful effects on the German health system and the politics of health care in the late 1970s, '80s, and '90s. As prosperity blossomed, so did pressure to expand both cash benefits (sick pay) and health benefits—decisions that would haunt Germany and its neighbors during later economic downturns. To meet increased expenses, more and more Germans were brought into the statutory sickness funds by periodic increases in the minimum income threshold at which citizens could opt out and buy private insurance. (After 1971, this threshold was automatically pegged to increases in the national wage level to avoid political battles.) Nevertheless, payroll deductions and employers' contributions for health coverage rose steadily.

Meanwhile, structural changes in the German workforce were altering the topography of health insurance. By the mid-1900s, white-collar workers were the fastest-growing segment of the workforce—from about one in five workers before 1950 to nearly two in five in 1965 and almost one out of two by 1985. Since salaried employees in German historically have had the choice of the *RVO*, or statutory, sickness funds and the substitute funds, or *Ersatzkassen*, this employment trend had the effect of ballooning the number of *Ersatzkassen* members and drawing better-paid (and lower-risk) participants from the statutory funds. This trend, in turn, fed the widespread perception that the *Ersatzkassen* were more prestigious and their members enjoyed a higher standard of care—a perception that the *Ersatzkassen* fully exploit for competitive reasons. But more importantly, in terms of future political tensions, the trend drove a wedge between statutory and substitute funds on the fundamental issue of diverging contribution rates. A simultaneous trend was a steady erosion in the number of factory-based sickness funds, or *Betriebskranken*, which are basically self-insurance funds based in medium- to large-sized firms. Though still the most numerous type of statutory sickness fund, with 700 funds insuring 11 percent of the population, the number is shrinking, not growing. The net impact of these developments is a steadily diminishing number of funds of increasing size.

Cost Control: The 30-Year Struggle

The Germans' struggle to control health costs began inauspiciously in the early 1960s, when Christian Democrat-led governments tried to introduce patient copayments for doctors' services and state control over physicians' fees. After a bruising and unsuccessful battle, Chancellor Konrad Adenauer remarked that it was "extraordinarily difficult" to enact a law against the wishes of 70,000 doctors who each saw 30 patients a day.[60]

Nonetheless, Adenauer's attempt launched a series of health care reforms that have accelerated in frequency between 1972 and 1993. With the overall intent of controlling costs and, thus, keeping sickness fund contribution rates within politically acceptable bounds, the general strategy embodied in these reforms has been to set various kinds of limits on system capacity and spending. So far, the available evidence suggests that Germany has been successful in setting these limits without imposing health care rationing or other constraints on access to care or technology unacceptable to either patients or health care providers.

These cyclical reforms are one of the most striking features of the (West) German health care system in its latest incarnation. Critics sometimes cite periodic health reform laws as evidence of the system's troubles and impending doom. At a minimum, the need for periodic political intervention, and for a steadily increasing role for government monitoring and legislative prescriptions, suggests that the sickness funds by themselves have not been up to the task of restraining health care costs. Some see this as a predictable result of decisions made since the 1920s that strengthened doctors' role and weakened that of sickness funds. In the postwar preference for free-market solutions and "self-regulation" in health care (and other sectors), Rosenberg and Ruban noted in 1986,

> ...One might have expected that the social security agencies, especially the sickness funds, would fill the power vacuum and try to exercise control over suppliers. This was not the case. Indeed, sickness funds are still unable to formulate uniform health policies, to organize scientific counseling preparatory to negotiations, or to enforce their legitimate rights of supervision and control. In this political climate, it was easy for physicians, hospitals, and the pharmaceutical industry to pursue their own interests without opposition, and this has led to malfunctions detrimental to consumers.[61]

Nevertheless, the record suggests that Germany's periodic reforms of health care—which have actually been, up to this point, course corrections rather than restructuring—probably account for the for the remarkable flexibility and durability of the system compared to all others.

References and Notes

1. Leibfried, S and Tennstedt, F (1986). "Health-Insurance Policy and *Berufsverbote* in the Nazi Takeover" in *Political Values and Health Care: The German Experience*, ed. DW Light and A Schuller. Cambridge, MA: The MIT Press, p. 129.

2. Ibid.

3. Arnold, M (1992). "Protection Against Health Risk in the Federal Republic of Germany: Social-ethical and Historical Aspects," a talk delivered at the Goethe Institute of Boston, October 16, 1992.

4. Stone, DA (1980). *The Limits of Professional Power: National Health Care in the Federal Republic of Germany*. Chicago: University of Chicago Press, p. 21.

5. Glaser, WA (1991), p. 115.

6. Ibid, p. 14.

7. Rosenberg, P (1986). "The Origin and the Development of Compulsory Health Insurance in Germany," in *Political Values and Health Care: The German Experience*. Cambridge, MA: The MIT Press, p. 110.

8. Ibid, p. 106.

9. Reinhardt, KF (1961). *Germany: 2000 Years*, Volume II. New York: Frederick Ungar Publishing, p. 518.

10. Carr, W (1991). *A History of Germany, 1815-1990*. London: Edward Arnold/Hodder & Stoughton, p. 136.

11. Rosenberg, P (1986), p. 110.

12. Ibid, p. 111.

13. Raff, D (1988). *History of Germany from the Medieval Empire to the Present*. Oxford: Berg, p. 158.

14. Public assistance for the poor was enacted in 1924 and unemployment insurance in 1927.

15. Arnold, M, 1992.

16. Widgery, AG (1950). "Classical German Idealism, the Philosophy of Schopenhauer and Neo-Kantianism," in *A History of Philosophical Systems*, ed. Vergilius Ferm. New York: The Philosophical Library, p. 296.

17. Starr, P (1982). *The Social Transformation of American Medicine*. New York: Basic Books, p. 239.

18. Glaser, WA (1991), p. 69.

19. Carr, W (1991), p. 137.

20. Rosenberg, P (1986), p. 112.

21. Reinhardt, KF (1961), p. 517.

22. *Daten des Gesundheistwesens, 1991*. (*Health Care Data, 1991*) Bonn: Bundesministeriums für Gesundheit, p. 171.

23. Rosenberg, KF (1986), p. 115.

24. Stone, DA (1980), p. 49.

25. Ibid, p. 85.

26. Rosenberg, KF (1986), p. 112.

27. Schulenburg, J-M (1989). "The West German Health Care Financing and Delivery System: Its Experiences and Lessons for Other Nations," presented at an International Symposium on Health Care Systems in Taipei, Taiwan, Republic of China, unpublished.

28. Stone, DA (1980), p. 49.

29. Stone, DA (1986), p. 50.

30. Ibid, p. 50.

31. Rosenberg, KF (1986), p. 117.

32. Stone, DA (1980), pp. 44-51.

33. Rosenberg, KF (1986), p. 117.

34. Stone, DA (1980), p. 51.

35. Carr, W (1991), p. 273.

36. Rosenberg, KF (1986), p. 118.

37. Stone, DA (1980), p. 53.

38. There is some dispute over who was responsible for establishment of the *kassenärztliche Vereinigungen*—the Weimar government or the successive Hitler government of the National Socialists. While Webber (1992) includes it as part of the Weimar Settlement of 1931, Stefan Kirchberger of Münster University (in *Political Values and Health Care: The German Experience*, 1986, p. 209) asserts that the *KV*s were established in law by the Nazis, which physician groups postdated to 1932 "in order to avoid the stigma of National Socialist ideas." Kirchberger does acknowledge, however, that the *KV*s resulted from "interim regulations" dating from the final, crisis-ridden years of the Weimar Republic.

39. Webber, D (1992). "The Politics of Regulatory Change in the German Health Sector" in *The Politics of German Regulation*. Aldershot, England: Dartmouth Publishers, p. 211.

40. Light, DW (1986). "State, Profession, and Political Values" in *Political Values and Health Care: The German Experience*. Cambridge, MA: The MIT Press, p. 6.

41. Webber, W (1992), p. 210.

42. Stone, DA (1980), p. 54.

43. Kirchberger, S (1986). "Public-Health Policy, 1945-1949" in *Political Values and Health Care: The German Experience*. Cambridge, MA: The MIT Press, p. 210.

44. Sauerborn, M (1953). Kassenärzterecht in der Entwicklung, in *Bundesarbeitsblatt*, No. 8, pp. 205-215. Quoted in Douglass Webber, *The Politics of German Health System Reform: Successful and Failed Attempts at Reform from 1930 to 1984*.

45. Rosenberg, KF (1986), p. 119.

46. Leibfried, S and Tennstedt, F (1986), pp. 127-138.

47. Zimmerman, H (1938) "25 Jahre AOK Nürnberg." *Die Ortskrankenkasse* 26(12):388, cited in *Political Values and Health Care: The German Experience*, p. 137.

48. Leibfried, S and Tennstedt , F (1986), pp. 164-165.

49. Dr. Friedrich Hansen of Hamburg, personal interview, March 10. 1991.

50. Leibfried, S and Tennstedt, F (1986), p. 186.

51. Ibid., p. 131.

52. Rosenberg, P and Ruban, ME (1986). "Social Security and Health-Care Systems" in *Political Values and Health Care: The German Experience*, ed. Donald W. Light and Alexander Schuller. Cambridge, MA: The MIT Press, p. 276-277.

53. Kirchberger, S (1986), p. 196

54. Baum, R (1986). "Out of the Rubble: Political Values and Reconstruction," in *Political Values and Health Care: The German Experience*, ed. DW Light and A Schuller. Cambridge, Massachusetts: The MIT Press, p. 242.

55. Kirchberger, S (1986), p. 205.

56. Muthesius, H. (1947), quoted in Kirchberger, S (1986), p. 206.

57. Webber, D (1992), p. 212.

58. Glaser, WA (1991), p. 32.

59. Webber, D (1992), p. 212.

60. Ibid, p. 212

61. Rosenberg, P and Ruban, ME (1986), p. 281.

CHAPTER 3

Paying for Health Care: The German Formula

By Richard A. Knox and Christopher Straub, MD

I f the German method of financing health care appears complicated, it is largely due to two things: unfamiliarity and comparison to Canada, the United Kingdom, and other nations that rely on single-source—virtually all-government—funding. In fact, Germany's system for paying health care bills is simpler than those of European neighbors such as France and Switzerland in terms of multiplicity of payers, benefits, and relationships among payers, providers, and patients. And the U.S. system makes Germany's pale in any objective comparison of incoherence. There is ample reason to think that the labyrinthine complexity of the U.S. system, with its resulting lack of accountability, is a major factor in its higher costs, and in America's conspicuous lack of success in controlling health care costs compared to Germany. (Table 3.1)

Two Systems of Financing Care

Consider the following U.S. health care attributes and the corresponding German situation.

Determining who is eligible for health insurance in America is exceedingly difficult. The U.S. system is characterized by multiple payment sources without uniform criteria relating to employment status, residence, age, income level, medical need, or group affiliation. Instead, an individual's or family's insurance status derives from capricious and shifting criteria that include

- employers' discretion, employees' political influence, labor markets, and macroeconomic trends such as the shift to a service-based economy that relies more on a transient, less unionized, often less highly skilled workforce;
- state policies governing private insurance and eligibility for public programs;

□ medical disqualifications for preexisting conditions and health risks, applied to individuals seeking coverage;

□ group exclusions—for instance, certain types of businesses considered as posing high insurance risks or groups perceived to be at high risk of expensive diseases, such as AIDS; and

□ above all, the ability of individuals to afford premiums that are the world's highest and are rising at an annual rate of 10.1 percent in 1992, more than triple the general inflation rate.[1]

As a result of this tattered patchwork of coverage, nearly one in six Americans lacked health coverage in 1992,[2] and nearly two-thirds of the uninsured reside in families supported principally by a full-time worker.[3]

Eligibility for health insurance in Germany is based almost solely on one criterion: residency status. Everyone who resides within the nation's borders may have health coverage, and 99.8 percent do.[4] (Table 3.2) The criteria

---

Table 3.1

Growth in Health Insurance Costs: Germany vs U.S., 1986-91 in Dollars of Total Plan Cost Per Employee*

Year	Germany		U.S.		Ratio U.S./Germany
	Cost	Difference from prior year	Cost**	Difference from prior year	
1986	$1,480	---	$1,857	---	1.26
1987	1,553	+4.98%	1,985	+6.9%	1.28
1988	1,695	+9.2	2,354	+18.6	1.39
1989	1,653	-2.5	2,748	+16.7	1.66
1990	1,785	+8	3,217	+17.1	1.80
1991	1,936	+8.5	3,605	+12.1	1.86

Avg. annual increase, 1987-91
Germany = 5.6% U.S. = 14.3%

*Using OECD purchasing power parity conversion rates.
** Includes employer and employee costs for indemnity and managed care plans, dental plans, vision/hearing plans, and perscription drugs.

Sources: Jahresgutachten 1992, Sachverstandigenrat für die Konzertierte Aktion im Gesundheitswesen; Health Care Benefits Survey: *Medical Plans, Foster Higgins, 1993.*

determining how one receives coverage are clear, nationally consistent, and well-understood by individuals, employers, providers, and policymakers. For health insurance purposes, the German population is divided into

- employed people with incomes under an annually revised ceiling (DM 61,200, or about $29,300, in 1992)[5], who must belong to one of eight different types of sickness funds depending on type of employment;
- those with incomes above this ceiling, who may join a statutory sickness fund—as two-thirds do—or buy private health insurance;[6]
- pensioners, who are insured either by the same sickness fund they belonged to as active workers or by private for-profit insurers, depending on their income and personal choice;
- self-employed people, who may buy coverage privately or from a sickness fund (if they have previously been sickness fund members);
- civil servants, including public school teachers and university professors as well as government bureaucrats, whose medical costs are covered by their respective government employers, by private insurance, or by a combination of both;
- police and military personnel, who are covered by government;
- unemployed workers, who remain in the same sickness fund they belonged to while employed as long as they are on unemployment compensation benefits (up to one year), with their premiums paid by the Federal Labor Administration and local welfare offices; and
- welfare recipients—chronically unemployed or unemployable people receiving income assistance from local communities—who are either enrolled in local sickness funds with their premiums paid by welfare agencies or have their medical expenses paid directly by local agencies.

In the U.S., health insurance benefits are almost infinitely variable, from one plan to another and over time. This situation is confusing to consumers, frustrating for health care providers, and costly to administer for insurers and government payers. Although a thorough description of the universe of health insurance benefits in the U.S. is beyond the scope of this report, the variations lie along a number of axes, including but not limited to:

- the amount of out-of-pocket expenses (deductibles) that consumers must pay before coverage kicks in;
- the share of ongoing costs (copayments) that consumers must pay;
- the maximum limits of coverage;
- benefits and limits particular to hospital care, outpatient physician care, diagnostic procedures, laboratory tests, and other services, such as home care;
- coverage (if any) for prescription drugs, dental care, and medical aids and appliances, from eyeglasses to wheelchairs;
- the degree of choice subscribers or beneficiaries have of doctor, hospital, pharmacy, or other providers;
- inclusions, exclusions, waiting periods, and special rules for innovative, high-cost, and transitional medical technologies (those between purely research and clearly mainstream); and
- preventive services, such as well-child care, immunizations, vision and hearing examinations, routine physicals, Pap smears and mammograms, and colonoscopy.

Table 3.2

Health Insurance in Germany: An Overview

Year	Total Population	without coverage	%	with coverage	%
1970	60,924	648		60,240	
1976*	61,542	223		61,319	
1980	61,516	237		61,379	
1985	60,987	215		60,772	
1990	63,062	97	0.2%	62,965	99.8%

Individuals Per Type of Coverage, in 1,000s

Year	Statutory insurance		Private insurance		Other coverage**	
1970	5,3531		5696		1013	
1976	5,5577		4482		1260	
1980	5,5565		4611		1203	
1985	5,4447		5135		1190	
1990	5,4361	86.2%	6935	11%	1669	2.6%

* No survey of health insurance coverage was conducted in 1975.
** Includes social welfare, private charity, and the wealthy who self-pay.

Source: Sachverständigenrat für Konzertierte Aktion im Gesundheitswesen, 1992.

"Anyone familiar with the offerings of the Federal Employees Health Benefits Program or other multiple-choice systems knows how quickly the eyes glaze over when confronted by page after page of coverage variations among alternative plans," comments Linda A. Bergthold of William M. Mercer, Inc., a national benefits consulting firm. The disadvantages of such disarray, she notes, are serious:

> When each health plan is allowed to vary its benefits, consumers cannot easily make price comparisons. They may be reluctant to choose plans with lower prices for fear those plans have hidden exclusions buried in the fine print....If plans can vary their benefits, they likely will modify them to attract low-risk enrollees and avoid those with higher risks.[7]

Health care benefits in Germany are very broad and nationally uniform, with only minor variations among plans. The generous catalogue of benefits goes a long way toward explaining why the system has such strong support among both beneficiaries and providers. Near-uniformity of benefits among payers (including private insurance plans) eliminates confusion about what is covered for both consumers and providers, facilitates political debate about benefit changes, and makes cost-comparisons among plans feasible. Differences in contribution rates (premiums) among sickness funds are not due to difficult-to-quantify variations in benefits but to other readily identifiable factors, such as inter-plan differences in wage levels and members' average age. Policymakers can readily track expenditures by type. (Figure 3.1)

Regardless of one's plan, statutory health insurance in Germany provides

- virtually free choice of doctors, unlimited physician visits (including house calls), preventive checkups, and total freedom from out-of-pocket payments for physician services;*
- unlimited acute-hospital care, with only nominal copayment—DM 11 per day (about $5.26) for the first 14 days of hospitalization, a maximum of about $74;
- prescription drug coverage, with a copayment of DM 3-7 ($1.44-$3.35) as of January, 1993;
- dental benefits more comprehensive than any nation,[8] encompassing routine preventive care, restorative care (fillings and crowns), periodontal services, dentures and other prostheses, and orthodontia. Copayments range from 25 to 40 percent of claims depending on the service, and discounts of up to 15 percent are granted to patients who have had regular checkups;[9]
- vision and hearing exams, eyeglasses, hearing aids, prostheses, wheelchairs, and other "healing and helping" aids;
- inpatient psychiatric care and outpatient psychiatric visits (although mental health benefits are widely considered inadequate);
- monthly home care allowances for the chronically ill ($191 for family caregivers and $359 for professional caregivers in 1991), plus four weeks annual respite care;
- liberal maternity benefits, including 14 weeks of employer-paid income replacement for employed women, lump-sum payments at the time of birth for employed and unemployed women, cash incentives and total coverage for complete prenatal care, household assistance following birth, and monthly cash allowances for mothers of children under the age of one year;

□ up to five days of full pay for parents of sick children under eight years of age;

□ disability pay after six weeks of illness (during which the employer pays full wages), providing 80 percent of full pay for a maximum of 78 weeks; and

□ four- to six-week stays every three years (on the advice of a physician) at *Kurkliniks*, resort spas which offer mineral baths and other restorative treatments, physical therapy, exercise regimens, and rehabilitation.

Relations among U.S. payers, providers, and patients are highly fragmented, variable, unpredictable, and confusing. In recent years, as the U.S. market for private health insurance has become increasingly competitive, it has splintered into a proliferating array of new entities and types of plans—prepaid staff-model health maintenance organizations (HMOs), independent practice associations (IPAs), preferred-provider organizations (PPOs), point-of-service plans, and self-insuring employee groups, as well as traditional indemnity plans. Benefits and restrictions vary considerably from one plan to another, as do billing requirements and forms, prior-approval rules, and utilization controls. In the volatile market that has resulted, there has been much "churning" of subscribers as employers and beneficiaries switch from one insurer to another in response to price increases.

This turmoil and complexity has its price for all involved. By one estimate, total U.S. health administration costs jumped 37 percent, in inflation-adjusted dollars, between 1983 and 1987.[10] During this period, insurance overhead—the cost of administration, claims processing, marketing, and expenses other than paying for care—rose from 4.4 to 5.1 percent of total U.S. health spending.[11] The American hospital workforce has grown by 20 percent in administrators and 71 percent in marketing specialists between 1983 and 1989, compared to only 13 percent in nursing staff.[12] Figuring out ways to shift costs to payers with less clout has become a major (and widely acknowledged) preoccupation of hospital managers. Except for the Medicare system, the fees of physicians and the prices charged by hospitals are virtually unique to each doctor and hospital, a chaotic situation that makes prices and price comparisons meaningless.

The "hassle factor" may have displaced the threat of medical malpractice litigation as the leading complaint of American doctors. A recent cross-national survey of physicians conducted by Robert J. Blendon of the Harvard School of Public Health and colleagues found that 78 percent of U.S. physicians reported "excessive delays or disputes in processing insurance forms or receiving payment for services rendered." This was twice the proportion of West German doctors with that complaint.[13]

For U.S. health care consumers, and for their employers' benefit managers who offer employees whatever choices they have, the current marketplace is confusing. Few people can decipher exactly what their escalating premium dollars buy. Both competition and public debate is muddled by the lack of consistent benchmarks; it is impossible to compare one group's premiums or trends with another's, or to track health costs except at an aggregate level that has little meaning for individuals or specific groups.

Finally, despite an ideology that favors privately funded and administered programs over public ones, the proportion of the total U.S. health care dollar that flows through government budgets is more than twice as high as in Germany. (Figure 3.2)

Figure 3.1

German Statutory Health Insurance Outlays by Type of Benefit, 1990

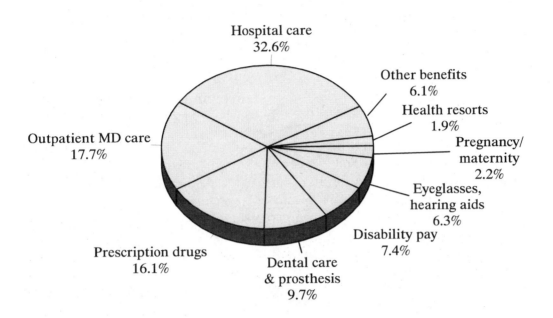

Benefit	Expenditure	
	DM	$$
Hospital care	49.0	23.6
Outpatient MD care	26.7	12.8
Prescription drugs	24.4	11.7
Dental care and prostheses	14.6	7.0
Disability pay	11.4	5.4
Eyeglasses, hearing aids, etc.	9.5	4.6
Pregnancy/maternity	3.3	1.6
Health resorts	2.9	1.4
Other benefits	9.1	4.4
TOTAL	150.9	72.5

Source: Kassenärztliche Bundesvereinigen, Düsseldorf, 1992.

Figure 3.2

Paying for Health Care

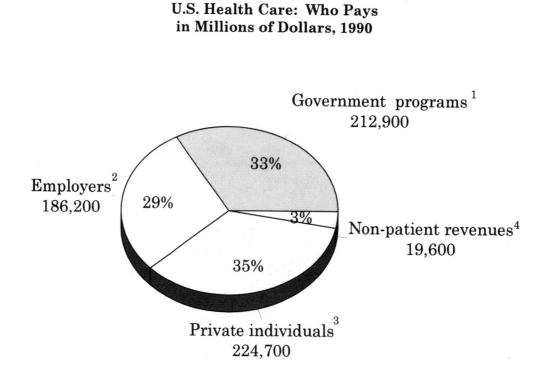

U.S. Health Care: Who Pays
in Millions of Dollars, 1990

Government programs [1]
212,900

Employers [2]
186,200

Non-patient revenues [4]
19,600

Private individuals [3]
224,700

[1] Includes only general-revenue federal and state government sources: Medicaid, some Medicare, premiums for government employees, U.S. Departments of Defense and Veterans Affairs, Bureau of Indian Affairs, school health programs, public health activities.

[2] Includes employer contributions to health insurance premiums, mandatory contributions to Medicare, Workers' Compensation medical premiums, temporary disability medical insurance, industrial in-plant medical services.

[3] Includes private contributions to health insurance premiums, contributions, and premiums to Medicare, out-of-pocket payments to cover copayments, deductibles, and services not covered by insurance.

[4] Includes philanthropy; income from gift shops, cafeterias, parking lots, education programs, interest, dividends, rents.

Source: Levit, KR and Cowan, CA, Health Care Financing Review, *Vol. 13, No. 2, Winter 1991, pp. 83-92.*

Figure 3.2, continued

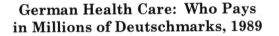

German Health Care: Who Pays
in Millions of Deutschmarks, 1989

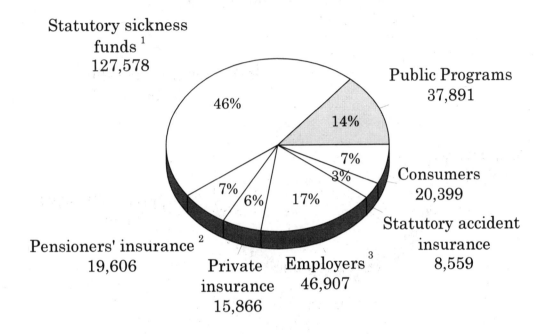

Statutory sickness
funds [1]
127,578

Public Programs
37,891

46%

14%

7%

3%

7%

6%

17%

Consumers
20,399

Pensioners' insurance [2]
19,606

Private
insurance
15,866

Employers [3]
46,907

Statutory accident
insurance
8,559

[1] Premiums are paid 50/50 by employees and employers.
[2] Paid jointly by pensioners, pension funds, and sickness funds through cross-subsidy payments among funds depending on share of retired members.
[3] Primarily in the form of sick pay in first 6 weeks of illness.

Source: Sachverständigenrat für Konzertierte Aktion im Gesundheitswesen, 1992.

Relationships among German payers, providers, and patients are highly structured, orderly, predictable, and well-understood by all parties. While no one could characterize these relationships as simple, payers and providers in Germany deal with each other in an organized fashion, and can count on a high degree of stability. Health benefits, being essentially uniform, are not an arena for dispute or complicated accounting for either providers or payers.

The pivotal point of German payer-provider relationships is the round of annual negotiations that set budgets for the coming years. Groups of sickness funds negotiate with individual hospitals; sickness funds negotiate with physician collectives with statutory authority to bargain for doctors in a given region and to act as the payment intermediary. Prices and cost-sharing for pharmaceuticals and other medical goods are set centrally.

Perhaps most crucially, Germany's method of financing health care is uniform across all the sickness funds that make up the statutory health insurance program: the rules of compulsory membership are nationally uniform, as is the method of calculating the premium (called the *Beitragssatz*, or "contribution rate"), and all employers and employees split the contributions evenly. (The worker's portion is not considered as taxable income.) "This contribution rate is the beacon that politicians, unions, employers, and the media watch to track health care costs," says Uwe E. Reinhardt, PhD, a Princeton University economist and authority on the German health system. "Sharp increases in that rate usually trigger tough new cost-control measures. It is a simple number, easily tracked, and well understood by all parties."[14]

Administrative costs in the German system appear to be lower than in the U.S. system, although data are sparse and there are conflicting interpretations of available data. One recent cross-national comparison of health administration costs by Jean-Pierre Poullier of the Organization for Economic Cooperation and Development found that U.S. per capita administrative costs in 1990 were nearly 50 percent higher than Germany's.[15] However, Poullier's per capita administrative expense calculation for the U.S.—$149—is much lower than that estimated by Steffie Woolhandler and David U. Himmelstein of Harvard Medical School, who calculated an all-inclusive U.S. administrative cost in 1987 of $400 to $497 per capita.[16] (Woolhandler and Himmelstein did not estimate an administrative cost for Germany.) Whatever the exact figures, Poullier's analysis suggests that the U.S. and Germany, along with the Netherlands, "could be in a league of their own" in terms of administrative cost, since these nations' reported administrative burdens are substantially higher than the single-payer systems of Canada, the United Kingdom, or Sweden. "These data confirm that countries with segmented sources of insurance pay for their flexibility through higher administrative costs," Poullier writes.[17] In addition, Germany has recently stepped up monitoring of health providers for quality, utilization, and efficiency—a step that entails what some call a "planned increase" in administrative costs. "However, if recent German experience is any indication," Poullier concludes, "a stable ratio of health expenditures to GDP [gross domestic product] can be maintained along with a high level of services, even with increasing administrative costs."[18]

Statutory Insurance: Who Must Belong, Who May Opt Out

Germany's 1,340 statutory sickness funds comprise the central feature of the nation's health financing system. For 86 percent of the population, sickness funds are the pipelines that channel money from workers, employers, retirees, pension funds, and government welfare programs to those who provide health care goods and services. (Table 3.3) The term "statutory" as applied to these entities has real force: It means they are quasi-public institutions, or "bodies of public law," required or entitled by statute and court rulings to

Table 3.3

Germans Covered by Statutory Health Insurance, 1985-90

Numbers by category of insureds in thousands and percent by category

Year	Obligatory members		Dependents		Voluntary members		Pensioners		Total
	#	percent	#	percent	#	percent	#	percent	
1985	21,105	37.9%	19,507	35%	4,481	8%	10,632	19.1%	55,716
1986	21,386	39	18,433	33.6	4,412	8	10,652	19.4	54,883
1987	21,559	39.3	18,144	33.4	4,446	8.1	10,713	19.5	54,862
1988	21,838	41	16,200	30.5	4,372	8.2	10,791	20.3	53,201
1989	21,885	41.3	15,726	29.7	4,441	8.3	10,904	20.6	52,956
1990	22,426	41.7	15,973	29.7	4,418	8.2	11,010	20.4	53,827

Source: Bundesministeriums für Gesundheit (1991). Daten des Gesundheitswesens. *Baden-Baden: Nomos Verlagsgesellschaft, p. 171.*

□ collect mandatory contributions from employers and workers to finance their operations;

□ guarantee their members access to the most advanced medical care;[19] and

□ bargain with health care providers over budgets and prices.

In addition to these legal requirements, statutory sickness funds are forbidden from altering the basic benefit package (though they may supplement it), and may not engage in medical underwriting, or the exclusion of members on the basis of medical or actuarial risk. Because of these statutory prerogatives and obligations, German sickness funds occupy a space in between government-run insurance programs like those in Canadian provinces and private-sector U.S. insurers such as Blue Cross-Blue Shield and commercial companies. Reinhardt suggests that Germany's statutory sickness funds be considered "a private-sector extension of the government's will."[20]

Membership in a sickness fund is compulsory for only about 70 percent of working-age Germans—those whose income is below a statutory ceiling. The ceiling rises each year as the average income increases; in 1992, it was about $29,300.

Of the higher-income population, 30 percent select statutory sickness fund membership voluntarily in large part because there are clear financial incentives for them to do so rather than buy private health insurance. All members of a given sickness fund pay the same contribution rate, a percentage of their income up to the statutory ceiling. For that contribution, they get the full benefits regardless of their family status; there is no separate, higher contribution required for a family plan. (If both parents in a family work, and their individual income is below the income ceiling, they both pay the mandatory contribution and their children's coverage comes from the parent with the higher income.[21]) For most German families, statutory health insurance is a favorable deal.

By contrast, private insurers in Germany charge a separate, age-related premium for each member of a family. Obviously, this makes private insurance more attractive for single adults and unmarried couples whose incomes are high enough to allow them to opt out of the statutory health insurance program. If they choose sickness fund membership, they will pay the maximum contribution (on average about $3,800 a year, or $320 a month, in 1992), which includes an implicit subsidy of families. If they buy private coverage, they pay only for themselves. This premium structure results in risk selection that works against statutory sickness funds. For example, nearly two-thirds of privately insured Germans had monthly incomes over $1,050 in 1985, compared to only 15 percent of statutory fund members.[22] However, policymakers recognize the risk to the statutory system of people switching back and forth from the sickness funds to private insurance based on their financial advantage and medical needs. To prevent rampant adverse selection, German law bars individuals from returning to the statutory system once they have left it for private coverage, except in unusual circumstances such as a dramatic decline in income.

The Sickness Fund Structure

German sickness funds are grouped into two main divisions and 8 types. (Table 3.4) This structure reflects the system's historical origins as an occupation-based scheme focused initially on manual laborers. Six of the eight funds are known as **State Insurance Regulation funds** (*Reichsversicherungsordnung* or *RVO* funds), which are governed by boards composed equally of employer and elected member representatives. The *RVO* funds are subject to tight federal regulation. (The six thick volumes containing the much-amended *RVO* law of 1911 are prominently displayed on the bookshelves of all sickness fund managers.) Virtually all German workers whose incomes fall below the statutory ceiling must belong to an *RVO* fund. Those who work fewer than 50 days per year are exempted. Many have no choice of funds. For instance, all blue-collar employees who work for a company with its own fund must join it. These so-called *Betriebskrankenkassen* are equivalent to self-insurance plans in the U.S.; in Germany a company must employ at least 450 people to set up its own fund. Similarly, tradesmen who belong to a craft union which has a sickness fund, called an *Innungskrankenkasse,* must join. Farm workers, miners, and seamen must belong to their respective funds. Many workers with incomes below the

Table 3.4

German Sickness Funds and Their Membership Shares, 1990

Type of fund	Number of funds	Number of members and dependents	Percent of total	Percent of pop.
RVO FUNDS				
Local	267	23,277,000	42%	27%
Company-based	692	7,028,000	13%	11%
Craft-affilliated	152	3,058,000	5%	5%
Agricultural workers	19	1,342,000	2%	2%
Miners	1	1,378,000	2%	2%
Seamen	1	N.A.	N.A.	N.A.
SUBSTITUTE FUNDS				
Blue-collar substitute	8	1,097,000	2%	2%
White-collar substitute	7	18,577,000	33%	29%
All statutory funds	1,147	55,832,000	100%	89%

Sources: Jahresgutachten 1992, Sachverständigenrat für die Konszertierte Aktion im Gesundheitswesen; Bundesministeriums für Gesundheitswesen.

statutory ceiling, as well as unemployed people and welfare recipients, have nowhere to obtain coverage except their local sickness fund, or *Ortskrankenkasse*. These catch-all local funds, similar in some ways to the Blue Cross-Blue Shield plans of the 1960s before they became more commercially oriented, cover nearly 40 percent of the German population.

White-collar employees have more choice. They may be eligible to join a company sickness fund or a trade-based fund. Local funds are always open to them. Or they may choose one of seven white-collar **substitute funds**, called *Ersatzkassen,* as two-thirds of white-collar workers do. In general, these plans operate nationally and are open to all professional, managerial, and clerical workers. (One substitute plan is available only in a limited geographical area, and some specialize in certain occupational categories, such as engineers and technical workers.) Even though substitute funds offer the same benefits as *RVO* funds, membership carries a certain cachet, certifying the higher social status of white-collar workers. Substitute funds have a different governance structure; instead of sharing authority with employers, the substitute funds are totally governed by their members, reflecting a time when they were mutual funds operating outside the *RVO* system of compulsory insurance.

Some blue-collar workers can join a substitute fund. Eight such funds for manual laborers exist, but their membership is limited to certain geographic areas or trades. In 1990, these "workers' substitute funds" enrolled just over one million members, or about 2 percent of the sickness fund population.

Covering German "Welfare Recipients"

About 14 percent of the German population in 1990 were not working--the recently unemployed, the chronically unemployed, those residing in institutions, and those receiving "social aid," who would be called "welfare recipients" in the U.S.[23] The system makes special allowances for these populations, hewing as closely as possible to the employment-based insurance model and minimizing the amount of government subsidy. For instance, jobless people who are still receiving unemployment compensation benefits (which last up to 1 year) continue as members of the sickness fund that covered them while they were working. Their premiums are paid by a national unemployment insurance fund, but the absolute contributions are lower than for the average employed sickness fund member. Thus, employed sickness fund members and their employers pay a hidden subsidy to continue health coverage for unemployed members. Since the unemployed are concentrated in the *RVO* funds, and especially the local funds, this burden falls more heavily on members of these funds, who have lower incomes than members of substitute funds or private insurance subscribers.[24] (Table 3.5)

Local governments, which have responsibility for social aid, pay the sickness fund contributions of the poor, or, in some locales, directly pay for medical and hospital care on their behalf. However, the contribution is pegged to the lowest amount paid by self-employed individuals, about $38 a month in 1991.[25] Since this is significantly below the average cost of coverage, it means that sickness fund members—again, especially local funds whose members have the lowest average incomes—are implicitly subsidizing the poor through their premiums. Elliot K. Wicks, PhD, of the Center for Health Policy Development in Washington, D.C., remarks that this was not a burning issue in

Table 3.5

Health Coverage for the Unemployed in Germany: Concentration of Unemployed in *RVO* Sickness Funds, 1985

(Type of insurance in thousands)

Employment status	*RVO* sickness funds	Substitute funds	Private insurance
Employed	14,954	7,563	2,430
Unemployed	1,057	349	28
Ratio of unemployed to employed	1:14	1:22	1:87

Source: Wysong, J, and Abel, T, The Milbank Quarterly, *1990.*

Germany when he interviewed authorities about it in early 1991, since "welfare" recipients make up only about 2 percent of sickness fund members. By comparison, Wicks notes, the U.S. Medicaid program covers about 8 percent of the total population, and still falls short of encompassing all those officially considered to be in poverty.

What To Do About the Self-Employed

About 4 percent of the German population is self-employed[26] compared to nearly 10 percent of the U.S. workforce.[27] All nations with employment-based health insurance systems have difficulties with this individualistic group, and Germany is no exception. "The self-employed consistently resist paying rates exceeding their actuarial costs," observes William A. Glaser, PhD, professor of health services management at the New School for Social Research in New York City. "Social solidarity is the philosophy of the labor movement, not theirs."[28] Only the lowest-income self-employed are required to buy health insurance in Germany, and until 1989 they could join sickness funds. Under current law, those who have previously belonged to a sickness fund may continue with that fund when they become self-employed.[29] They must pay the entire contribution according to a schedule of 10 income ranges that is designed to impose a payment equivalent to the rate of employed people with the same income. Most self-employed people, however, must buy private insurance. The usual income threshold that entitles most workers to buy private coverage is waived for the self-employed. "Much of the competition among carriers in the [private] health insurance market is over the self-employed," Glaser reports.[30] Consistent with the rest of German society, very few self-employed people go without coverage, perhaps partly because their access to coverage in retirement depends on participation in some form of insurance while they are active earners.

The Retiree Problem

The U.S. addressed the problem of retirees' health costs three decades ago with Medicare, an employer-mandate program funded by payroll taxes and general revenues. But, as of 1993, the U.S. had yet to extend secure coverage to the working population or many of the poor. Germans went at it the other way around. They started 110 years ago with an employer mandate and payroll tax to fund workers' health coverage, and added retirees to the general system in 1941. Yet, as recent years have shown, neither nation has solved the problem of funding elders' medical costs. Medicare spending more than tripled during the 1980s, rose another 36 percent between 1990 and 1993, and is expected to shoot up another 78 percent between 1993 and 1998.[31] Germany's statutory sickness funds doubled their spending for pensioners' health benefits between 1980 and 1990.[32] German policymakers are also anxious about the future burdens of retirees on the working population, and the impact of this ineluctable trend on the viability of their social insurance system.

An Aging Population. The demographic trends are indeed worrisome. West Germany's life expectancy rate has increased substantially since the 1960s while the fertility rate fell by 50 percent between 1964 and 1984. The result is a projected population decline and a ballooning of the dependent elderly population. Germany's dependency ratio (the proportion of the population under age 19 and over age 65 compared to the working-age population) was 58 percent in 1988, the most recent OECD figure. This is considerably lower, and thus more favorable in terms of social insurance financing, than the U.S. ratio of 70 dependent persons for every 30 workers. However, this comparison is misleading, because the U.S. has a higher percentage of young dependents who will become workers, while Germany already has 25 percent more elders, and 37 percent more people over 80 years old, as a proportion of its population. Moreover, the accumulation of elder Germans will inevitably increase over the next three decades, a trend that will only be partially offset by German reunification and the flow of refugees from former Soviet bloc countries. J.-Matthias Graf von der Schulenburg, professor of insurance economics at the University of Hannover, points out that

> The number of elderly will increase over the next 40 years, which will increase the demand for health services and for nursing care....The number of people in the workforce will decline. Because social security is financed by pay-as-you-go premiums of the employees and their employers, the contribution rates are increasing and will increase due to the change of population structure....It is clear that future generations will not be willing to finance this burden.[33]

Paying for Elders' Care. The funding of German retirees' health care comes from three sources:

1. the government social security pension fund, which contributes a nationally uniform percentage of the retiree's pension that matches the combined average contribution rate of all active workers and their employers—13.1 percent in 1993;[34]

2. private pension income, which individual retirees must remit as a percentage of their pension check equal to the average sickness fund contribution rate;

3. subsidies from each sickness fund, raised by a tax on all active workers' base wages (the tax rate 2.93 percent in 1990[35]) plus whatever additional contributions are necessary to pay for retirees' health benefits out of general sickness fund revenues.

The funds from pension funds and individual retirees amount to less than half the money needed to pay for retirees' health benefits—48 percent in 1990. This requires active workers and their employers to subsidize the rest through their 3 percent retiree payroll tax, divided equally between workers and employers, plus a portion of their regular contributions to their respective sickness funds. No general tax revenues are used to make up the difference. Retirees stay with the same sickness fund that insured them when they were in the workforce, and a 1989 law requires those who were privately insured while working to remain privately insured when they retire, paying the entire premium themselves.[36]

Because some sickness funds have higher proportions of retirees than others, a 1977 reform law established a mechanism to redistribute money from those with lower retiree burdens to those with higher pensioners' costs. This program, called **Health Insurance for Pensioners** (*Krankenversicherung der Rentner*), set up an incentive for sickness funds to spend more on pensioners' care so they would draw from the equalization pool rather than pay into it. "It might grant frills that please subscribers but lack medical value—such as trips to spas and...extra fees to doctors," Glaser explains.[37] To ward off such waste, Parliament passed laws requiring sickness funds to limit costs to medically necessary care, mandating audits of sickness fund cost reports for retiree-related expenditures, and requiring funds to absorb the first 10 percent of any above-average retiree spending.[38,39]

The Politics of Long Term Care. Politicians are aware that measures will have to be taken to control the cost of caring for elders. A long term care insurance plan, long contemplated as a way of moving elders out of acute care hospitals into cheaper settings, may finally be pursued in earnest in the mid-1990s. Martin Pfaff, PhD, a University of Augsburg economist and member of Parliament from the Social Democratic Party, says that long term care is one of the handful of issues "that move people greatly," along with such issues as financing the costs of reunification and restrictions on political asylum-seekers. "We recognize it is only going to get worse," Pfaff said in an interview in late 1992, referring to the costs of caring for the aged. The issue of controling health care costs in general transcends long term care, he explained:

> The incomes of the retired are based on an increase in net wages, and net wages are depressed by higher contribution rates [for health insurance generally and pensioners' health care]. The prospects for the next few years is a real purchasing power loss among pensioners. The election year of 1994 is certainly one factor politically.[40]

At the same time, Germany conducted extensive political debate about a long term care insurance program in the mid-1980s, and many expected such legislation to pass before the federal elections of 1987, but the issue was derailed because of factional politics.[41]

Social Solidarity vs Sickness Fund Classism

From the beginning, there has been a built-in tension in Germany's health insurance system between its two cardinal features:

1. social solidarity, the willingness to subsidize others in need in the expectation that the favor will someday be returned; and
2. stratification among sickness fund members and other members of society according to their occupation, income, and social class.

Despite Germany's durable commitment to solidarity in sickness fund financing, there are many examples of discrimination against blue-collar workers. Until 1969, manual laborers' sick pay was much less generous than office workers'. It was not until 1989 that blue-collar workers with incomes above the sickness fund assessment ceiling were given the same choice to opt out of the *RVO* funds and buy private insurance that white-collar workers had always enjoyed.[42] However, the principal tension between solidarity and classism is inherent in Germany's method of sickness fund financing.

Solidarity is built into the method of calculating contributions. Individuals pay a percentage of their gross wages, up to the nationally defined income ceiling. The percentage is the same for all members of a given sickness fund, whatever the individual member's family status or medical needs, but the absolute contribution varies with the worker's income. As Wolfgang Schmeinck, director of the National Association of Company Sickness Funds, explains:

> The insured pay according to their economic situation. However, they receive benefits according to their medical needs, independent of their contribution....The result is [an] equalization of burdens which takes care that better-off members also pay higher contributions; that younger members support older members with numerous diseases, that single members support those with numerous dependents, etc.[43]

At the same time, even German workers with identical incomes can pay considerably different percentages of their wages, as well as varying absolute amounts, for the same package of health benefits. (Figure 3.3) This is due partly to the sickness fund system's architecture, which has compartmentalized people by their occupational and income status since the beginning, and partly to outside forces only minimally under the sickness funds' control.

Is the Sickness Fund Structure Out of Date?

It is no accident that the structure of Germany's sickness funds reflects an array of occupational categories that no longer seem to fit the nation's modern workforce profile. There are separate funds for miners, craftsmen, manufacturing workers, seamen, and farmers. Off to one side, organizationally almost an

Figure 3.3

Varying Contribution Rates Among German Sickness Funds, 1990

Average, highest, and lowest rates, as percent of gross wages under about $27,000.

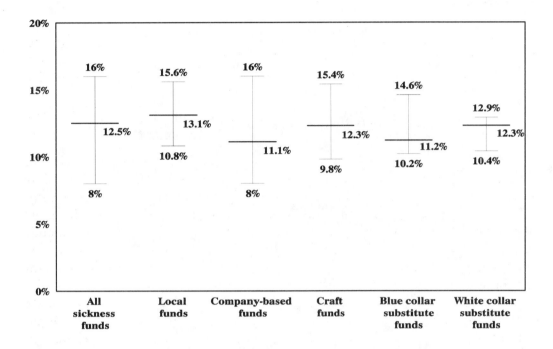

Source: Sachverständigenrat für die Konsertierte Aktion im Gesundheitswesen, 1991.

afterthought, are the substitute funds made up mostly of office personnel, salespeople, civil servants, and managers.

Chancellor Otto von Bismarck conceived and designed the statutory insurance system in 1883 to benefit the common laborer—the tradesman and wage-earner. This burgeoning social class clearly needed the state's help; Bismarck, the conservative aristocrat, realized that if they didn't get it from Germany's fledgling government, laborers would support the socialists' offers of aid. Salaried employees, those who worked in offices and shops, could take care of themselves. Moreover, civil servants and white-collar workers made up only 6 to 8 percent of the workforce in the 1880s and 1890s, while blue-collar workers accounted for 55 to 60 percent.[44] The political priorities were clear.

As Jere A. Wysong of the State University of New York in Fredonia and Thomas Abel of the University of Marburg (Germany) point out, the contemporary German workforce is virtually a mirror image of the one in Bismarck's day. By 1950, civil servants and white-collar workers made up one-quarter of the workforce. Laborers were still barely in the majority, but the self-employed had declined by half, from 28 to 14.5 percent of all workers. By 1985, white-collar workers were the largest group, 48 percent of all workers, while blue-collar laborers had declined to 39 percent. By the mid-1980s, the Federal Republic of Germany "clearly had become a middle-class society," Wysong and Abel note.[45]

This shift has major implications for contemporary sickness funds. White-collar workers, who tend to have higher incomes and lower health risks than manual laborers, are largely segregated in the substitute funds. This leaves the *RVO* funds, especially the local funds, with members who have lower incomes and more costly health needs. In addition, as discussed above, the local funds enroll most of the unemployed, the disabled, and the poor—groups which must be subsidized by the local funds' working members. Since the sickness fund system is pay-as-you-go, it does not accumulate reserves, and deficits cannot be made up by government subsidies. Therefore, to remain solvent the local funds must requisition a higher percentage of their members' wages, on average, than the substitute funds.

Substitute fund managers vigorously dispute the allegation that their members have lower health risks, but it is taken as axiomatic by many German health care authorities. For one thing, the *RVO* funds have a disproportionate number of older workers, those between 50 and 65.[46] A 1988 survey of sickness fund members also found that members of local funds and company-based funds had a higher average number of chronic diseases than members of substitute funds or private insurance subscribers. Local fund and company fund members were also significantly less likely to report that their health was good or very good, according to the survey.[47]

Most telling, the benefit outlays of community-based and company-based sickness funds are significantly higher per member than the substitute funds', and their claims costs have been growing faster. (Table 3.6) The differences are most striking in hospital expenses. Wysong and Abel found that community-based funds used 33 percent more hospital days per 100 members than white-collar substitute funds in 1985, and their yearly outlays per member for hospital care were 32 percent higher. Moreover, the local funds' hospital costs grew by 710 percent between 1965 and 1985, while the white-collar funds' hospital outlays rose by 600 percent.[48]

Locally based funds, which enroll three-fifths of all workers,[49] also reflect local health care costs. If a region has a costlier than average medical care system, due to a greater density of physicians, higher-cost hospitals, greater utilization of services, or any combination of factors, its regionally-based sickness funds must charge higher contribution rates to workers and employers. Year-to-year increases in health care costs must also be passed through to contribution rates, which thus become barometers of both regional cost variations and health care inflation. "Increases as small as half a percentage point in the cost of services, hospital care, therapeutic drugs, technology, hospital construction, and salaries and wages of hospital workers present serious financial implications for both [the statutory insurance system] and the total national health budget," observes Christa Altenstetter, professor of political science at the City University of New York.[50] For the same reason, individual funds' contribution rates will reflect demographic variations in member characteristics; older age, poorer health, and larger average numbers of dependents will increase a particular fund's contribution rates.

The percentage of income devoted to most sickness funds' contributions also depends directly upon a region's economy. If average wages are depressed, or if a higher proportion of people are unemployed, the burden of health care coverage falls more heavily on the average wage and on those who are employed. The 277 local sickness funds (the number of *Ortskrankenkassen* in all of Germany in 1992) are most sensitive to their regional economies, because they reflect the number of unemployed, urban poor, and other high-risk members in their service areas who have nowhere else to turn for coverage.

How the "Elite" Funds Compete

The blue-collar/white-collar division built into the German health system fuels competition among sickness funds that has intensified in recent years. The growth of the white-collar sector of the economy means that a larger and larger share of the population may choose between an *RVO* fund and a substitute fund. As the sickness fund of the white-collar class, the substitute funds start out with a marketing advantage rooted in snob appeal. The substitute funds have exploited this head start by fostering an elite image as the funds that provide better benefits. "They try to get their members the status of private patients," says Peter Rosenberg, Dr.Rer.Pol., policy analyst in the Federal Labor Ministry. For instance, their advertising hints that substitute funds give more lenient access to month-long "cures" in resort spas than the *RVO* funds. Most potently, they have developed a pattern of paying physicians considerably higher fees, implying in their marketing efforts that this buys their members favorable treatment.

Table 3.6

Sickness Fund Benefit Costs per Member* in Dollars, 1990 and Six-Year Average Annual Increase in Per-Member Costs, in Percent

Sickness fund type	Benefit outlay/ member	Average yearly increase 1985 through 1990
Local *Ortskrankenkassen*	** $1,443	3.42%
Company-based *Betriebskrankenkassen*	1,513	2.77%
Substitute/blue-collar *Ersatzkassen der Arbeiter*	1,339	2.07%
Substitute/white-collar *Ersatzkassen der Angestellten*	1,340	2.33%

* Excluding pensioners.
** In purchasing power parities.

Source: Bundesministerium für Gesundheit, 1991.

Physicians take advantage of this competition to play one set of funds off against the other in annual bargaining sessions over payments. As Deborah Stone, PhD, a Brandeis University political scientist, explains:

> The *RVO* funds...are constantly running from the popular charge that they provide second-class medicine. Physicians can wield a great deal of influence in shaping public demand for higher fees and greater benefits in the *RVO* system, simply by hinting to their *RVO* patients that the low payment levels and benefit coverage of *RVO* funds prevent patients from getting care that would be given to substitute fund or private patients.[51]

Stone and others believe that this competition has hindered efforts to control costs. Since *RVO* funds are legally mandated to provide their members access to all care that is "necessary and effective," the substitute funds provide a *de facto* standard of what that means by providing coverage for the latest diagnostic test or procedure. "The standard of care provided to private and substitute fund patients naturally becomes the standard that courts use for *RVO* funds," Stone reports.[52] When a major federal cost-control act was passed in 1977, the substitute funds' list of covered services and physician fee schedules were adopted as the standard for all sickness funds. "The substitute funds have consistently exercised a dominant influence over patterns of reimbursement, benefits, and fee schedules," conclude Wysong and Abel.[53] One example is the way the substitute funds scuttled a modified capitation method of physician reimbursement used until the early 1960s. The method was unpopular with physicians, and after substitute funds abandoned it in favor of a fee-for-service system, the *RVO* funds were forced to follow suit.[54]

As a marketing tactic the strategy has paid off. Between 1960 and 1990, membership in community funds (*Ortskrankenkassen*) grew by 6.5 percent while substitute funds (*Ersatzkassen*) enrolled 270 percent more—a difference not accounted for merely by the increase in the number of white-collar workers during that period. However, German observers say the actual difference between substitute funds and other sickness funds, in terms of the deference health providers show to fund members, is more apparent in advertising than in reality. "I don't think there is a difference," says Christian Zimmermann, director of the *Allgemeine Patienten Verband* (Patients' Defense Union), a consumer advocacy group based in Marburg. "A little bit, maybe, but not much."[55]

Fairness: Engine of Continuous Reform

The fact that sickness funds' contribution rates can and do vary is central to an understanding of the political dynamics of German health care. The idea of social solidarity requires fairness. It offends the German ideal of fairness if some are paying considerably more of their income for a standard package of health benefits simply because they happen to live in an economically depressed or medically high-risk region, or because they belong to a group with higher than average insurance risk.[56] While such variations are bound to occur in any system that groups people by occupation or region, they set up tensions that increase with the degree of divergence between the upper and lower bounds of contribution rates.

That is what has been happening in recent years in Germany. In 1990, average contribution rates among all statutory sickness funds varied two-fold, from 8 to 16 percent. (See Figure 3.3) Among sickness fund types, the degree of variance differed considerably: 200 percent for company-based funds, 57 percent for craft funds, 44 percent for local funds, and only 24 percent for white-collar funds. The 13.1 percent average contribution rate among local funds was the highest.

Containing the *Kosten-Explosion*

Between 1970 and 1992, the average "bite" that sickness fund contributions took out of German workers' wages and salaries increased by 60 percent. (Figure 3.4) This trend sparked much political debate and gave rise in the 1970s to the term *Kosten-Explosion* which, though it sounds like hyperbole to American ears, is still heard frequently on the lips of German politicians. The rise in sickness fund contributions was an "important catalyst," according to Michael Arnold, MD, professor of health services research at the University of Tübingen,[57] for the health system reforms that began in 1977 and continued on an almost annual basis for the next 15 years. It is the duty of politicians, explains Gerhard Schulte, Germany's deputy minister of health, to maintain "some sort of social equilibrium" in the health system. "But this is only possible," he adds, "if the statutory health insurance system is not jeopardized by excessively high contribution rates."[58]

Most of the cost containment measures enacted since 1977 have been targeted at health care providers and the suppliers of health care goods, such as pharmaceutical manufacturers, rather than at sickness funds. The exceptions, up until very recently, have been relatively minor. For instance, in 1981, Parliament ruled that visits to "cure resorts" could be granted only once every three years—an apparent response to the competition over such perquisites that was drawing more affluent members away from local sickness funds to the substitute funds. There has been a series of measures requiring sickness funds to impose minor cost-sharing burdens on their members, intended to make consumers more cost-conscious, but these did not fundamentally alter the sickness fund structure or their way of doing business.

At the same time, the reforms undertaken since the late 1970s did amount to a step-by-step departure from the principle of self-government (*Selbstverwartung*) that has been at the heart of the German system of health care financing. Under that principle, the countervailing powers of workers, employers, and health care providers are supposed to produce a sort of "golden mean" compromise that works for all parties with a minimum of government interference. By its increasing pace of intervention, the federal government has implicitly declared that sickness funds were not strong enough to prevail over the cost pressures generated by providers. Therefore, Parliament considered it necessary to set up, in 1977, the **Council for Concerted Action in Health Care**—an attempt to set the parameters of each year's negotiations between sickness funds and providers. That measure, the most visible and oft-cited example of government's "steering" role, has had mixed success. For instance,

Figure 3.4

Sickness Fund Contributions: Average Percentage of Wages, 1970-90

Percent of Wages

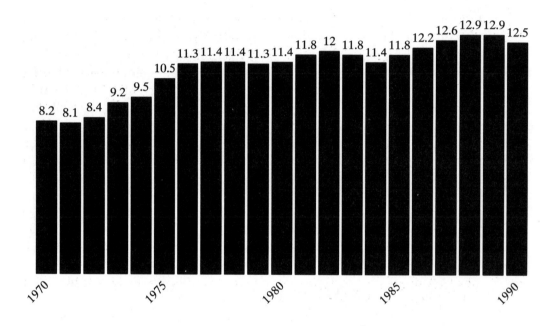

Source: Sachverständigenrat für die Konzertierte Aktion im Gesundheitswesen, 1992.

Christa Altenstetter points out that in 1986 the Concerted Action panel recommended that hospital spending increases be limited to 3.25 percent, but the sickness funds and hospitals negotiated increases of 7 percent or more.[59] In subsequent reforms, the parliament shored up sickness funds' bargaining position in dozens of ways, often involving minute aspects of the system's functioning.[60]

The 1989 reform of Labor Minister Norbert Blüm (whose portfolio then included health care) represented a departure—its long list of measures included several directed at sickness funds. The most important of these was a statutory directive that the stability of contribution rates be a "prerequisite in all contracts"; though unenforcable, the provision was a shot across the bow indicating that government was getting serious about the continuing increase and variation in sickness fund contributions despite previous interventions against providers. In addition, sickness funds were also empowered in 1989 to cancel contracts with inefficient hospitals and step up monitoring of doctors and hospitals for inefficiency and overutilization. To reduce adverse selection, the statute also tightened conditions for voluntary sickness fund membership among people with above-average medical needs.[61]

1993 Reform: Toward Real Structural Change?

On January 1, 1993, a *Health Care Structural Reform Act* took effect in Germany. This legislation was passed in reaction to mounting deficits in the statutory sickness fund system. (The 1992 deficit was estimated at DM 11 billion, about $5.3 billion.) The 1993 reform law contains the most sweeping changes in many years—some say since the system's beginnings. Public attention in Germany has focused primarily on the law's budgeting of prescription drug costs and its curtailing of doctors' freedom to practice wherever they choose. However, the statute contains the seeds of major changes in the ways statutory sickness funds are financed, the way they operate, and perhaps even whether there will continue to be multiple sickness funds. The changes are concentrated in two areas.

1. An attempt will be made to design a mandatory "basic benefits" package to replace the current comprehensive menu of sickness fund benefits, with the aim of financing benefits outside the basic package through voluntary private insurance. Health Minister Horst Seehofer, in late 1992, announced formation of an expert committee to determine what should be included in a basic benefits package.[62]

2. A method will be devised to equalize risk among sickness funds--that is, provide for transfers of money between funds to reflect differences in the risk profiles of their respective memberships—as a precondition to giving consumers free choice among funds and permitting the funds to compete freely for members. The risk equalization methodology is scheduled to be in place by 1994, while the "free choice" provision is supposed to take effect in 1996.[63]

The Basic Benefits Package

Those who advocate the narrowing of sickness fund benefits insist it is necessary to increase personal responsibility. They argue that German consumers have become spoiled by their first-dollar, comprehensive coverage. This, combined with the anonymity of today's large sickness funds, has distorted the original meaning of social solidarity, they say. The old idea that the healthy should pay for the sick has been replaced by a get-what-you-can ethic, what economists call **moral hazard**. "The insured individual tries to exploit the system to regain at least what he had to pay into it," says University of Tübingen's Arnold, who until recently chaired the Concerted Action's expert advisory council. Arnold is among those who would like to redefine which health benefits should be guaranteed collectively and which should be considered individuals' responsibility.

The idea of replacing comprehensive coverage with basic benefits, however, faces a steep uphill battle. While the principle is favored by neoconservative economists and the Free Democratic Party, which is a member of virtually any German coalition government, it is likely to be opposed strongly by the Social Democrats, who already feel that consumers have borne a disproportionate burden under the Blüm and Seehofer reforms, and that health care providers should sacrifice more in order to preserve the full-coverage system. Moreover, German "basic benefits" advocates face a problem that confronts their American counterparts: no one has yet defined what should be left out of a "basic benefits" package, or demonstrated that a stripped-down package that would save significant amounts of money could be publicly or politically acceptable.[64]

Risk Equalization

The risk equalization scheme, which resembles the system of inter-fund transfers already in place to finance pensioners' coverage, appears to have a somewhat better chance of coming to fruition, though it, too, faces political obstacles. It represents the uneasy marriage of ideologically opposed ideas:

1. the concept that solidarity should be practiced across the sickness fund spectrum rather than merely within each fund, (as advocated by the leftist Social Democratic Party); and

2. the idea, promoted by the neoconservative.[65] Free Democratic Party, that the market should be given freer rein in health insurance as a mechanism of cost control; once the playing field is leveled by inter-fund transfers of money according to the risk profiles of their respective members, it is assumed, true competition will be possible among the sickness funds.

Because these advocates have such disparate motives and values, they expect diametrically opposed outcomes from opening up sickness funds to competition. The Free Democrats hope for a more vigorous market that will preserve and enhance the multiple-payer aspect of German health care. The Social Democrats are widely suspected of harboring a desire for convergence of all sickness funds into one single fund, which would at last have decisive leverage over health care providers and would be practically equivalent to a single-payer government-sponsored system.

If this is the Social Democrats' aim, it will not be the first time German leftists have pushed for a single big sickness fund. After World War II, the German Trade Union Federation, which had historical ties with local health insurance funds, agitated for a single health or social insurance fund. If the unions had succeeded, it "would have been tantamount to a takeover of the substitute, company, and other smaller insurance funds by the local funds," observes political scientist Douglas Webber of the European Institute of Business Administration. However, the trade unions were blocked by the German White-Collar Workers' Union, for whom (Webber notes) "the maintenance of the substitute insurance funds is a *raison d`etre*."[66] While the sickness funds have longed shared the aim of strengthening their position *vis-a-vis* powerful provider interests, Webber adds, "competition among the insurance funds has tended to prevent them from making common cause against the service providers' organizations, either politically or in collective bargaining."[67]

The Kohl government's rationale for risk equalization (called *Finanzausgleich*) is "to facilitate fair competition among the health insurance funds," as Gerhard Schulte put it.[68] As he explains it, once the effects of differing risks are canceled out—by taking into effect sickness fund members' wage levels, number of dependents, age, and sex—sickness funds will be able to compete on the basis of "efficient administration and correct management of the diverse benefits being offered." On this new playing field, the consumer will be able to shop among different funds and the price of each, as represented by the contribution rate, will be an important "parameter of competitiveness."[69]

Others have their doubts it will work out that way. As Arnold and a colleague, Dominik von Stillfried, explained it in a *British Medical Journal* editorial: "Although the reformers claim to be generating equal conditions for competition between the funds prior to the introduction of unlimited choice between [statutory sickness funds], they have effectively standardized all areas of activity of the funds. This opens up the prospect of forming a single national sickness fund in the near future."[70]

Christian Zimmermann of the German Patients' Union believes the outcome could go either way, and foresees many pitched battles ahead. "If you have one big health care system there is the big danger of bureaucracy. On the other hand, if you have a lot of different health care companies, that costs more in administration," Zimmermann says. "Those are different positions in the ideological spectrum. It's not quite sure where the development will go, finally."[71]

References and Notes

1. Foster Higgins (1993). *Health Care Benefits Survey: Medical Plans*. Princeton: Foster Higgins.

2. Gordon, NM (1993). Testimony before the U.S. House Ways & Means health subcommittee, January 26, 1993. Figure is an estimate based upon data from Current Population Survey of March, 1992.

3. Employee Benefit Research Institute (1993). *Sources of Health Insurance and Characteristics of the Uninsured: Analyis of the March 1992 Current Population Survey*. Washington, D.C.: Employee Benefit Research Institute.

4. Sachverständigenrat für die Konzertierte Aktion im Gesundheitswesen (1992). Ausbau in Deutschland und Aufbruch nach Europa: Jahresgutachten 1992. Baden-Baden: MonosVerlagsgesellschaft, p. 187.

5. This and other conversions in this chapter from deutschmarks to dollars use purchasing power parities published by the Organization for Economic Cooperation and Development (OECD), eg. DM 2.09 = $1.00 in 1991.

6. Wicks, EK (1992). *German Health Care: Financing, Administration, and Coverage*. Washington: Health Insurance Association of America, p. 28.

7. Bergthold, LA (1993). Benefit Choices Under Managed Competition. *Health Affairs*, Vol. 12, Special Supplement, p. 100.

8. Glaser, WA (1991). *Health Insurance in Practice: International Variations in Financing, Benefits, and Problems*. Cambridge, MA: The MIT Press, p. 316.

9. Arnold, M (1991). *Health Care in the Federal Republic of Germany*. Köln: Deutscher Ärzte-Verlag, p. 50.

10. Woolhandler, S and Himmelstein, DR (1991). The Deteriorating Administrative Efficiency of the U.S. Health Care System. *New England Journal of Medicine*, Vol. 324: 1253-1258.

11. Ibid.

12. Center for National Health Program Studies (1991). *Monthly Labor Review*, quoted in *The National Health Program Chartbook*. Cambridge, MA: Center for National Health Program Studies, p. 92.

13. Blendon, RJ, et. al. (1993). "Physician Perspectives on Care for Patients in Three Different Health Systems." *New England Journal of Medicine*, Vol.328, No. 14, pp. 1011-1016.

14. Reinhardt, UE (1993). Reorganizing the Financial Flows in American Health Care. *Health Affairs*, Vol. 12, Supplement, p. 184.

15. Poullier, J-P (1992). Administrative Costs in Selected Industrialized Countries. *Health Care Financing Review*, Vol. 13 , No. 4, p. 170.

16. Woolhandler and Himmelstein (1991).

17. Poullier, J-P (1991).

18. Ibid.

19. Altenstetter, C (1987). "An End to Consensus on Health Care in the FRG?" *J of H Politics, Policy & Law*, Vol. 12, No. 3, p.520.

20. Reinhardt, UE (1990). West Germany's Health Care and Health Insurance System: Combining Universal Access with Cost Control. *Supplement to the Final Report of the U.S. Bipartisan Commission on Comprehensive Health Care* (the Pepper Commission). Washington, D.C.: U.S. Government Printing Office, p. 9.

21. Wicks, EK (1992), p. 21.

22. Wysong, JA and Abel, TA (1990). Universal Health Insurance and High-risk Groups in West Germany: Implications for U.S. Health Policy. *The Milbank Quarterly*, Vol. 68, No. 4, p. 542.

23. Unemployment has climbed since 1990, further straining the system. In the states of former West Germany, 8.3 percent of the workforce was unemployed in January, 1993, In the eastern states, unemployment was running 15.1 percent in early 1993.

24. Wysong, JA and Abel, TA (1990), pp. 540-541.

25. Wicks, EK (1992), p. 26.

26. Wysong, JA and Abel, TA (1990), p. 541.

27. Employee Benefits Research Institute, (1993), p. 47.

28. Glaser, WA (1991), p. 119.

29. Wicks, EK (1992), p. 25.

30. Glaser, WA (1991), p. 36.

31. Gordon, NM (1993). Congressional Budget Office testimony before the subcommittee on health, U.S. House Ways & Means Committee. January 26, 1993.

32. Sachverständigenrat für die Konzertierte Aktion im Gesundheitswesen (1992), p. 222.

33. Schulenburg, J-M (1989). The West Geman Health Care Financing and Delivery System: Its Experiences and Lessons for Other Nations. Given at an International Symposium on Health Care Systems. Tapei, Taiwan, December 18-19, 1989.

34. Henke, K–D; Murray MA; and Ade, C (1993) Berman Global Budgeting of Physician Expenditures: Lessons for the Reform of U.S. Health Care. Unpublished paper, February, 1993.

35. Sachverständigenrat für die Konzertierte Aktion im Gesundheitswesen (1992), p. 222.

36. Wicks, EK (1992), p. 26.

37. Glaser, WA (1991), p. 209.

38. Ibid.

39. Wicks, EK (1992), p.26.

40. Pfaff, M (1992). Personal interview, December 6, 1992.

41. Altenstetter, C (1987), pp. 520-521.

42. Schneider, M (1991). Health Care Cost Containment in the Federal Republic of Germany. *Health Care Financing Review*, Vol.12, No. 3, p. 91.

43. Schmeinck, W (1992). "Statutory Health Insurance: Its Role, Structure and Way of Functioning." Talk at a conference on German and American Health Care Systems, Goethe Institute of Boston, October 15, 1992.

44. Wysong, JA and Abel, TA (1990), p. 537.

45. Ibid.

46. *Daten des Gesundheitswesens* (1991). p. 32.

47. Infratest, Gesundheitsforschung (1988). Chronic Illness of the Cardiovascular System and Perceived Health by Health Insurance Membership in the Federal Republic. Internal report to the Enquette Commission. Munich: Infratest. As quoted in Wysong and Abel (1990), p. 548.

48. Wysong, JA and Abel, TA (1990), pp. 545-547.

49. Sickness funds that are locally or regionally based—that is, they draw on local populations rather than from the nation as a whole—include the local sickness funds (*Ortskrankenkassen*), company-based sickness funds (*Betriebskrankenkassen*), craftsmen's sickness funds (*Innungskrankenkassen*), and agricultural workers' sickness funds (*Landwirtschaftliche Krankenkassen*). Together these funds enrolled 60 percent of the 27.1 million active workers enrolled in statutory sickness funds in 1990, according to the Federal Ministry of Health.

50. Altenstetter, C (1987).

51. Stone, D (1987). *The Limits of Professional Power: National Health Care in the Federal Republic of Germany*. Chicago: University of Chicago Press, p. 150.

52. Ibid.

53. Wysong, JA and Abel, TA (1990), p. 544.

54. Ibid.

55. Zimmerman, C (1993). Personal interview.

56. About four out of five Germans pay the average sickness fund contribution (13.1 percent in 1992), according to Michael Arnold, professor at the University of Tübingen. Nevertheless, the extreme rates cause political concern because, Arnold explains, they "represent undue hardship for those [who] must pay more for the same range of benefits." (Arnold, 1991, p. 30).

57. Arnold, M (1991), p. 28.

58. Schulte, G (1992). "Problems of Health Care in the Conflict Area between Market Economy and Governmental Economic Control," a talk at the Goethe Institute of Boston, October 16, 1992.

59. Altenstetter, C (1987), p. 518.

60. For lists of some of the particulars, see articles on German health care reform by Jeremy Hurst and Markus Schneider in *Health Care Financing Review*, Vol. 12, No. 3, Spring 1991.

61. Schneider, M (1991), p. 91.

62. Schmeinck, W (1992).

63. Pfaff, M (1992). Personal interview, December 6, 1992.

64. The state of Oregon is a possible exception to this statement, since officials there have designed a new catalogue of Medicaid benefits that excludes some assumedly cost-ineffective medical interventions. However, the Oregon program's principle architect, state Sen. John Kitzhaber, MD, acknowledged in an interview that it was considered politically unacceptable to impose the proposed Medicaid benefit package on state employees and legislators.

65. In Germany, the Free Democratic Party is considered "liberal," in the classical economics usage of that label. Many of its positions are akin to the neoconservitive ideas of the University of Chicago school of economics.

66. Webber, D (1988). "The Politics of German Health System Reform: Successful and Failed Attempts at Reform from 1930 to 1984." Typescript of a paper prepared for workshop in policy change, University of Bologna/Rimini, Italy, April, 1988.

67. Ibid.

68. Schulte, G (1992).

69. Ibid.

70. Arnold , M and Stillfried, D (1993). What's Happening to the Health Care in Germany? *British Medical Journal,* vol. 306, No. 6884, pp. 1017-1018.

71. Zimmerman, C (1993).

A Closer Look:
Paying for Health Care

The Role of Private Health Insurance in Germany

Despite its historical emphasis on equity in health insurance, Germany does tolerate a two-tier system. More prosperous Germans—those who earn more than about $30,000 a year—are permitted to opt out of the statutory health insurance scheme and purchase private health insurance that buys them certain advantages over the great majority of Germans who must belong to statutory sickness funds. However, Germany has carefully limited the latitude of private health insurers to prevent them from undermining the fiscal soundness of the social insurance system.

About 7 million Germans were insured privately in 1990, 11 percent of the total population.[1] Approximately three times that number were eligible to purchase private coverage. Another 4 million people purchase private supplemental coverage to pay for private or semiprivate hospital rooms, access to leading specialists, and other amenities not covered by statutory health insurance.[2] Altogether, private insurers pay about 6 percent of Germany's total health bill[3], a disparity that probably reflects the lower-risk nature of the population covered by private insurance.

Those who purchase comprehensive coverage from one of Germany's 50 private insurance companies can be divided into four main groups.

1. People who earn more than the income ceiling (which varies annually with the increase in average wages) and choose not to be members of statutory sickness funds.
2. Senior-level civil servants, university professors, and teachers, who account for more than half the private insurance market.
3. Self-employed people, who could formerly be members of statutory sickness funds but, as of 1989, must be privately insured.
4. Pensioners who were privately insured when they were working.

In deciding whether to buy private insurance, each of these groups (except the pensioners, who have no choice) has to weigh a different set of incentives and disincentives. In general, high-income people may find private premiums lower than the contributions they would have to pay to sickness funds—especially those who are young, enjoy good health, and have no dependents. This is because private companies insure each person in a family individually and base premiums on the age of subscribers when they sign up, their gender, and their health status. But even if a private premium is advantageous at a given moment, the childless young adult must consider whether he or she might want a family later. As of 1989, Germans who "go private" cannot generally return to the statutory insurance system once they have left it. As a further barrier to desertion of the statutory system by high-income young adults, the 1989 health reform law doubled the premiums of children who are insured through the statutory sickness funds if their parents are insured privately.[4]

The decision to buy private insurance is more clear-cut for most civil servants, 75 percent of whom are privately insured. (The other one-quarter generally are lower-wage bureaucrats who, until 1989, were required to join a sickness fund.) Government agencies pay from 50 to 95 percent of the medical costs of their employees, according to the number of dependents they have, and the employees typically buy private insurance to pay the remainder. Self-employed people must now insure privately, paying the entire premium themselves with only limited tax-deductibility. Yet very few self-employed people choose to go without insurance.[5] As for pensioners, they must generally continue to purchase private coverage if they were insured privately when they were younger, paying the entire premium out of their own resources. This 1989 requirement was designed to prevent elders with higher-cost medical problems from switching back to the statutory insurance system upon retirement, where contribution rates are lower than private premiums because actively employed sickness fund members subsidize retirees. "The reform was one of the measures enacted to protect the social insurance sector from the drawbacks of a competitive market," notes William A. Glaser, Ph.D., professor of health services management at the New School for Social Research in New York City.[6]

The Lure of Preferential Treatment

Other than an advantageous premium for some people, the leading allure of private insurance is the extra physician attention it purportedly buys subscribers. Private insurers pay physicians on a government-set fee schedule that is, on average, double the remuneration of sickness funds. For instance, doctors can (and generally do) bill private patients 2.3 times as much as sickness fund patients for personal services, and 1.8 times higher for laboratory tests. With written justification, the doctor can charge even more. In contrast to the statutory system, in which no money changes hands between patients and doctors, privately insured patients are expected to pay the bill and seek reimbursement from the insurer, an arrangement that some speculate also induces physicians to pay them more attention.[7] Though studies confirming this differential care are sparse, it is widely believed to be true. One concrete advantage for private patients is guaranteed access to the hospital department chiefs, while sickness fund patients generally are treated by doctors lower on the hospital totem pole.

Private insurers pay hospitals directly on the basis of the per diem rates negotiated regionally between hospitals and statutory sickness funds. Five percent is subtracted to allow for private patients' separate reimbursement of hospital-based physicians that normally is built

---

Table 3b.1

Growth of Private Health Insurance in (West) Germany, 1970-90

Year	Total Population	No. Privately Insured	% Privately Insured
1970	60,924,000	5,969,000	9.3%
1975	61,542,000	4,482,000	7.3
1980	61,516,000	4,611,000	7.5
1985	60,987,000	5,135,000	8.4
1990	63,062,000	6,935,000	11.0

Source: Sachverstandigenrat für die Konzertierte Aktion im Gesundheitswesen, 1992.

---

into the per diem rate. In addition, private insurers pay hospitals a private-room surcharge of about 50 percent.[8] Hospitals generally make a "profit" on privately insured patients.[9] The total costs per hospital case are about twice as high for private patients.[10] Private carriers pay the same for prescription drugs as statutory sickness funds. Medical providers of all types appreciate the fact that private insurers do not engage in utilization review. "If physicians are following accepted standards of medical practice, the insurer generally pays even if the procedure is of questionable appropriateness in a particular situation," says Elliot K. Wicks, Ph.D., of the Center for Health Policy and Development in Washington, D.C.[11]

Except for the additional perquisites mentioned above, private health insurers cover the same services as sickness funds—as they must in order for employers to contribute the same 50 percent share of the premium they bear for workers insured through sickness funds. The principal difference in private insurance benefits is in cost-sharing. Unlike the statutory insurance system, most private insurance policies require subscribers to pay a portion of their outpatient medical costs and many also have deductibles that can range as high as DM 3,000 a year ($1,435).[12] German insurers offer a long menu of cost-sharing options that can essentially be customized to each customer's tastes, with concomitant differences in premiums. However, each plan offered must be approved by government regulators for actuarial soundness.

Life-Long Level Premiums

Private health insurance in Germany is financed by a method quite unlike its U.S. counterpart. American health insurance premiums are based on the actuarial risk of an individual or group for a limited term, usually one year, taking into account such volatile factors as the previous year's actual experience and rising health costs. But German insurers calculate each individual's lifetime actuarial risk—the amount of expected pay-out—for the age group in which the individual finds himself when he first enrolls.[13] (Age groups are calculated in five-year increments.) Theoretically this yields a flat premium that is weighted heavily toward the early years of enrollment in order to build up sufficient reserves to pay for the costs the subscriber will incur in his advanced years. This is the reason that private insurers in Germany had revenues of DM 21.2 billion ($10.1 billion) but paid out only DM 15.2 billion ($7.3 billion).[14]

In practice, the Germans have found it necessary to permit increases in these flat-rate premiums to keep up with inflation in health costs—which has been 65 percent higher throughout the 1980s for privately insured Germans than for sickness fund members.[15] To qualify for inflation adjustments, health costs must exceed 10 percent of projections and be approved by state regulators. Inflation adjustments are usually spread unequally to spare elder subscribers from excessive burdens.

Flat-rate premiums for health insurance originated in Germany in the 1930s and later spread to other European countries, such as Switzerland. Borrowed from level-premium life insurance, the system was devised to avoid steep premium increases for elderly subscribers who could not turn to statutory sickness funds when their private insurance premiums became unaffordable, because they had never been sickness fund members. "The insurance companies needed to demonstrate they could provide the same lifetime protection as the sickness funds, making unnecessary the enactment of universal obligatory health insurance," writes Glaser.[16] A company called Deutsche Krankenversicherung A.G. (DKV) became Germany's largest private insurer, with a market share of about 19 percent, in large part because it was one of the first to offer level premiums, which had strong appeal for a postwar population with great anxiety over future security.[17]

The level premium is a powerful incentive for subscribers to stay with one insurer for a lifetime. If they switch to another company, they will leave behind all the reserves they have accumulated, and they will pay a substantially higher premium to their new insurer because they will be entering at a more advanced age. Not only has this reduced competition among private insurers, Glaser points out, but it has helped stifle experimentation with new modes of insurance coverage and service delivery such as health maintenance organizations (HMOs), because such innovations would require private subscribers' willingness to abandon their previous coverage.[18]

Another unusual feature of private health insurance in Germany, from an American point of view, is the practice of giving subscribers' rebates for not submitting claims. The incentive can be considerable. "One company...will rebate half of the premium if no claims are made for six years," Wicks reports. "Since for employed people the employer pays half the premium, this amounts to a full rebate for the employee's share."[19] In 1988, private insurers gave rebates amounting to about 10 times aggregate profits.[20]

Selling and writing health insurance on a totally individual basis is an expensive way of doing business. The administrative costs of private insurers are more than triple the reported administrative costs of sickness funds. Sickness funds spend about 4 to 5 percent of their revenues on administration, compared to 16 percent among private insurers in 1987—4.4 percent for "pure" administrative costs (such as claims processing) plus 11.6 percent for marketing and other "closing costs" associated with setting up new policies.[21] By comparison, the reported overhead costs of private insurance in the U.S. amounted to 14.2 percent of private health insurance premiums in 1990. Taking into account the administrative costs of public medical coverage and philanthropic organizations, the overall average administrative cost in the U.S. was 5.8 percent of total national health expenditures in 1990.[22]

The Future of Private Insurance in Germany

The market for private health insurance grew moderately between 1970 and 1990, posting a 22 percent gain during a period when the West German population grew by 3.5 percent.[23] During that period, the proportion of (West) Germans who were privately insured increased from 9.3 percent to 11 percent. This overall trend masks a significant drop in private insurance market share during the 1970s, despite German prosperity at that time. That decline was due in large part to the government's action to keep more workers in the statutory system by increasing the income threshold beyond which people could opt out and buy private coverage. The private market recouped in the late 1970s and 1980s, according to Glaser, "largely because the civil service grew and because young and healthy salaried employees were attracted by cheap policies with benefits limited to large bills."[24]

Wicks, on the basis of his 1991 interviews with German insurance executives, concludes that "rapid continued growth seems unlikely, for political reasons." Rapid growth in private insurance "would be viewed as a potential threat to the future of [the statutory system] and would probably provoke government action to limit growth," he writes.[25]

Wicks also foresaw a serious threat to the future of German private health insurance stemming from European economic unification. European Economic Community (EEC) rules forbid member nations from perpetuating regulations that would bar foreign companies from competing for domestic markets. German insurance executives have worried that this would enable foreign insurers to sell policies with premiums geared to subscribers' ages rather than the level premiums that domestic insurers must charge. If this occurred, foreign competitors could substantially undercut premiums for the younger segment of the German market. German insurers have also been apprehensive about foreign competitors who would be free of restrictions against subsidizing health insurance with other lines of business, as they are strictly prohibited from doing.

By 1993, these worries seemed to have lessened. The reason reveals much about the interdependence of statutory and private health insurance in Germany. Basically, Germany has declared private insurance to be an integral part of its social insurance system, exploiting a provision of the EEC treaty that protects each nation's social security programs from competition. The government of Chancellor Helmut Kohl did not need much persuading to let private health insurers shelter under the umbrella of the Social Code, according to German observers.

"It is not against all logic," comments Michael Arnold, MD, professor of health systems research at the University of Tübingen. "But it is very interesting to see how these people who are supposedly for competition are now against the market!"[26]

References and Notes

1. *Daten des Gesundheitswesens 1991*, Bundesministerium für Gesundheit, p. 31. Baden-Baden: Nomos Verlagsgesellschaft

2. Wicks, E (1992). *German Health Care: Financing, Administration, and Coverage*. Washington, D.C.: Health Insurance Association of America.

3. Sachverständigenrat für die Konzertierte Aktion im Gesundheitswesen (1992). *Jahresgutachten 1992*. Baden-Baden: Nomos Verlagsgesellschaft, p. 189.

4. Hurst, JW (1991). Reform of Health Care in Germany. *Health Care Financing Review*, Vol. 12, No. 3, p. 81.

5. Wicks (1992), p. 25.

6. Glaser, WA (1991). *Health Insurance in Practice: International Variations in Financing, Benefits, and Problems*. San Francisco: Jossey-Bass Publishers, p. 505.

7. Wicks (1992), p. 32.

8. Reinhardt, UE (1990). West Germany's Health Care and Health Insurance System: Combining Universal Access with Cost Control. *Supplement to the Final Report, U.S. Bipartisan Commission on Comprehensive Health Care*. Washington, D.C.: U.S. Government Printing Office, p. 11.

9. Wicks (1992), p. 32.

10. Schneider (1991), p. 99.

11. Wicks (1992), p. 32.

12. Wicks (1992), p. 31.

13. German private insurers practice medical underwriting, accepting or refusing applicants because of health risks or preexisting conditions, or excluding covering for specific conditions. The only exception to this rule are civil servants, who are guaranteed acceptance. However, even competing private insurers in Germany practice a form of industry solidarity: if one company's portfolio includes an unusually high-risk group of civil servants, its competitors will share some of the burden. (Wicks, 1990, p. 28)

14. Sachverständigenrat (1992), pp. 266-267.

15. Schneider, M (1991), p. 99.

16. Glaser (1991), p. 164.

17. Glaser (1991), p. 165.

18. Ibid.

19. Wicks (1992), p. 31.

20. Ibid.

21. Reinhardt (1990), p. 11.

22. Levit, KR et.al. (1991). National Health Expenditures, 1990. *Health Care Financing Review*, Vol. 13, No. 1, p. 36.

23. Sachverständigenrat (1992), p. 187.

24. Glaser (1991), p. 505.

25. Wicks (1992), pp. 32-33.

26. Arnold, M (1993). Personal interview.

CHAPTER 4

Doctors in Germany: Balancing Autonomy and Regulation

G ermany owes much of its relative success in controlling health care costs during the 1980s to constraints on physicians—specifically, office-based doctors. By adopting nonbinding expenditure targets in 1978 and then enforceable budgetary caps in 1986, Germany reduced inflation-adjusted spending on ambulatory physician care by as much as 17 percent from projected levels between 1977 and 1987, according to a 1991 study by the U.S. General Accounting Office (GAO).[1] (Figure 4.1) While U.S. nominal spending on physician care increased 300 percent between 1980 and 1990,[2] Germany's physician spending grew by 60 percent.[3] By contrast, there is no evidence that Germany has been able to slow hospital inflation[4] and, indeed, the Germans expect to spend much of the 1990s addressing that problem. Recent data show that German hospitals are consuming an ever-larger portion of the health care dollar, while physicians' share is relatively flat. (Table 4.1)

Ironically, Germany's achievement in slowing physician expenditures stems from associations of doctors set up in the 1930s at the insistence of the medical profession to preserve doctors' autonomy. The genius of these mechanisms, from the profession's point of view, is the way they combine independent medical practice and fee-for-service payment with the power of collective bargaining. Membership in regional associations of sickness fund-authorized physicians (*kassenärztliche Vereinigungen* or *KV*s)[5] is "designed to symbolize the doctors' professional independence from the lowly insurance clerks," says William A. Glaser, professor of health services management at the New School for Social Research.[6] Formal and legally binding economic relationships between physicians and sickness funds are enshrined in German law, but government plays the role of referee, scorekeeper, and occasional rule-revisor.

Not until a half-century after the establishment of the *KV*s was there any thought of using such structures against the medical profession, to curb its costs. When the time came, however, Germany found that the time-honored relationships between payer and provider were easily adapted to the needs of cost

Figure 4.1

Effect of Budget Controls on Physician Care Spending in Germany

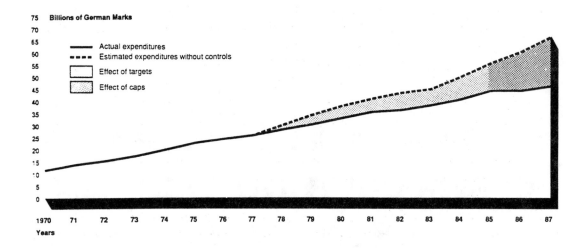

Source: U.S. General Accounting Office, 1991

Table 4.1

Changes in German Statutory Health Insurance Spending By Type of Service, 1980-90

Type of service	1980 share	1990 share	% change in share
Ambulatory physicians	17.9%	18.2%	1.7%
Hospitals	29.6	33.2	12.2
Prescription drugs	14.6	16.3	11.6
Dentists	6.4	6.1	-4.9
Dentures	8.6	3.6	-58.6
Eyeglasses, hearing aids	5.7	6.3	10.5
Sick pay	7.7	6.5	-15.6
Preventive	1.0	0.9	-10.0
Pregnancy care and cash benefits	3.5	2.4	-54.2
Other benefits	5.0	6.5	30.0
	100%	100%	

Source: Bundesministerium für Gesundheit, Daten des Gesundheitswesens 1991.

control; clearly they have been the key to whatever success Germany has achieved in constraining physician spending. Conversely, the absence of concentrated authority over doctors' fees in America—except for parts of the system such as Medicare, which pays for only one-quarter of physicians' services[7]—is perhaps the biggest problem the U.S. faces in putting effective brakes on its costs. Reviewing the experiences of Germany, France, Canada, and the U.S. in setting physicians' fees, Victor G. Rodwin of the Advanced Management Program for Clinicians at New York University and his colleagues observe that the absence of a national health insurance system "deprives [the U.S.] of the monopsony power of a sole payer with concentrated financing."[8]

Germany does not have a "sole payer;" it has more than 1,300 separate payers. But the *KV*s do concentrate the financing for ambulatory physician care in each region, and the regional negotiations are coordinated within a national policy framework. A system designed to preserve physician autonomy has become a method of controlling the size of the financing stream.

The Hegemony of Private Practice

The shape of contemporary German medical practice, which preserves the private-practice, fee-for-service mode to a far greater degree than in America, owes everything to what Glaser characterizes as "decades of dispute" between doctors and sickness funds.[9] Before 1931, Germany's growing sickness funds often employed physicians in "closed panels," hiring only as many doctors as they needed, dictating the terms of employment, and freezing independent practitioners out of statutory health insurance practice. The medical profession resorted to collective action—including frequent, prolonged, and acrimonious strikes—to protect itself against divide-and-conquer tactics and what it considered to be intolerable exploitation of individual physicians by the sickness funds (see Chapter Two). The profession eventually prevailed with the establishment of *KV*s in 1933, organizations which gave their physician members a monopoly franchise over all ambulatory care in their respective regions. All physicians who wish to treat sickness fund subscribers must belong to the local *KV*, which has legal standing as a "body of public law" with special prerogatives and duties.

The Purview of the KVs

The *KV*s negotiate with sickness funds over the collective reimbursement levels of their members. They also serve as fiscal intermediaries, collecting quarterly bills from the independent fee-for-service practitioners and distributing the money that flows from the payers. In return, the *KV*s have the legal duty to assure sickness fund members adequate access to high-quality and efficient medical care at all times. Money does not change hands between doctor and patient. "Physicians and patients meet each other not as individual buyers and sellers in a market, but rather as members of large organizations that engage in collective bargaining," writes Deborah A. Stone, professor of law and social policy at Brandeis University.[10]

After World War II, German physicians were threatened with the prospect of a single social insurance fund for all health, pension, and unemployment insurance—the brainchild of a coalition of Social Democrats, trade unions, and locally based sickness funds. Such a single payer would have been a far more formidable bargaining partner than the divided and competitive sickness funds the *KV*s had been accustomed to dealing with (and playing off against one another). To fend off this proposal, maintain their exclusive franchise for ambulatory care, and ratify their right to govern their own economic affairs, German office-based doctors in 1955 forfeited their right to strike.[11]

In the process of fighting for independent practice, the doctors ultimately succeeded in killing not only "closed panels" but virtually all group practice in Germany. So bitter and protracted were the early 20th-century disputes between sickness funds and organized medicine that even now there are strict prohibitions against salaried practice (in outpatient care), against doctors forming group practices unless they practice the same specialty, and against sharing the care of individual patients among a group of colleagues.[12] German doctors may not "be subject to the instruction of nonphysicians in the practice of medicine," according to Article 10 of the *Professional Medical Code*, a detailed body of regulations developed and occasionally revised by the German Medical Association (*Bundesärztekammer*) that has the force of law. A 1955 law appeared to open a door to the establishment of sickness fund-operated outpatient clinics with salaried physicians; however, the law required *KV* approval of such clinics, and such approval has never been given.[13] When the nation was partitioned after World War II, East Germany reinvented multispecialty, salaried group practices along Soviet lines; but the power of organized medicine in West Germany was undiminished. When reunification occurred in 1990, western doctors succeeded in reimposing the old structure.

A Wall Between Doctors

The struggle between sickness funds and organized medicine had another far-reaching effect on the structure of German medical care: It cemented the strict division between fee-for-service ambulatory medical practitioners and salaried hospital-based physicians originally caused by a historical accident. This wall is nearly absolute. In all but a few circumstances, hospital doctors are not allowed to encroach on the turf of doctors with the sickness fund franchise for ambulatory care. Until a sweeping reform law in December, 1992, designed in part to breach this wall, ambulatory physicians had been successful in maintaining strict rules against even preadmission testing and post-surgical follow-up care by hospital-based colleagues. At the same time, office-based physicians may not practice in hospitals unless they get special dispensation from their local ambulatory physicians' association. Only about 7 percent of all sickness fund-authorized physicians have such privileges, and the proportion is not growing.[14] About 10 percent of hospital-based doctors are authorized to provide outpatient services.[15]

Office-based doctors and hospital-based doctors have their own largely separate organizations for promoting their economic interests. Office-based doctors belong to the *Hartmannbund*, founded in 1900 as a trade union to counter the power of sickness funds. Hospital-based physicians and salaried public health officials belong to the *Marburgerbund*, which functions largely as a trade union to negotiate salaries and working conditions.[16] Office-based physicians tend to dominate the politics of health care in Germany,[17] even though they make up a shrinking minority of all German physicians. By 1989, hospital-based doctors outnumbered office-based practitioners by more than 30 percent. (Table 4.2) Between 1970 and 1989, the number of hospital-based doctors doubled while the number of beds declined by 2 percent. The greater prestige of office-based practice is manifest in the career trajectory of most German physicians, who view hospital-based practice as a second-best, transitory career—a way-station *en route* to independent practice. The very term for office-based physician, *niedergelassene Arzt*, means "settled-down doctor."

Table 4.2

Physician Practice Settings in Germany*: Trends in Office-Based and Hospital-Based Practice, 1970-90

Year	No. office based physicians	No. hospital-based physicians	Ratio of office:hospital physicians
1970	46,302	46,550	1:1.01
1975	49,928	60,635	1:1.21
1980	56,138	72,540	1:1.29
1985	63,694	83,082	1:1.30
1989	69,861	91,895	1:1.32

* Does not include physicians in public health, occupational health, research, administration, nonmedical settings, inactive, retired, and unemployed.

Source: *Sachverständigenrat für die Konzertierte Aktion im Gesundheitswesen, 1992.*

Duty, Self-Regulation, and the Force of Law

German physicians enjoy a degree of clinical autonomy that might be envied by their U.S. colleagues, who increasingly complain of tedious and conflicting rules, prior-approval requirements, and second-guessing of medical decisions by third-party payers. German doctors "have virtually no government or payer intrusion into clinical practice," note Rodwin and his coauthors.[18] They cite this as an instance of "Reinhardt's irony," after the German-American professor of political economy Uwe E. Reinhardt of Princeton University. As Reinhardt explains it,

> The less tightly society controls the overall capacity of its health system and the economic freedom of its providers to practice as they see fit, the more direct appears to be the private or public payer's intrusion directly into the doctor-patient relationship— the less clinical freedom at the level of treatment will payers grant providers.[19]

Reinhardt's observation is another way of saying that societies tend to regulate health care either at a macroeconomic level, through such mechanisms as limiting capacity or setting global budget limits, or at a microeconomic level, by attempting to police what individual providers do. Germany has elected for many years to follow the former strategy, but not in a simple and undeviating way. There are departures from this "macro" strategy which are necessary to understand for a complete picture of the tradeoffs that German payers and providers have made. Two major exceptions:

1. Physician capacity, the total number of practitioners admitted to the profession, has not been controlled in Germany—a policy lapse with major implications for future cost control and for the profession's well-being that will be addressed later in this chapter;

2. German physicians are subject to a great deal of detailed regulation which U.S. physicians might consider intrusive; however, this regulation does not constrain clinical decision making, and it does not emanate from government or other third-party payers but from **physicians' chambers**—government-chartered organs of physician self-government.

Licensure

As a condition of licensure, every German physician must belong to his respective state physicians' chamber (*Ärztekammer*) and abide by its elaborate code of professional conduct. In addition, the typical physician belongs to an array of other organizations, both compulsory (i.e., a *KV* for office-based practitioners) and voluntary (specialized societies representing every conceivable subgrouping of physicians, from general practitioners to the Society of Female Physicians, the Central Society of Naturopathic Doctors, and the German Society of Physician Drivers). This is a reflection of the corporatism that pervades Germany society, but physicians take such group-forming behavior to extremes. They constitute "the most highly organized profession in German society," observes J.-Matthias Graf von der Schulenburg, professor of insurance economics at the University of Hannover.[20]

Regulating the Physician

The regulation that German doctors face is partly related to the privileges and obligations they assumed when they promised to provide accessible, high-quality, uninterrupted health care to all sickness fund members. Those freedoms and duties are generally embodied in a federal *Medical Profession Law* and further articulated in *Professional Medical Codes* in each of the German states. The federal law declares medicine to be "by nature a profession" rather than a business or trade — an important distinction won by physicians in 1935 that exempts them from laws regulating businesses or tradesmen. The pivotal prerogative the law guarantees is "freedom of professional discretion." As professionals, doctors are also expected to renounce commercial competition.[21]

At the state level, physicians' chambers, which are "bodies of public law," formulate doctors' prerogatives and duties more fully in state *Professional Medical Codes*. Under these codes, for instance, a German doctor must

- keep regular hours that can be specified by the state chamber to meet the needs of a local population or limited to prevent competition among physicians;
- participate in an after-hours emergency duty plan, from which duty they may be relieved duty only for "grave reasons," such as personal injury;
- seek permission to add paramedical personnel to his or her practice or hire a temporary replacement while on vacation;
- not bill sickness fund patients for payment beyond the fees received from sickness funds (through the *KV*);
- not engage in any kind of direct or indirect advertising or self-promotion, though he or she may inform other doctors of special diagnostic or therapeutic services offered;[22]

In a sense the state physician chambers are analogous to state medical licensure boards in the U.S., but they are explicitly and solely physician groups with delegated state powers—not agencies of state government with appointed physician representatives sharing power with nonphysicians.

Daily medical practice is also hedged about with myriad regulations governing which services, out of approximately 2,500 separate items, a German physician may and may not bill for. For instance, in a given patient visit the physician may not bill more than 200 "points" for any combination of 29 routine laboratory tests. In a given quarter-year and a given patient, a physician may not bill twice for an extended consultation (*Beratung*). If particular services are considered duplicative or mutually exclusive for a given diagnosis, the bill will not be honored. While doctors and their office assistants grumble about all the billing rules, the regulations appear to be relatively well accepted, partly because the rules and forms are uniform for the vast majority of payers and patients—and because they emanate from physician-dominated organizations rather than from insurers.

Participation Makes All the Difference

Many students of the German system stress this physician involvement, as embodied in the *Ärztekammer* and the *KV*s, as critical in understanding the acceptance that makes the system work. Explaining the term **body of public law** as applied to the *Ärztekammer* and *KV*s, Stone writes: "To the extent that a regulatory agency has been captured by its regulatees, it could be said to resemble a body of public law. But this situation is a long way from the German system, in which the blending of private interests and public authority is sanctioned in both political ideology and administrative law." As a result of this blend, she adds, the German medical profession "is more directly integrated into the structure of policymaking than the American and has access to more formal channels of influence."[23]

Paying the Doctor: Capitated Budgets, Fee-for-Service Payments

The German system of physician reimbursement involves four basic elements.

1. A regional budget for ambulatory care, determined on a capitation basis in negotiations between sickness funds and associations of sickness fund-authorized doctors, or *KVs*;
2. A national fee scale that sets the relative value of each medical service in points;
3. A conversion factor, couched as X deutschmarks per point, to transform each doctor's billings (in points) to actual monetary reimbursement; and
4. A system of vouchers, called *Krankenschein*, distributed by sickness funds to their members, given by patients to doctors as their "ticket" to purchase services, and conveyed by doctors to the *KVs* as billing forms itemizing the services provided.

Although German doctors are paid on a fee-for-service basis, the system "bears only a remote resemblance to the fee-for-service system" of the U.S., comments Simone Sandier of the *Centre de Recherche d'Etude et de Documentation en Economie de la Santé* in Paris. "Under Germany's statutory health insurance scheme, neither the patient nor the doctor knows at the time of treatment the exact amount the doctor will be paid. The patient, moreover, will never know."[24] (One might ask, however, how many U.S. patients actually know the size of their doctors' fee.)

The *Kopfpauschale* System

When the associations of sickness fund-authorized doctors, or *KVs*, were set up in the early 1930s, a system of pooled financing was devised between each sickness fund and the corresponding *KV* in each region. Under this system, the sickness fund and the *KV* negotiate annually over the size of a prospectively fixed sum of money to cover ambulatory care services for all the sickness funds' members. Negotiations start with a **capitation rate** for each sickness fund member, called a *Kopfpauschale*. Once this "lump sum per head" is agreed upon, it is multiplied by the total number of sickness fund members to derive the **aggregate budget**. The *KV* negotiates separately with each sickness fund in its region, so that capitation rates for each payer may differ according to the financial situation of each fund and how hard a bargain it was able to drive— or, in the case of the nationally based substitute funds (*Ersatzkassen*), how much more they were willing to give as an inducement for better physician service. All sickness funds in a given region did not pay the same capitation rate. "A fund with predominantly low-income members would have a lower capitation rate than a fund with fewer low-income members," explains Bradford Kirkman-Liff, Dr.P.H., professor of health administration and policy at Arizona State University. "This structure allowed an implicit cross-subsidization between 'wealthy' funds and 'poor' funds."[25]

The system has advantages for both sides; it greatly simplifies the daunting process of arriving at reimbursement rates for a multiplicity of payers and providers, while it also allows for sensitivity to the differing economic conditions of each sickness fund and region. It relieves sickness funds of the burden of claims processing and the politically sensitive task of policing deviant doctors. Equally significant, the process was controlled by the parties who were directly affected, so it avoids the imposition of rates by government bureaucrats.

As William Glaser points out, the *Kopfpauschale* system functioned as a fixed ceiling on annual expenditures between its inception and the mid-1960s. Cognizant of this expenditure cap, doctors competed with one another to maximize their incomes within the aggregate allotted amount. Fees were not nationally uniform during this period, and varied considerably from one place to another.

Introducing the Fee-for-Service Method

In 1955, federal law was modified to allow use of other methods of calculating the annual pool of physicians' payments besides the *Kopfpauschale*, such as fee-for-service, fee-per-visit, or mixed methods. Initially few sickness funds departed from the old capitation method.[26] However, partly because of criticism that the *Kopfpauschale* system motivated doctors to deliver unnecessary services, work sloppily, and even bill fraudulently,[27] the KVs persuaded sickness funds in the late 1960s to switch to a uniform fee-for-service scheme, with payment levels determined retrospectively. One political factor behind the change, according to Stone, was the switch to a retrospective fee-for-service method by the white-collar substitute funds (*Ersatzkassen*). This led to the popular idea, encouraged by physicians' groups, that substitute-fund members got better care while members of the sickness funds which stuck to the old capitation method had to settle for bargain-basement medicine. Pure fee-for-service payment became "the prestigious method," Stone reports. "The whole issue of determination of the pool became in the public debate one of two-class medicine."[28]

Under the fee-for-service method, doctors' fees are set in advance using a fee schedule, but the size of the payment pool is determined at the end of the year, by multiplying the volume of services rendered by the respective fees. In essence, Germany abandoned prospectively determined fixed budgets in favor of open-ended, retrospectively determined reimbursement. To put it another way, Germany exchanged expenditure caps for expenditure targets. By promising doctors a consistent and full fee for each service, sickness funds hoped physicians might forego their frenzied income-maximizing habits. It didn't work. Instead, the sickness funds "eventually had to achieve...discipline by postulating their own expenditure targets and driving hard bargains in the annual financial negotiations with the provincial KVs," Glaser writes.[29]

Limiting Spending On Physicians

Expenditure targets, which set a hoped-for goal rather than an absolute limit on spending, are inherently more permissive than expenditure caps. However, physician spending in the 1970s and early 1980s did not rise dramatically under the expenditure target system. Between 1976 and 1985 nominal spending for ambulatory physician services by statutory sickness funds rose by only 7.2 percent per year on average. This may have been partly due to an element of self-restraint operating on annual negotiations between sickness funds and *KV*s, since this was a time of growing public concern over a health care "cost explosion." Responding to the threat of cost-control legislation, the sickness funds and *KV*s in many German states agreed on a self-disciplinary device that prefigured a subsequent reform: a uniform national relative value fee schedule, which took effect in 1978. Point values were assigned to each of 2,500 separate procedures, and the capitation pool—set according to each year's expenditure target—was distributed according to the number of points individual physicians billed and a negotiated conversion factor. If doctors were found to be spending at a rate that would exceed the current year's expenditure target, the *KV* would prorate its doctors' fees downward in the final quarter of the year.

Despite these voluntary efforts, Germany would not stick with retrospective fee-for-service reimbursement for long.

Tightening the Screws

The mid-1970s in Germany brought severe recession in the wake of the "oil shock" of 1973. General economic troubles coincided with mounting concern over health costs, which had been growing at 10 percent a year in the 1960s and 20 percent between 1971 and 1975. The combination sparked a periodic cycle of health care cost control reforms that has stretched into the 1990s.

These reforms have attracted international attention because of their success. Germany's growth in real health spending between 1980 and 1989 was lower than that of Canada, Japan, France, and the United Kingdom—and less than half that of the United States.[30] Constraints on Germany's office-based doctors have been the most successful of the dozens of specific cost-control measures Germany has employed since 1977. In the 1980s, for instance, no increases would have been necessary in the contributions of German wage-earners to health insurance "if cost increases in other sectors had been as low as those for doctors' fees," comments Douglas Webber of the European Institute of Business Administration in Fountainebleau.[31]

The Trial-and-Error Approach to Cost Constraint

Germany's relative success in controlling office-based physicians' spending resulted from a series of trial-and-error actions that spanned more than a decade. In the mid-1970s, beset by a recessionary slump in their revenues, sickness funds pressured doctors to accept yearly increases in line with growth in the sickness funds' budgets—which were dependent, in turn, on growth in the average German wage. Under the economic pressure of the times, there was some voluntary compliance with this plea, and in 1978 the idea was formalized by the federal government in a policy of **physician expenditure targets**. The targets were supposed to take into account demographic changes, increases in morbidity, improvements in technology, and changes in the wage base of sickness fund members. When spending exceeded the target, spending for the subsequent year was to be rolled back. However, the rollback policy was not enforced.[32]

Because spending consistently exceeded targets, Germany in 1986 reverted to prospectively determined expenditure caps on physician expenditures.[33] The 1986 reform explicitly ties annual increments in ambulatory physician spending to the increase in the average German wage, a concept that has the advantage of being both simple to understand and socially equitable. (If the average worker is making only X percent more, according to the implicit logic, why should doctors do better?) Another far-reaching aspect of the 1986 reform was the **flexible fee schedule**.

Under a flexible fee schedule, doctors' fees for each service are adjusted downward if their aggregate billing volume exceeds the budgeted amount. It puts doctors collectively at risk for the billing behavior of individual physicians, and it guarantees that expenditures stay within the agreed-upon ceiling. The strategy does appear to be holding down aggregate physician costs. According to the 1991 GAO study, physician spending for outpatient services rose at 7 percent per year between 1977 and 1985, when expenditure targets were in place. But it slowed to only 2 percent a year after expenditure caps and flexible fees were imposed.

The **expenditure caps** adopted in 1986 were more sophisticated than the 1965 pre-*Kopfpauschale* version. In determining the prospective budget for each *KV*:[34,35]

- each German state has its own *Kopfpauschale*, or capitation rate, taking into account regional price differences and economic circumstances;
- pensioners, whose care is more expensive, have their own capitation rate, separate from the standard rate for each employed person and his or her dependents;
- payments from sickness funds to *KV*s are made quarterly, and close watch is kept to ensure that *KV*s do not exceed quarterly allowances; and
- "substitute" funds (*Ersatzkassen*) were brought into the "flexible fee" system, closing a loophole that historically allowed more liberal treatment of white-collar patients.

In addition, capitation rates are determined separately for different types of services so that excess volume in one area does not "steal" funding from other service types. The service categories are:

- **basic services**, including consultations and physical examinations;
- **general laboratory services**, the routine physical chemistry tests such as complete blood count and urinalysis that account for about 88 percent of all laboratory tests in Germany;[36] and
- **other services**, such as more specialized lab tests, injections, allergy tests, bandaging, and proctological exams.

Moreover, about 20 percent of ambulatory services are excluded from the overall payment cap. They are largely preventive services, such as Pap smears and routine checkups (including electrocardiograms), which are not intended to be constrained by a fixed budget.[37]

The Circle Closes

Thus, the Germans have come full-circle in their approach to reimbursement of office–based physicians—from prospectively determined, capitation-based budgets to open-ended, retrospectively determined payments, and back again. (The cycle continues: The 15 "substitute" funds, which insure 31 percent of the population who are mainly white-collar workers and their dependents, removed spending caps on physician services in 1991. Data on the impact of this step were not available in early 1993.) It is clear that the basic structure set up in 1931, by providing coherent channels for physician payment streams, has permitted this kind of experimentation without complicated and politically difficult upheavals accompanying each change of course (which is not to say that there was not spirited controversy). The current system appears to work well, but it is not without problems. From the doctors' point of view, the overriding issue is the amount of work they must do to meet their income targets.

German Style of Practice

Rushed...

The flexible fee system is explicitly designed to address a problem that has plagued German medicine since the establishment of the original capitation payment scheme in the 1930s. In a fixed-budget system that pays doctors on a fee-for-service basis, each physician has an incentive to increase the volume of services he provides in order to garner a larger share of reimbursement. Under the original *Kopfpauschale* system, German doctors "developed a practice style of long hours, the use of labor-saving equipment and auxiliaries, and rapid work," Glaser reports. "Many itemized services were provided, each fee was low, but the doctor's total income could be high."[38]

This "hurry-up" practice style is apparent in international studies of physicians' workload as well as in interviews with German doctors and patients. In a 1989 study, Simone Sandier found that general practitioners in Germany spend 9 minutes per patient visit on average compared to 14 minutes in the U.S. and France and 15 minutes in Quebec. General practitioners in the United Kingdom and Netherlands spend even less time: 8.2 minutes and 5 minutes per patient, respectively.[39] (Figure 4.2)

Sandier did not have data for the average annual number of office visits seen by a German general practitioner. In recent interviews by this author, one German GP, who said he practices a conservative and relatively leisurely style of medicine, reported he has about 10,000 patient visits per year. Another German generalist said he has about 7,400 patient-visits a year. A third GP reported "up to 2,000 patients per quarter."[40] Although obviously not a scientific sample, these highly reputable doctors all had more patient visits than the average of 6,723 visits Sandier reports among U.S. general practitioners, even though American generalists said they work about four more hours a week than Germans reported.[41]

German patients often complain about feeling rushed. "In order to run their practices economically, German doctors have to treat as many patients as possible as quickly as possible," says Christian Zimmerman of the German Patients' Union, a consumer advocacy organization. "It has led to what people call 'three-minute medicine.' They're very unhappy with the short term they get with the doctor but it's difficult to do something about it."[42] This perception is (and has long been) exploited by private health insurers, who imply by their marketing that by paying doctors more than twice as much as statutory sickness funds their subscribers will get more time and attention from physicians.

Figure 4.2

Number of Patient Visits Per General Practitioner Per Year, Average Duration of Visits, and Number of Hours Worked Per Week, 1979-87

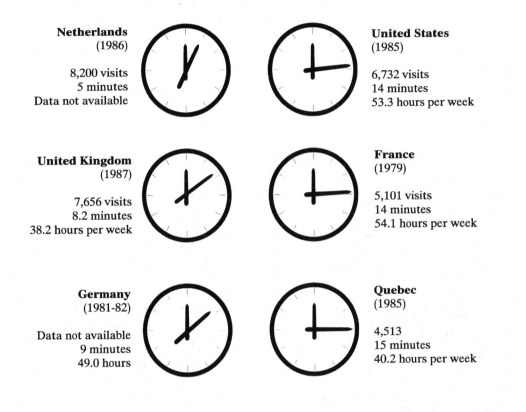

Netherlands
(1986)

8,200 visits
5 minutes
Data not available

United States
(1985)

6,732 visits
14 minutes
53.3 hours per week

United Kingdom
(1987)

7,656 visits
8.2 minutes
38.2 hours per week

France
(1979)

5,101 visits
14 minutes
54.1 hours per week

Germany
(1981-82)

Data not available
9 minutes
49.0 hours

Quebec
(1985)

4,513
15 minutes
40.2 hours per week

Source: Health Services Utilization and Physician Income Trends, Simone Sandier, Centre de Recherche d'Étude et de Documentation en Economie de la Santé, Paris. Health Care Financing Review, *Annual Supplement, 1989, p. 38.*

...But Intensive

While German doctors appear to spend less time with each patient, they also see each patient more often—a long-standing pattern that may reflect both cultural preferences and, at least implicitly, a desire by German physicians to increase reimbursements. The average German patient sees a physician nearly 11 times a year, twice as often as the 5.4 physician contacts of the average U.S. patient and considerably more frequently than citizens of other industrialized nations except Japan. (Figure 4.3) Outpatient visit rates have been fairly constant for many years in both the U.S. and Germany.[43] However, the most recent data hint at an increasing visit rate in Germany. One study reported in a German daily physicians' newspaper in 1992 found a rate of 16 visits per year in a study of 8,000 patients, with 88 percent of the survey population seeing the physician at least once.[44] A separate 1991 study found visit rates of 8 to 20 visits per year among Germans aged 25 to 69, with women having more frequent physician contacts than men.[45]

Germans also see specialists more often (5 times a year on average) than Americans (3.7 times), Canadians (2.5 times), or the British (1.2 times). This is interesting, since Germany has a smaller proportion of specialists among its physician population, and since access to specialists in Germany constrained more than it is in the U.S. Technically in order to see a specialist a German patient must obtain a referral from her primary care physician or a separate sickness certificate from his or her sickness fund. Anecdotally, German doctors and patients report this is not much of an obstacle. This is backed up by the statistics. In addition, some data suggest that German general practitioners refer their patients to specialists somewhat more often than U.S. generalists do.[46]

Figure 4.3

Utilization of Physician Services, 1981-86

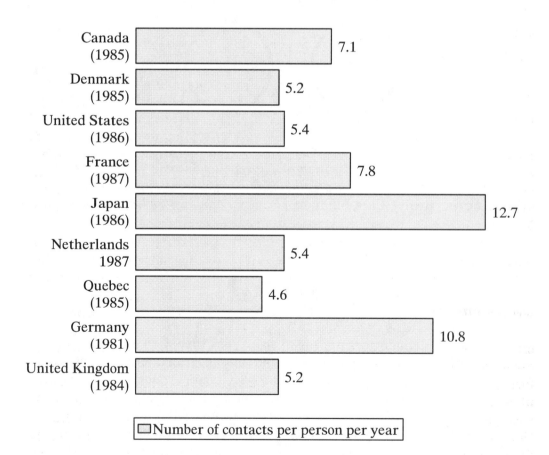

Source: Simone Sandier, Health Care Financing Review, *1989.*

Because German patients visit the doctor more often, it appears that they accumulate about the same amount of time each year with their physicians as Americans do—it is merely chopped up into smaller pieces. "The total amount of time spent with physicians of all types [per year] would appear to be about 1.5 hours in Germany and the United States and roughly 2 hours in France," Sandier comments.[47]

What Happens Behind the Office Door?

Once in the doctor's office, a German patient may receive more and somewhat different kinds of services than an American patient. Comparative studies on the content of outpatient care are lacking. There is little effort in Germany "either to analyze patterns of medical care utilization or to evaluate the appropriateness, let alone effectiveness, of medical care," Rodwin and his colleagues observe.[48] However, available evidence suggests that the intensity of services in Germany is not lower than in the U.S. German doctors prescribe nearly twice as many medicines per person as American doctors[49] and one-third more than the European average.[50] Per capita prescription drug spending is substantially higher—$257 in Germany versus $210 in the U.S., $230 in France, $179 in Japan, $175 in Canada, and $93 in the United Kingdom.[51] A study in doctors' waiting rooms found that 84 percent of patients expect to receive medications, and only 1 percent were disappointed.[52] By comparison, 60 percent of U.S. physician visits resulted in a prescription in 1989—but American patients went to the doctor only half as often, so their annual chances of receiving a prescription were undoubtedly substantially lower.[53]

The German fee schedule disproportionately rewards procedure-based services as well, despite efforts to reform it to place more emphasis on cognitive and consultative services.[54] For instance, though the percentage of office visits involving electrocardiograms is the same in the U.S. and Germany (about 2.9 percent in Germany versus 2.7 percent in the U.S.), Germans are more likely to have an EKG in a given year because they go to the doctor so much more often. According to one study, as many as 1 in 5 Germans may have an EKG each year.[55] To put this in context, EKG is a service widely considered to be seriously overused and overpriced in the U.S., where 8 percent of all office visits for elderly Medicare patients involved performance of an EKG in 1988.[56]

Moreover, German doctors routinely perform services that are either not part of American medical practice or are restricted to specialty situations. A list of the top 20 service charges of all German doctors (Figure 4.4) includes many that would not appear on a similar U.S. roster, such as microwave treatment, writing a "certificate of disablement," house call, and "electrostimulation."

Diagnostic ultrasound machines are commonplace in German doctors' offices, and they are routinely used in a wide variety of clinical situations. By one estimate, there are more than 16,000 ultrasound machines in the states of former West Germany—one for every 4,000 people or one for every dozen active physicians.[57] In the U.S., ultrasound is largely restricted to specialty practices such as obstetrics and cardiology and to a narrower set of indications. But in Germany, indications for ultrasound have expanded to include the "early diagnosis of tumors," general internal medicine, ear-nose-and-throat problems, routine gynecology and urology, and orthodontics. "This development has been mirrored in an increase in [ultrasound] benefits" paid by sickness funds "of 840 percent between 1979 and 1989," according to a German expert panel's 1991 report. "Because of the simplicity of the methods (but also because of the special fascination of the patient with the pictures) one could suspect a medically unjustified increase in sonography procedures," the report comments.[58]

Utilization Review and the "Fund Lions"

Germans have long been aware of the problems of over-utilization and fraudulent billing among fee-for-service physicians. Unlike third-party payers in the U.S., sickness funds are not in a position to do much about it directly because German physicians have jealously guarded their clinical autonomy. As Glaser notes, "The sickness funds must pay all doctors regardless of practice style."[59] The task thus falls to the *KV*s, which as physician-controlled organizations have the legal and moral authority to conduct utilization review of their members. Under a prospective budgeting system, the *KV* has an interest in preventing its individual members from over-billing, since the excess comes out of the pockets of more conservative (or honest) colleagues. An individual *KV* member does not have a right to payment in full for all the services he has billed, even though these charges serve as the basis for the collective payment from sickness funds to the *KV*. Instead, the individual doctor is entitled to be included in a fee distribution plan, developed by *KV* associations, that is designed to prevent "extreme expansion of the volume of gainful activity [by] a single...physician." This provides the legal basis for utilization review (UR) and "regression" of fees by the *KV*s, which are also mandated by federal law to monitor doctors.

Let Sleeping Lions Lie

The *KV*s have had UR programs for decades. Long before the advent of computers, clerks employed by the *KV*s and supervised by physicians reviewed all the quarterly sickness certificates (*Krankenschein*) submitted by participating physicians to compare doctors on their billing activity and watch for statistical outliers. Until recent years, these reviewers, known as *Kassenlöwen* or **fund lions**, could not disaggregate doctors' billings by type of procedure or compile sophisticated time series. This type of physician profiling also cannot detect petty fraud or **upcoding** (billing for more remunerative services than actually provided) unless the physician is so indiscreet as to submit an especially large number of claims.[60] It is widely suspected among doctors themselves that many of their colleagues engage in this kind of fraud. Often doctors sit with their office clerks (who are often their spouses) for a couple of days at the end of each quarter and fill out billing forms to be sent to the *KV*, explained one general practitioner. "Those are the best two days of the quarter," he said with a wink. "More than that I don't want to say."[61]

With the advent of computerized monitoring, *KV*s routinely provide very detailed information to their members on how they compare with their peers in billing activity. In addition, many doctors reportedly use computer software to keep track of their own billings and warn them when they are at risk of waking a *Kassenlöwen*.[62] Dr. Peter Helmich, a general practitioner who left his 32-year

Figure 4.4

The 20 Most Common Billings* by Office-Based Doctors in Germany, Third Quarter of 1979

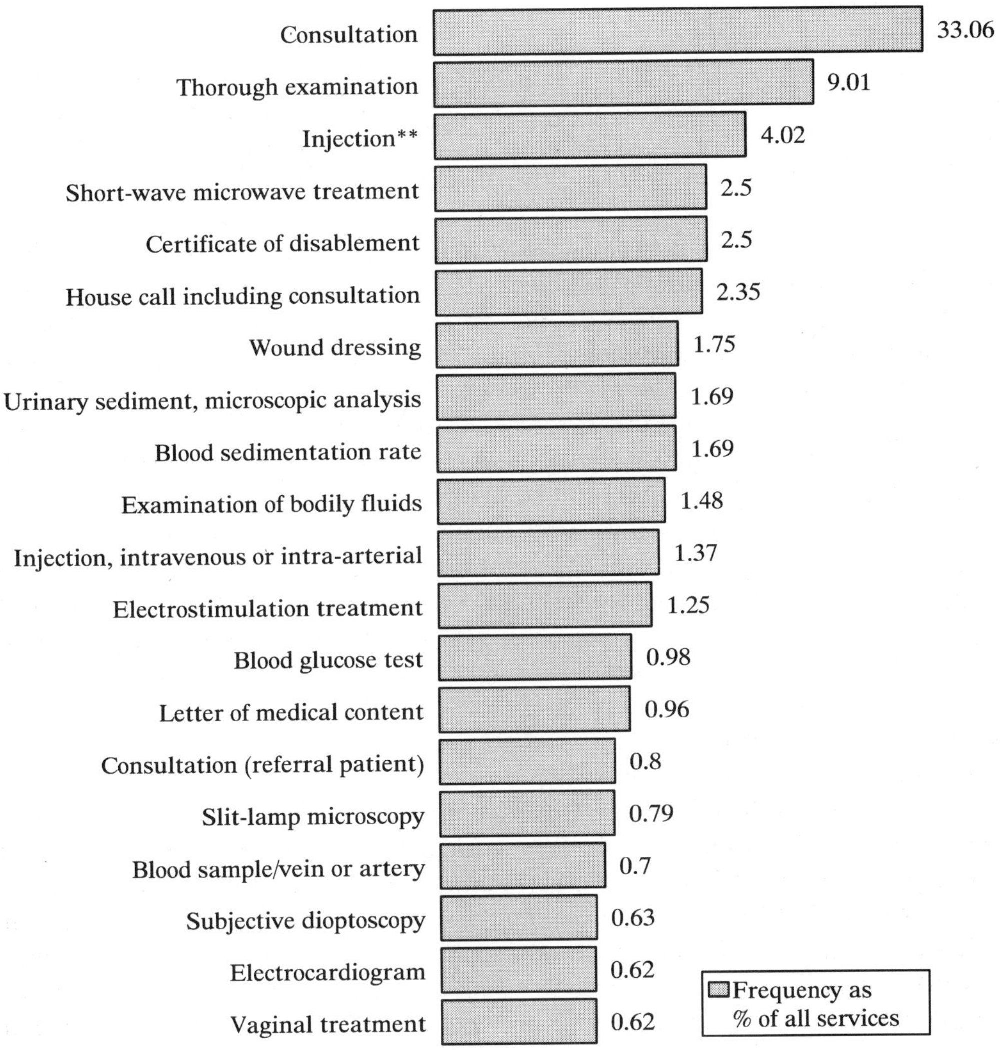

Billing	Frequency as % of all services
Consultation	33.06
Thorough examination	9.01
Injection**	4.02
Short-wave microwave treatment	2.5
Certificate of disablement	2.5
House call including consultation	2.35
Wound dressing	1.75
Urinary sediment, microscopic analysis	1.69
Blood sedimentation rate	1.69
Examination of bodily fluids	1.48
Injection, intravenous or intra-arterial	1.37
Electrostimulation treatment	1.25
Blood glucose test	0.98
Letter of medical content	0.96
Consultation (referral patient)	0.8
Slit-lamp microscopy	0.79
Blood sample/vein or artery	0.7
Subjective dioptoscopy	0.63
Electrocardiogram	0.62
Vaginal treatment	0.62

*Based on all doctors' charges.
**subcutaneous, submucosal, intracutaneous, intramuscular.

Source: Kassenärztliche Bundesvereinigung (National Association of Sickness Fund-Authorized Physicians).

practice in 1992 to teach family medicine at the University of Düsseldorf, explains the kind of feedback physicians get:

> The *KV* gives us a paper every quarter and you can see exactly what your costs are broken down by consultations, house visits, EKGs, laboratory services, and so forth. For example, our third-quarter data show that my partner and I exceeded the regional norm for routine consultation by 25 percent. But other doctors do 89 percent more "consultation outside normal hours" and 100.3 percent more "extensive consultations," which have higher point values. Others do 514.6 percent more "full body exam, including full history, consultation, and documentation." Others do 442 percent more "plaster of Paris casts" and 418 percent more "compression bandages." I do 195.7 percent more nursing home visits, but there's no test billing possible and therefore no doctor wants to go there. The tax man tells me "You are a very crazy fellow. You have to work more. You and your partner could make 100,000 more deutschmarks a year." Well, the way we do it is terrible for the money but it's good for the patient.[63]

The utilization review process conducted by each *KV* is paid for jointly by the *KV* and the sickness funds and supervised by a joint committee whose chair alternates between the two parties. In reviewing individual cases of abuse, the chair casts the deciding vote, but most decisions reportedly are unanimous.[64] The process is explicitly premised on the assumption that the vast majority of physicians are efficient and honest. Hospital physicians are not subject to UR because nearly all of them are salaried and thus have no financial motive to overutilize, and because they are strictly supervised (more so than in U.S. hospitals) by department chiefs, who are assumed to exercise control over inappropriate utilization.

The threshold for intensive review of an office-based physician's practice pattern varies from one region to another. Physicians whose utilization rates exceed 40 percent of the regional norm are notified of an automatic reduction in reimbursement for the excessive elements unless they can convince the "fund lions" that there is a valid reason for the disparity, such as an unusually high number of elderly patients. This threshold results in about 7 percent of physicians being called on annually to explain their practice patterns, with the burden of proof on them to justify it. About 2 percent actually have payment reductions.[65,66] Habitual offenders are monitored by regional committees on an ongoing basis.

To take the example of one regional *KV* in southwestern Germany, about 300 or 15 percent of the association's 2,000 doctors are reviewed each quarter and about a third of these, or 100 doctors, are required on the basis of this review to have a "consultation" with the monitoring committee about problem areas, such as their prescribing habits. Perhaps 30—1.5 percent of the total *KV* membership—actually have their fees reduced or be ordered to pay money back. In one extreme case in 1992, a physician was required to pay back DM 80,000 (about $38,000) for overutilization of prescription drugs—an amount lowered on appeal from DM 140,000 (about $70,000). The *KV*'s officials say the UR program does not bring in as much as it costs, about DM 400,000 a year ($191,000). "When all is accounted for, if you talk in terms of fees returned, the program does not pay for itself," one official said. "But you can't calculate the sentinel effect."[67] A sickness fund official in the same region agreed that "the sentinel effect is generally very important for the individual doctor," but he added that "there are of course strategies to circumvent regression [fee reduction] and still increase your volume."[68]

Both physician groups and sickness funds have been unhappy with physician UR as it has historically been practiced. For more than 15 years some doctors have sought, depending on their point of view, a more palatable alternative or a more effective one. While many see the process of **economic monitoring**, as it is called, as merely a nuisance, others complain that it is ineffective because it relies on identifying doctors with utilization above the average, when the average itself is arguably too high.[69]

Negotiating the Bavarian Contract

One widely known result of discontent with the usual mechanisms of cost control was an experiment launched in 1979 called the **Bavarian Contract**, which sprang out of a reaction among conservative physicians in the south of Germany to what they saw as a growing centralization of authority in health care. The concept behind the Bavarian Contract was to relieve doctors from a ceiling on physician spending if they could demonstrate savings in other sectors subject to their control. "The theory was that greater savings could be obtained if the sickness funds shifted their focus from reducing physician incomes to working with them to control more expensive hospital costs, since physicians generated by their actions and decisions 80 percent of costs," Kirkman-Liff explains.[70] Specifically, the agreement called on doctors to:

- reduce hospital admissions;
- prescribe fewer medications and medical appliances;
- limit the number of sickness certificates (excusing patients from going to work and qualifying them for sick pay); and
- reduce the use of physical therapy.

The Bavarian Contract was judged a failure. "Overall, there appeared to be no substitution effects and no cost savings," reports Kirkman-Liff. "While ambulatory care increased, hospital care also increased. Ambulatory surgery increased, but not at a higher rate than it had before the Bavarian Contract."[71] Various commentators agree that the explanation "is that the financial incentives in the scheme were designed to work only at an aggregate level, leaving open the possibility of 'free rider' behavior by the individual physician," as Jeremy W. Hurst of the British Department of Health puts it.[72] This collective incentive was basically a threat that had little meaning for individual physicians: if the experiment failed, physician income would be budgeted. Also, notes Christa Altenstetter, professor of political science at the City University of New York, successful cost reduction would have required the cooperation of a wide variety of actors—hospital physicians, social security offices, sickness funds, disability programs, patients, and their families. "Another reason the contract did not attain its goals is that community-based, coordinated networks of health and social support are not available in all regions and cities in Germany," Altenstetter writes. For instance, to reduce hospitalization requires more nursing home and alternative housing options than many communities have.[73]

Using MSOs

More recently, Germany has inaugurated other measures to reduce unnecessary utilization. A major federal reform law in 1989 created **Medical Service Organizations** (MSOs) in all states somewhat along the lines of the U.S.

Professional Review Organizations (PROs). Funded by an assessment on sickness funds, their general purpose is to ensure that medical care is appropriate, high-quality, and efficient. For instance, they are to develop new UR standards, advise on regional peer review efforts, and assess the appropriateness of such services as *Kurkliniks*, or medical resorts. They are also empowered to do some concurrent review of hospital stays.[74] Since then, another federal law has required regional UR boards to sample 2 percent of all physicians randomly to assess the appropriateness of their services. Both the MSOs and the random sampling measures have been established too recently to assess their impact.

Doctors' Earning Power: Mirror of Cost Control

Germans would be the last to claim success in optimizing cost-effective physician care. Yet the data show that global budgeting of ambulatory doctors has had a real constraining effect, possibly abetted by utilization review. In the 1950s, spending for ambulatory physician care was increasing at an annual average rate of more than 14 percent.[75] Between 1970 and 1985, a period of much public discussion about the "explosion" in health costs and, after 1977, of yearly physician expenditure targets, average annual inflation in statutory sickness fund spending for physician care was 9 percent. After the enactment of an expenditure cap and flexible fees in 1986, the yearly average rate was nearly halved, to 4.4 percent.[76] (Figure 4.5) By comparison, U.S. nominal spending on physician services grew by an annual average of 26 percent in the 1960s, 31 percent in the 1970s, and 30 percent in the 1980s.[77] On an inflation-adjusted basis, using constant 1982 dollars, the corresponding U.S. growth rates were 16 percent, 14 percent, and 14 percent.[78] The German expenditure cap system enacted in 1987 "has been effective in radically reducing the growth of ambulatory care costs," summarizes Kirkman-Liff.[79]

Not only is physician inflation lower, but German physicians account for a significantly lower proportion of national income than their counterparts in the U.S. — though their share is higher than Canadian doctors'. In 1980, ambulatory physician services consumed for the same share of gross national product in both the U.S. and Germany. But in 1990, doctors consumed less than 1.4 percent of Germany's GNP compared to 2.4 percent in the U.S. German doctors' share of GNP had actually declined slightly during the 1980s, while U.S. physicians' share rose by nearly 76 percent.[80] (Figure 4.6) This trend is mirrored in physicians' claim on the contributions that most Germans must pay for statutory health insurance. As German physician lobbyists like to point out, the doctors' share—1.64 percent of the average German's gross wages—has remained unchanged since 1970, while the share for hospital care grew from 1.59 to 2.22 percent of gross wages between 1970 and 1990.[81]

Not surprisingly, Germany's success has been reflected in its physicians' earning power. In 1987, the average office-based physician in Germany netted DM 209,400 before taxes ($95,600 on a purchasing power parity basis) on a gross income of DM 454,800 ($207,700).[82] The corresponding Figures that year for an American doctor were $132,300 net income on total revenues of $256,000.[83] In other words, U.S. physicians took home 38 percent more.

The disparity was not always so large. In 1971, German doctors' net pretax earnings were 6.5 times the national average wage—among the highest in the world.[84] (Many analysts consider this ratio, rather than absolute monetary amounts, to be the most meaningful index of physicians' economic status within a given society.) In 1984, German doctors were still the world's second best-paid doctors—after Japanese and before American physicians—in terms of this ratio. In that year, the average net pretax earnings of Japanese physicians was 7.3 times the national average; German doctors' net earnings were 4.4 times the average; and for American doctors the ratio was 3.9.[85]

Since 1984, however, German doctors' earnings have slipped to 3.5 times the average wage-earners'.[86,87] Sandier finds this narrowing of the gap between physicians' earnings and general wage-earners' in a number of industrialized nations, but notes that the ratio stabilized elsewhere after 1983 and even

Figure 4.5

Yearly Inflation in Physician Spending: Increase in Outlays by Statutory Sickness Funds, 1971-90

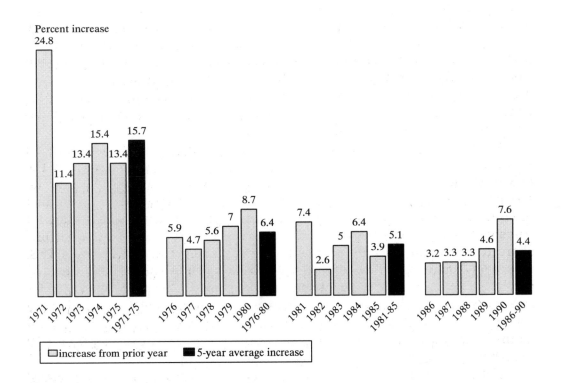

Source: Sachverständigenrat für die Konzertierte Aktion im Gesundheitswesen, 1992.

Figure 4.8

Doctors' Share of National Income in Three Nations, 1980-90

(Physician spending as percent of gross national product)

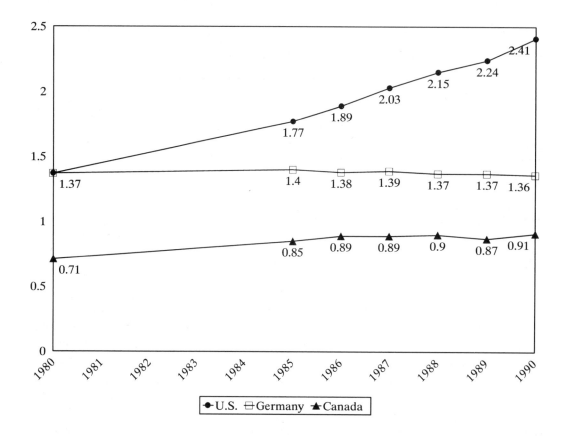

Source: BASYS (Beratungsgesellschaft für angewandte Systemforschung), Augsburg, 1992.

reversed slightly in the U.S. during the 1980s. "Germany is the only country [among 6 surveyed] where this trend has continued," Sandier reports.[88] Between 1985 and 1989, for instance, German doctors' income grew by about 6.6 percent, while private-sector compensation increased almost twice as much—about 13 percent.[89]

The continued decline in German doctors' earning power since 1986 largely reflects the reimposition of an expenditure cap on office-based physician services in 1986, along with the "flexible fee" enforcement mechanism.[90] While total physician income has been depressed, German doctors' practice costs increased 40 percent between 1981 and 1989, according to the National Association of Sickness Fund-Authorized Physicians;[91] professional expenses currently consume 56 percent of the average physician's gross income.[92] Even though American physicians pay much higher malpractice insurance premiums, their practice costs are not as onerous, averaging 49 percent of gross income among self-employed U.S. physicians in 1989.[93]

The Exceptions To The Rule

Hospital department chiefs, especially in teaching hospitals, are a small but important exception to this general picture of physician earnings. These chief physicians, who constitute about 11 percent of hospital-based doctors,[94] have the exclusive franchise for the hospital care of privately insured patients. Consequently, their income is on a different plane from all other German doctors. Academic chiefs in many fields command seven-Figure incomes and wield unchallenged institutional authority. "Department chief is a rank somewhere among the angels," explains one teaching hospital administrator. "But academic hospital department chiefs are also German professors. Now they *are* gods!"[95] Nevertheless, under a health care reform law that took effect in January 1993, hospital chiefs are required to pay a sizable proportion of their private-patient income to the hospital, a step the hospital official calls "very, very unwise politically."

Slicing Up the Fee-for-Service Pie

Both German and U.S. office-based physicians work in a fee-for-service world. Like their German colleagues, American doctors have become accustomed by Medicare to the idea of a relative value scale and conversion factors that transform relative values into fees (and may change from year to year). But, as Sandier has commented, the resemblances between U.S. and German fee-for-service medicine are only superficial. One major divergence is in the fees themselves.

U.S. and German Fees: There's No Comparison

Recent comparisons of what doctors actually receive for given services in the two nations reveal enormous disparities, nearly always in American physicians' favor. An initial examination of a new patient, for example, was worth only about one-fifth to one-quarter as much to German physicians in 1987. A routine consultation brought a German doctor as little as one-twentieth as much, while an electrocardiogram fee was 34 to 44 percent of the U.S. equivalent. Interestingly, technical diagnostics, such as computerized tomography and even routine x-rays, fetched more nearly equal remuneration.[96] (Table 4.3) A 1991 comparison of gastroenterology fees found similar divergence. An upper-GI tract endoscopy paid the doctor $57.42 in Germany (using purchasing power parity conversion) versus $217 under the U.S. Medicare mean charge, or $244 with a biopsy. Colonoscopy with examination of the terminal ileum brought the Germany physician $96 and his American colleague $281 to $303.[97]

Such comparisons indicate a clear difference in how doctors in the two systems are paid, but they do not tell the whole story. When treating most patients German doctors do not know until the end of the year exactly what fee a given service will bring them. If doctors in a given region collectively bill more than the budgeted amount for that service category (basic services, laboratory tests, other services), the conversion factor will be reduced and every doctor's reimbursement for services in that category will go down. An analysis of these conversion factors (or "point values" as they are known) shows they have fluctuated from one quarter to the next in recent years, but the general trend has been flat or downward. This means that the unit price of services in each category has not kept pace with inflation. (Figure 4.7) There are disparities from one region to another, reflecting the financial situation of regional sickness funds (and thus their overall budgets for physician care) as well as the billing activity and physician supply in each area. (Table 4.4)

Obviously, a flat unit price provides a strong incentive for German physicians to increase the volume of services they provide in order to keep pace with

Table 4.3

Fees for Selected Physician Services in Germany and the U.S.*

Service	German fee range 1989				U.S. Medicare 1987		Ratio G–U.S.
		High		Low			
Initial exam	DM	27.21	DM	19.53	DM	95.92	.20–.28
	$	12.89	$	9.26	$	43.80	
Followup exam	DM	18.04	DM	7.55	DM	50.14	.15–.36
	$	3.58	$	8.55	$	22.89	
Home visit	DM	43.05	DM	26.85	DM	91.56	.29–.47
	$	20.40	$	12.73	$	41.80	
Consultation	DM	18.04	DM	7.81	DM	154.78	.05–.12
	$	8.55	$	3.70	$	70.68	
Chest x-ray	DM	82.74	DM	46.86	DM	61.04	.77–1.36
	$	39.21	$	22.21	$	27.87	
CT head scan	DM	553.51	DM	229.42	DM	327.00	.70–1.69
	$	262.87	$	108.73	$	149.32	

*DM-to-$ conversions based on OECD purchasing power parity for the respective year: 2.11 for 1989, 2.19 for 1987.

Source: Markus Schneider, et.al., BASYS, Augsburg, 1993.

inflation in their practice expenses and to support personal lifestyles and obligations. This is apparently what has occurred, despite the well-known disincentive inherent in the system—that if many doctors increase volume, everyone's remuneration will be depressed. As the Bavarian Contract experiment showed, collective incentives may not be very effective in changing individuals' behavior. "Although rational behavior would motivate physicians to reduce, collectively, the number of their services so as to be compensated at a higher rate, individual physicians are motivated by what [Gerhard] Brenner calls 'irrational behavior patterns' (in a collective sense) to increase their volume," write Rodwin and his colleagues.[98] Based on interviews with physician leaders in 1987 and 1989, Kirkman-Liff concludes that

Figure 4.7

Changes in National Average Point Values (Conversion Factors), 1989-92, In German Pfennigs

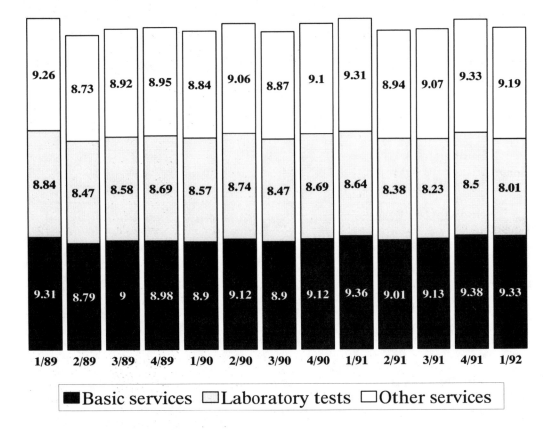

Source: *Kassenärztliche Bundesvereinigung, 1993.*

Table 4.4

Point Values for Basic Ambulatory Physician Services in Regional Associations of Sickness Fund-Authorized Physicians, 1991

State	Average Point Value
Schleswig-Holstein	8.4697
Hamburg	8.9627
Bremen	8.7380
Niedersachsen	8.7071
Westfalen-Lippe	9.0745
Nordrhein	9.0266
Hessen	9.1615
Koblenz	9.4323
Rheinhessen	10.3038
Pfalz	9.9238
Trier	10.3424
Nordbaden	10.2674
Südbaden	9.3061
Nord-Württemberg	10.3332
Südwürttemberg	9.6612
Bayerns	9.6112
Berlin	7.9768
Saarland	8.2682
National Average	**9.2249**

*Values in pfennigs, includes only regions of former West Germany.

Source: *Kassenärztliche Bundesvereinigung, 1992.*

While the expenditure cap system restrains cost increases by definition, it is not clear that the system modifies physician behavior. Despite the fact that physicians bear some collective economic risk for their incomes...it was generally reported that physicians continue to practice as if they were paid on a conventional fee-for-service basis. Both physician and nonphysician interviewees felt that as long as the payment rates to physicians were similar to what they were in the past, sickness fund physicians will have little concern about the methodology used for paying their association.[99]

An increase in volume helps explain why sickness funds' total annual outlays for physician care increased steadily by as much as 7.6 percent (in 1990), and outlays per insured person grew an average of 6 percent annually between 1985 and 1990[100]—even though there has been almost no increase in individual physicians' incomes from caring for sickness fund patients during the 1980s.[101] However, the principal reason why German physicians' pie is being sliced thinner is that the number of German physicians is growing faster than the pie.

German physicians' incomes in recent years presents a stark contrast to the experience of U.S. doctors. "After a stagnant period in the late 1970s to early 1980s, [U.S.] physicians' real income rose handsomely in the late 1980s," report Gregory C. Pope and John E. Schneider of the Center for Health Economics Research in Waltham MA. Average real physician income grew by a strong 24 percent form 1982 ($125,500 in 1989 dollars) to 1989 ($155,800). Almost all of this increase occurred in the latter four years, 1986 to 1989."[102] This increase in earning power occurred in the face of strong inflation in office expenses and malpractice premiums, and despite a 5.8 percent decline in the number of patient contacts per physician between 1982 and 1989. Pope and Schneider estimate that 42 percent of office-based physicians' increased income was derived from a greater number of services provided per physician and 58 percent from higher profit margins per unit of service.[103]

Physician Oversupply: Germany's Achilles' Heel?

A large and growing oversupply of physicians is a first-tier health care policy challenge for Germany in the 1990s and beyond—equal to the issues of reducing fiscal disparities among sickness funds, reforming hospital payment methods, and even upgrading of former East Germany's health infrastructure.

"Manpower supply growth is the German medical profession's greatest long-range concern, and Germany's most visible problem," comments Dale A. Rublee, PhD, policy analyst at the American Medical Association's Center for Health Policy Research.[104] The problem of excess physicians and its corollary, increasing overspecialization, has the potential of unraveling much of the enviable success Germany has enjoyed in the 1980s in controlling health care costs.

As Germany well understands, physicians drive the entire system's costs. Office-based practitioners generate more than 5 times the health care outlays that they themselves are paid, according to a 1992 analysis by an expert advisory committee to Germany's Concerted Action in Health Care Council.[105]

Moreover, each 1 percent increase in the supply of physicians induces a 1.1 percent increment in health care spending, according to another analysis.[106] Federal health officials point out that health expenditures within Germany correlate closely with regional physician supply—or oversupply. For instance, Munich has one sickness fund-authorized physician for every 611 inhabitants, compared to rural Middle Franconia, which has one doctor for every 867 residents and Hof, a medium-sized town in northern Bavaria, which has one panel doctor for every 1,051 inhabitants. Spending for ambulatory physician services in Munich were found to be 17.5 percent higher than in Middle Franconia and 46 percent higher than in Hof. "This example shows the connection between the number of physicians and...emphasizes the need to limit the number of doctors," says Gerhard Schulte, assistant secretary in the Federal Health Ministry.[107]

Not only is physician oversupply worrisome from the perspective of the system's total spending, but adding a steady stream of new doctors to a system in which physician outlays are constrained generates severe pressures—on each physician who is competing for a share of the "pie," and ultimately on the politicians and private-sector managers to lift the lid on physician spending. It is remarkable that Germany has resisted these mounting pressures as successfully as it has since 1986, when the expenditure cap was imposed. Moreover, in 1993 parliament succeeded in imposing *another* fiscal constraint on doctors by making them liable for a portion of overspending a new budget on prescription drugs, as will be discussed below. (One lapse in this otherwise rigorous constraint on physician spending, as mentioned above, was the doctors' 1991 success in persuading the "substitute funds," which cover 31 percent of those in the statutory insurance system, to lift expenditure caps.)

The Doctor Explosion

Germany's growth in physician supply since the 1960s far surpasses the United States' and possibly any other nation's. The physician-population ratio of Germany is higher than the average of 7 European nations (Belgium, France, Germany, Ireland, Netherlands, Spain, and the United Kingdom).[108] The population of West Germany remained essentially flat between 1970 and 1990 while the number of physicians nearly doubled. (Table 4.5) America rapidly expanded its physician output in the 1960s and 1970s, adding to supply at a rate three-and-one-half times faster than total population growth.[109] Nevertheless, a comparison of physician supply per 100,000 population reveals that Germany outpaced the U.S. during each decade since 1960. On a per-population basis, Germany has almost one-third more doctors than the U.S. (Table 4.6) Moreover, the supply is projected to increase by 50 percent between 1989 and 2000.[110]

Four out of five new doctors are being absorbed into the German health care system. But one German physician in five was "without medical employment" in 1990, a doubling of this category in the previous decade—on top of an earlier doubling between 1970 and 1980.[111] Michael Arnold, MD, professor of health services research at the University of Tübingen, points out that many of those without medical employment are "female physicians who have temporarily given up their profession to devote themselves to their families."[112] However, it appears that women, who make up nearly one in three German doctors, are more vulnerable to the tightening market for medical services. Female doctors

Table 4.5

Growth in West Germany's General and Physician Populations, 1980-90: Increase in Numbers, Physician Employment, and Percentage Change

Year	Total Pop. in 1000s	Total MDs	Practicing MDs	Office-based MDs	Hospital-based MDs	Adminis-trative MDs	MDs in other medical employment	MDsw/o medical employment
1960	55,433	n.a.	79,350	n.a.	n.a.	n.a.	n.a.	n.a.
1970	60,651	n.a.	99,654	n.a.	n.a.	n.a.	n.a.	n.a.
1980	61,658	164,124	139,452	59,777	67,964	6,944	4,767	24,672
1981	61,713	171,569	144,224	60,652	71,724	7,171	4,677	27,345
1982	61,546	178,119	148,720	62,418	73,420	6,981	5,901	29,399
1983	61,307	184,228	152,158	64,032	73,581	7,248	7,297	32,070
1984	61,049	191,771	156,593	65,780	75,750	6,906	8,177	35,178
1985	61,020	199,146	160,902	67,363	77,758	7,223	8,558	38,244
1986	61,140	206,934	165,902	68,698	79,216	7,279	9,822	41,919
1987	61,238	216,438	171,487	70,277	82,580	7,792	10,838	44,951
1988	61,715	223,664	177,001	71,751	85,150	8,018	12,082	46,663
1989	62,679	234,832	188,225	74,040	92,480	8,134	13,571	46,607
1990	63,726	242,578	195,254	75,251	96,203	8,356	15,444	47,324
% change:								
80/90	**3.4%**	**48%**	**40%**	**26%**	**42%**	**20%**	**324%**	**92%**
70/90	5.1%		96%					
60/90	14.9%		146%					

Sources: Sachverständigenrat für die Konzertierte Aktion im Gesundheitswesen 1992 and Health Care Financing Review *1992.*

predominate among those "without medical employment" in every age group, not merely among those of child-bearing age.[113]

A Growing Number of the Wrong Kind

"How physicians are distributed according to specialty," observes Steven Schroeder, MD, president of the Robert Wood Johnson Foundation, "has important implications for the medical marketplace—for what kinds of care are given, who receives it and where, and how much it costs."[114] In this regard, Germany has been relatively fortunate. Compared to the United States, Germany (like every other nation in the world) has a smaller proportion of specialists and a larger proportion of primary care physicians. In 1990, 40 percent of Germany's practicing physicians were classified as "without a specialty"; however, 8 percent of the total were "specialists in general medicine,"[115] so in American terms about half of German physicians might be called generalists.[116] In the U.S., more than 70 percent of physicians are specialists

Table 4.6

Practicing Physicians per 100,000 Population: U.S. vs Germany, 1960-90

Year	U.S.	% change/ prior 5-year period	Germany	% change/ prior 5-year period	Ratio Germany: U.S.
1960	136		143		105%
1965	150	10%	146	2%	97
1970	152	1	164	12	108
1975	171	13	192	18	112
1980	195	14	226	18	116
1985	216	11	264	17	122
1990	232	7	306	16	132
% change					
1990/80		19%		35%	
1990/70		53		87	
1990/60		71		114	

Source: Organization for Economic Cooperation & Development (OECD) Health Data File, 1992.

even if general internists and general pediatricians are counted as generalists.[117]

The unwavering trend in Germany, however, has been a rise in specialists and a decline in generalists. Between 1980 and 1990, the number of specialists rose by 25 percent while the number of generalists fell by 6.3 percent. The proportion of patients seen by specialists (including those certified as specialists in general medicine) was 52 percent in 1980, but a decade later 58 percent of all cases were being treated by specialists. Extrapolating from this trend, an expert advisory panel projected in 1992 that by the year 2000, 62 percent of all German doctors will be specialists and the same proportion of cases will be treated by specialists.[118,119]

As the market for physicians' services becomes increasingly competitive, and since doctors practice under a budget ceiling that constrains their collective income, becoming a specialist is one of the only ways the doctor can slice himself or herself a larger share of the "pie." As in the U.S., specialists tend to practice a more intensive and procedure-oriented style of medicine. Thus, for a given visit or a given case, they can bill more "points." Even if this increase in volume results in a depression of the value of each point, it redistributes remuneration from generalists to specialists. A 1990 study of six *KV* regions by the Research Institute of Local Sickness funds illustrated this phenomenon. Between 1988 and 1989,

☐ the number of "points" billed by specialists for each case increased 64 percent faster than those of generalists;

☐ the number of "points" per case for laboratory tests went up more than twice as much in specialist practices;

☐ total "points" per case increased 44 percent faster among specialists; and

☐ the rate of increase in total points per doctor was 50 percent higher among specialists.[120]

Physician Fee Reform

Recognizing the problem, Germany in 1987 implemented a major revaluation of physicians' fees. The revision "was intended to give greater emphasis to the role of the family physician and to personal medical services," explain Gerhard Brenner, managing director of the Central Institute of Sickness Fund Physicians in Cologne, and The American Medical Association's Rublee. "Fees for services requiring no medical consultation, especially laboratory services, were decreased relative to medical services with a high consultative content."[121]

The 1987 fee reform was a partial success. It narrowed the gap in physician incomes among specialties, but "the changes were far from dramatic," Brenner and Rublee note. "Germany's desire to give greater financial support to the family physician was only partly realized."[122] Ironically, specialists in "laboratory medicine" (pathologists in U.S. parlance) gained in income because specialized laboratory services were not devalued, although routine lab tests were. The biggest income "winners" were pediatricians and gynecologists; the biggest "losers" were radiologists. General practitioners had a slight gain in income. (Table 4.7) Table 4.8 gives a post-1987 picture of the 20 top revenue-producers in office-based billings, which together account for 43 percent of all procedures.

Professional Freedom vs Social Needs

Legal reasons play a major role in Germany's increasing physician and specialist oversupply. Decades ago, its Federal Constitution Court ruled that Article 12 of the postwar German constitution, which establishes "free choice of profession or occupation," guarantees every qualified applicant admission to medical school and freedom to practice medicine when qualified.[123] (In Germany, all medical schools and teaching hospitals are owned and administered by state governments, and there are no tuition charges.) In response, Germany developed an elaborate system of medical school admissions that stratifies applicants by test scores, premedical academic marks, and aptitude for medicine so the brightest are admitted sooner; but even the less-bright can get in if they wait long enough.[124]

Table 4.7

Impact of 1987 German MD Fee Reform: Income Changes and Percent of MDs With Higher Incomes, North Rhine Region

Specialty	%change in average MD income	% of MDs with higher incomes
All physicians	-0.8%	48%
General practitioners	1.3	52
Ophthalmologists	-4.3	32
Surgeons	-7.3	35
Gynecologists	11.5	74
Ear-nose-throat	-1.0	44
Cardiologists	-6.1	38
Internal medicine	-6.0	33
Pediatricians	17.8	84
Pathologists	2.0	42
Neurologists	-6.1	31
Orthopedic surgeons	-4.1	39
Radiologists	-13.3	15
Urologists	-2.3	43
Other specialists	5.3	59

Source: Bradford Kirkman-Liff after Brenner and Koch (1989), Central Institute of Sickness Fund Physicians, Cologne.

Table 4.8

Top 20 Revenue-Producers* in German Office-Based Medical Practice, 1990

Rank	Service	% of all office services
1	Thorough exam/single organ system	7.4 %
2	Short symptom-related exam/history	6.3
3	Extended consultation and advice	4.9
4	Discussion of therapeutic measures	4.3
5	Home visit	3.4
6	Exam of several organ systems/advice	2.6
7	Prescription renewal	1.8
8	Electrocardiogram (EKG)	1.4
9	Treatment of severe distress	1.2
10	Thorough exam/all organ systems	1.1
11	Intramuscular injection	1.0
12	Epigastric sonography	0.9
13	Spinal x-ray	0.9
14	Blood drawing	0.9
15	X-ray of an extremity	0.9
16	Cancer screening/female patient	0.8
17	Routine laboratory tests/maximum value per visit (includes bilirubin, total cholesterol, cholesterol fractions, triglycerides, uric acid, creatinine, alkaline phosphatase, liver enzyme tests, calcium, sodium, potassium, and other common tests, not including blood glucose)	0.8
18	Intravenous infusion	0.7
19	Saturday/Sunday/holiday visit	0.7
20	Preventive checkup	0.7

*Together, these services account for 42.7% of all billings.

Source: Kassenärztliche Bundesvereinigung, 1991.

In 1960, another bar to professional freedom was struck down when the Constitutional Court ruled, in a suit brought by the *Hartmannbund* and the Association of Sickness Fund-Authorized Physicians, that sickness funds could no longer exclude doctors from participation according to a formula of the number of doctors they needed to care for a population of given size. Sickness funds had generally used a 1:500 rule of thumb, a ratio 153 percent higher than Germany's ratio of practicing physicians to population in 1990. Since that decision, every licensed physician has been legally entitled to establish a practice and treat statutory sickness fund patients wherever he chooses.[125] As a result, the number of doctors admitted to sickness fund practice, particularly specialists, has soared. (Figure 4.8)

So Many Doctors; So Little Room

As the physician excess has worsened, policymakers, often at the instigation of alarmed medical leaders as well as sickness fund administrators, have made attempts to circumvent the court rulings. In 1986, a Need Planning Law authorized *KV*s and sickness funds to close regions to certain newcomers when they have determined there is a greater than 50 percent excess in their specialties. In addition, the statute authorized insurers and physicians' associations to "invite" doctors to retire early.[126] In the 1980s, medical schools successfully limited applicants on the basis of the physical capacity of lecture halls and their ability to maintain acceptable teaching standards.[127] Another deliberate strategy has been to increase the length of time medical graduates must spend in postgraduate training before entering the pool of full-fledged physicians. Between 1982 and 1990, the average time a newly minted doctor spends in hospital practice between licensure and establishment of an office practice has lengthened from 5.6 years to 6.4 years. The proportion of those who spend more than 4 years as junior hospital staff before "settling down" in an office practice, as the German phrase goes, increased from 50 to 66 percent.[128] As mentioned above, this has had the effect of ballooning hospital medical staffs, since hospital practice serves as a holding pattern for doctors until they are in a position to set up a private practice. Medical school applicants have gotten the message; their numbers peaked at nearly 68,000 in 1983 and by 1989 had dropped to fewer than 26,000. (Figure 4.9)

As in the U.S., German doctors are not always where they are needed, so physician groups have established a national counselling service for doctors seeking to establish an ambulatory practice, listing areas of greater need by specialty, the age of doctors by region (indicating future retirements), and the numbers of cases treated. If a given region has an undersupply in a particular specialty, the regional *KV* must advertise practice locations, guarantee applicants a certain level of gross billings, and grant loans to help doctors set up a practice.[129]

The Government Steps In

These marginal and voluntary measures have had little effect in the face of the burgeoning supply of new physicians. Therefore, a sweeping reform measure effective in January 1, 1993, confronted the issue head-on. The law

Figure 4.8

Trends in Sickness Fund Ambulatory Care Physicians, 1970-90: Specialists* and Nonspecialists

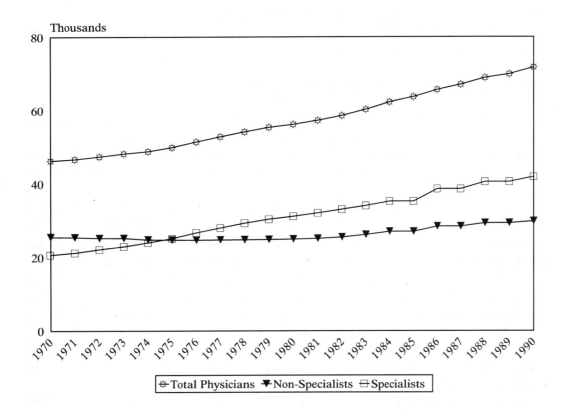

% Change	Total	Non-Specialists	Specialists
1980/70	21%	-2.2%	51%
1990/80	28%	19%	34%
1990/70	55%	17%	103%

* Specialists include those who are certified specialists in general medicine

Source: Sachverständigenrat für die Konzertierte Aktion im Gesundheitswesen 1992.

Figure 4.9

Medical School Places and Applicants in Germany, 1975-89

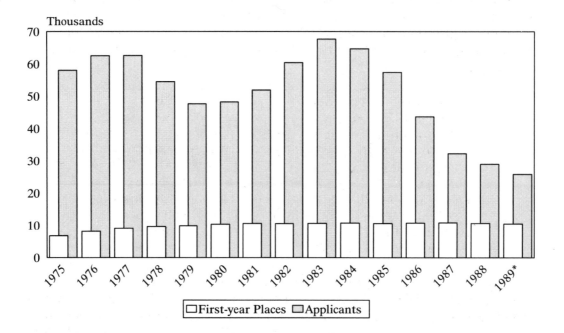

Year	First-year Places	Applicants	Ratio of Applicants:Place
1975	6,741	58,025	8.6:1
1976	8,119	62,515	7.7
1977	9,106	62,587	6.9
1978	9,652	54,553	5.7
1979	9,889	47,644	4.8
1980	10,335	48,228	4.7
1981	10,584	51,969	4.9
1982	10,551	60,414	5.7
1983	10,607	67,653	6.4
1984	10,712	64,707	6.0
1985	10,589	57,399	5.4
1986	10,718	43,665	4.1
1987	10,828	32,310	3.0
1988	10,637	28,965	2.7
1989*	10,470	25,859	2.5

* Preliminary estimates

Source: Sachverständigenrat für die Konzertierte Aktion im Gesundheitswesen, 1990.

establishes a mandatory retirement age of 68 for physicians.[130] Furthermore, beginning in March 1993, KVs have the option of refusing new applicants to statutory health insurance practice if they judge there are already enough doctors to serve the population in their region. (The standard is determined by each state's KV rather than the federal government.) That is just the first step toward what sounds like the pre-1960 days when sickness funds could set absolute population-based quotas for the number of doctors they would reimburse. Schulte, of the Federal Health Ministry, explains the federal aim in no uncertain terms:

> Starting in 1999 we shall be reducing the number of registered [statutory sickness fund-authorized] doctors and dentists providing outpatient medical and dental care to suit existing need. In the meantime, we will be organizing our planning for demand in such a way that regions in which too many physicians are already active now will be closed to new registrations. Physicians who wish to set up a private practice and be registered with the statutory health insurance [system] will then be obliged to move to regions where no oversupply as yet exists.[131]

Most policymakers expect these provisions to be challenged in court. In early 1993, the *Marburgerbund* (the association of hospital-based doctors) said it was exploring such a suit.[132] "There is a serious concern that it will be tested," says Martin Pfaff, a Social Democratic member of the *Bundestag* and a leading member of the health reform coalition.[133] "We are fully aware that such a legislative intervention in the right to the free exercise of one's profession is not easy against the background of our constitution," replies Schulte. "However, according to the consistent practice of the Federal Constitutional Court, the ability to finance our social security system is of such constitutional preeminence that even basic civil rights, such as the right to freely exercise one's profession, may be limited to maintain it."[134]

Hundreds of young physicians, deciding not to gamble that the reform will be overturned, have scrambled to put down roots before the March 1993 deadline, when KVs can start excluding new members. Some KV officials report that some doctors are cutting short postgraduate training and abandoning the goal of becoming specialists in order to get in under the wire. Projections of the number of new office practices for 1992 were 7,000 under the actual number, and officials report a similar surge in 1993.

"Before the reform was announced, we had about five new doctors a quarter who came into this area," one KV official in southern Germany, in a region with "about average" physician density, said in a December 1992 interview. "When it became clear that [Health Minister Horst] Seehofer's reform comprises a firm limit on the number of office-based doctors...we experienced a sharp increase in new doctors," he said. "We think we will have 500 new doctors by the end of March 1993."[135] That would be a 25 percent increase in the sickness fund-certified physicians in that region—an influx that poses a real threat to already-established doctors. "Yes, this is a problem," the official said. "Doctors overall will suffer a cut in incomes because the budget has not been increased by one-quarter."

Putting the
Physician
(More) at Risk

The 1993 reform contains other landmark provisions that have upset doctors because they intrude in dramatic new ways on the clinical autonomy German physicians have prized and guarded for generations. The new law attempts to apply the financial brakes on a collective yearly sickness fund deficit that was projected to reach DM 11.4 billion (about $5.5 billion in purchasing power parity terms) by the end of 1992. Under the reform law:

☐ all doctors will be held to a strict annual budget increase of approximately 4 percent per year between 1993 and 1995;

☐ physicians are directed to reduce spending for spas (*Kurkliniken*) by DM 350 million ($167 million) and other physical therapy by DM 200 million ($96 million);

☐ by late 1995 general practitioners are to be put on a flat-rate payment system (to be designed by the *KV*s) that reimburses them by diagnosis, by a global fee-per-case, or by some combination of the two, with exceptions that must be justified on a case-by-case basis;[136] and, most significantly,

☐ all doctors are put on a fixed budget for prescription drugs and collectively held liable for overspending.

Controlling Drug Costs

The drug budget is an outgrowth of the fixed budgeting system for doctors that has been successful in restraining physician spending since 1986--but with a major difference. It represents the first time German physicians have been put at financial risk for health spending beyond their own fees. The driving force behind it is Germany's relative lack of success in restraining pharmaceutical spending through a 1989 reform law; that statute increased patient copayments and attempted to clamp price ceilings on most prescription medications but fell far short of its goal. Between 1989 and 1991, drug expenditures in the western German states rose twice as fast as sickness funds' revenues. Federal health officials concluded that pharmaceutical price controls—the principal strategy of the 1989 reform—would be insufficient to halt the trend. Schulte notes that drug spending increased by 10.2 percent in 1991 while drug prices

> had risen by a mere 2 percent over the same period. Innovative drugs accounted for just 2.5 percent of the cost increase. The rise in the amount of drugs prescribed per insured person was consequently responsible for 5.7 percent of the increase. There is no medical explanation for this development. However, it is a fact that, over the same period, the number of doctors had risen by 3.5 percent, and it would seem that more physicians prescribe more drugs. The increasingly intense competition among doctors in private practice promotes a willingness to prescribe generously and thus uneconomically.[137]

The 1993 legislation sets a global budget for pharmaceuticals at the 1991 level of DM 24,485 billion (about $11.7 billion on a purchasing power parity conversion), less 1.6 percent. Without a limit, federal health officials estimate, pharmaceutical spending would have risen by DM 3.5 billion to about DM 28 billion ($13.4 billion) in 1993.[138] If physicians' national prescribing exceeds DM 24,093 in 1993, they will be collectively liable for the first DM 280 million ($134 million) of the excess. That is, it will come out of their own fee reimbursements. The pharmaceutical industry is responsible for paying the next DM 280 million.

An "Ugly Instrument of Torture"

Drug budgeting had German doctors up in arms in late 1992 when it was being debated. The German Society of General Medicine called the proposal an "ugly instrument of torture."[139] Leading national physicians' groups mounted an aggressive public relations campaign against the proposal that included television advertisements of doctors telling elderly patients they could no longer prescribe needed medication. Patients were confronted with fliers in doctors' waiting rooms and red protest postcards for mailing to the Health Ministry. Physician leaders gave angry public speeches and media interviews. Although doctors have long been acknowledged as one of the most politically potent groups in Germany, their campaign failed spectacularly — by common consensus because it was badly overplayed. "It backfired because it was cynical and excessive," comments one sickness fund official, who adds that the doctors' opposition to the reform will be more effective in the long run.[140]

"The doctors were foolish, foolish!" comments Michael Arnold of the University of Tübingen. "They tried to mobilize their patients. This failed totally. The propaganda in their ads was not true." During the height of the controversy in the autumn of 1992, the *Frankfurter Allgemeine Zeitung*, one of the nation's most prestigious newspapers, editorialized against the tactics of physicians, pharmacists, and pharmaceutical manufacturers.

> Whatever protest actions farmers might come up with to combat subsidy cuts, or miners devise to rescue their now unprofitable coal-pits, nothing can surpass the apocalyptic and drastic quality of the horror scenarios conjured up by the suppliers of services on the health care market. At the merest inkling, anywhere, that the massive sums flowing into their coffers threaten to decrease in the slightest, the lobby paints a picture of the ruin of prosperous industries, the withering of the research landscape, the impoverishments of the healing arts, and the agonizing wasting away of the population, in the grayest and blackest of tones.[141]

Were Needed Medications Denied?

After the reform bill passed Parliament over providers' objections, the German media in early 1993 carried frequent accounts of patients being denied vital prescriptions. The National Association of Local Sickness Funds threatened doctors with expulsion from sickness fund practice if they were found to be denying patients needed medication.[142] Part of the doctors' problem was uncertainty: Individual doctors had no way of knowing until the end of the year whether physicians collectively would exceed the budget limit and expose them to fee reductions, so many were said to be cutting back severely on prescriptions to be on the safe side. Pharmacists reported revenue losses of 20 to 60 percent, although some of this may have been due to the reportedly widespread practice of writing prescriptions for several months' supply of drugs in December 1992, before the reform took effect.[143] The actual risk to physicians may be less than it appears; by one estimate, after taking price cuts and copayments into account, doctors need to save about DM 600 million ($287 million), which works out to only DM 11,000 ($5,300), or 2.3 percent of the average DM 480,000 ($23,000) in annual prescribing costs for the average German physician.[144]

The Waning of Physician Influence

It will take some time for the dust to settle and the actual effects of the *Health Care Structural Reform Act of 1993* to be discernible. However, its very passage is a watershed in Germany's long history of health care politics. To doctors' shock and chagrin, it showed that German physicians could not count on broad public support when the chips were down and fundamental issues— clinical autonomy as well as threats to the pocketbook—were at stake. Not that doctors do not still wield considerable power and influence, nor that they might not regain the kind of absolute veto power over policy they once enjoyed. At this juncture, however, physicians are merely one voice in the clamor over how to control health costs without giving up Germans' cherished health benefits.

This waning influence was not a sudden development. In fact, there are striking parallels between the reform debate of 1992-93 and a debate 15 years earlier over another watershed health care cost control law. The 1977 reform act, which launched the modern cycle of health cost control efforts in Germany, also represented a severe defeat for doctors, who fought unsuccessfully against a proposal to hold physician spending to the increase in ordinary Germans' wages. Deborah Stone of Brandeis University, who has chronicled that debate, notes that it was preceded by a period of falling public sympathy for physicians. For instance, 2 out of 3 Germans at that time approved of a proposal to set a ceiling on prescription drug expenditures—the proposal that was finally enacted a decade and a half later. In 1977, as in 1992, physicians' tactics in opposing reform generated considerable public antipathy. Stone traces this feeling to a growing public perception that physicians were growing out of touch with common citizens:

> Although the medical profession in West Germany has consistently ranked at the top of all occupations in prestige with the general public, sympathy for physicians' economic plight declined dramatically in the 1970s. The level of physicians' incomes began to be publicized in the early 1970s, and popular knowledge about physicians' incomes became more accurate....And while only 20 percent of respondents of 1973 thought that physicians' incomes were "too high," this was the opinion of fully 60 percent in 1977.[145]

If the reform debates of 1977 and 1992 show anything, it is that the trust and goodwill most patients feel for their physicians can be overridden by concern over burgeoning costs—even when those costs are considerably less, relatively speaking, than those that afflict U.S. patients, families, workers, and employers.

References and Notes

1. General Accounting Office (1991). *Health Care Spending Control: The Experience of France, Germany, and Japan*, GAO/HRD-92-9. Washington: Government Printing Office, p. 46.

2. Levit, KR, Lazenby, HC, Cowan, CA, and Letsch, SW (1991). National Health Expenditures, 1990. *Health Care Financing Review*, Vol 13, No. 1, p. 45.

3. Bundesministerium für Gesundheit (1991). *Daten des Gesundheitswesens 1991*, p. 174. Baden-Baden: Nomos Verlagsgesellschaft.

4. General Accounting Office (1991), p. 48.

5. I have chosen to use the German acronym *KV* for these regional associations of sickness fund-authorized doctors. The term *kassenärztliche Vereinigung* is difficult to translate crisply, and different authors have used a variety of different English renderings and acronyms. In view of this, *KV* seems most likely to avoid confusion in comparing this text with others in English.

6. Glaser, WA (1991). *Health Insurance in Practice: International Variations in Financing, Benefits, and Problems*. San Francisco: Jossey-Bass, p. 229.

7. Physician Payment Review Commission (1992). *Annual Report to Congress 1992*. Washington: Physician Payment Review Commission, p. 6.

8. Rodwin, VG; Grable, H; and Thiel, G (1990). Updating the Fee Schedule for Physician Reimbursement: A Comparative Analysis of France, Germany, Canada, and the United States. *American Journal of Utilization Review Physicians*, Vol. 5, No. 1, p. 23.

9. Glaser (1991), p. 225.

10. Stone, DA (1980). *The Limits of Professional Power: National Health Care in the Federal Republic of Germany*. Chicago: University of Chicago Press, p. 75.

11. Webber, D (1992). The Politics of Regulatory Change in the German Health Sector. *The Politics of German Regulation*. Aldershot, England: Dartmouth, pp. 211-212.

12. Arnold, M, Brauer, H-P, Deneke JFV, and Fiedler, E (1982). *The Medical Profession in the Federal Republic of Germany*. Köln-Lövenich: Deutscher Ärzte-Verlag GmbH, pp. 68, 129, 130.

13. Kirkman-Liff, B (1990). Physician Payment and Cost-Containment Strategies in West Germany: Suggestions for Medicare Reform. *Journal of Health Politics, Policy and Law*, Vol. 15, No. 1, p. 77.

14. Sachverständigenrat für die Konzertierte Aktion im Gesundheitswesen (1990). *Jahresgutachten 1990*, Table T501.

15. Arnold, M (1991). *Health Care in the Federal Republic of Germany*. Köln: Deutscher Ärzte-Verlag, p. 35, and Sachverständigenrat für die Konzertierte Aktion im Gesundheitswesen (1992), p. 235.

16. The *Hartmannbund*'s association with sickness fund-authorized physicians persists, although a large fraction of the *Hartmannbund*'s members currently consist of salaried physicians working as public officials rather than exclusively office-based, fee-for-service practitioners. Thus, there is overlap and rivalry between the *Hartmannbund* and the *Marburgerbund*, with the *Hartmannbund* claiming to represent the interests of all German physicians. (Arnold et.al., 1982, pp. 177-179)

17. Schulenburg, J.-M (1989). The West German Health Care Financing and Delivery System: Its Experiences and Lessons for Other Nations. Typescript of paper prepared for an

International Symposium on Health Care Systems, December 18-19, 1989, Taipei, Taiwan, p. 9.

18. Rodwin et.al. (1990), p. 23.

19. Reinhardt, UE (1987). Resource Allocation in Health Care: The Allocation of Lifestyles to Providers." *Milbank Memorial Fund Quarterly*, Vol. 65, pp. 153-176.

20. Schulenburg (1989), p. 12.

21. Arnold, et.al. (1982), p. 60.

22. Arnold, et.al. (1982), pp. 63-68.

23. Stone (1980), pp. 31-32.

24. Sandier, S (1989). Health services utilization and physician income trends. *Health Care Financing Review*, Annual Supplement 1989, p. 34.

25. Kirkmann-Liff, B (1990). Physician Payment and Cost-Containment Strategies in West Germany: Suggestions for Medicare Reform. *Journal of Health Politics, Policy and Law*, Vol. 15, No. 1, p. 76.

26. Stone (1980), p. 93.

27. Glaser, WA (1993). How Expenditure Caps and Expenditure Targets Really Work. *The Milbank Quarterly*, Vol. 71, No. 1.

28. Stone (1980), p. 94.

29. Glaser, WA (1993).

30. General Accounting Office (1991), p. 18.

31. Webber, D (1992), p. 218.

32. General Accounting Office (1991), p. 43.

33. Ibid.

34. Glaser (1992), pp. 11-12.

35. The substitute funds still pay higher fees to physicians than other sickness funds, but since 1986 physicians have had to be equally disciplined not to exceed substitute funds' prospective budgets.

36. Brenner, G and Ruble, DA (1991). The 1987 Revision of Physician Fees in Germany. *Health Affairs*, Vol. 10, No. 3, p. 150.

37. Wicks, EK (1992). *German Health Care: Financing, Administration, and Coverage*. Washington: Health Insurance Association of America, p. 9.

38. Glaser, WA (1993). How Expenditure Caps and Expenditure Targets Really Work. *The Milbank Quarterly*, Vol. 71, No. 1.

39. Sandier (1989), p. 38.

40. Interviews with general practitioners in Brüggen, Bad Waldsee, and Eningen, Germany, March, 1991.

41. Sandier (1989), p. 38.

42. Zimmerman, C (1993). Personal interview, 1993.

43. Grogan, CM (1992). Deciding on Access and Levels of Care: A Comparison of Canada, Britain, Germany, and the United States. *Journal of Health Politics, Policy and Law*. Vol. 17, No. 2, p. 224.

44. Buxbaum, RC (1993). German Physicians' Prescribing Practices Lead to Calls for Reform. *American College of Physicians Observer*, January, 1993, p. 5.

45. Robra BP, Lu C, Kerek-Bodden HE, Schach E, Schach S, Schwartz FW (1991). Frequency of medical consultation as reflected in 2 representative surveys: German Cardiovascular Disease Prevention and Survey of Ambulatory Care. *Offentliche Gesundheitswesen*, Vol. 53, No. 5, pp. 228-232.

46. Sandier (1989), p. 39.

47. Sandier (1989), p. 37.

48. Rodwin et.al. (1990), p. 21.

49. Stone, D (1991). Brief History of the Health Care System of the Federal Republic of Germany. Paper prepared for the Massachusetts Health and Educational Facilities Authority Health Policy Forum.

50. Hurst, JW (1991). Reform of Health Care in Germany. *Health Care Financing Review*, Vol. 12, No. 3, p. 82.

51. Pharmaceutical Manufacturers Association (U.S.), (1993). Testimony submitted to the Subcommittee on Health and the Environment, Committee on Health and the Environment, U.S. House of Representatives, February 22, 1993. Dollar amounts are calculated in purchasing power parities for 1991.

52. Buxbaum (1993), p. 5.

53. American Academy of Family Practice (1991). *Facts about: Family Practice*. Kansas City: American Academy of Family Practice, p. 64.

54. Rodwin et.al. (1990), p. 22.

55. Payer, L (1988). *Medicine & Culture: Varieties of Treatment in the United States, England, West Germany, and France*. New York: Henry Holt and Company, pp. 82, 172.

56. Physician Payment Review Commission (1991). *Annual Report to Congress*. Washington: PPRC, p. 256.

57. Based on ratios calculated by the *Sachverständigenrat für die Konzertierte Aktion im Gesundheitswesen* for the number of ultrasound machines needed in the new eastern states in order to bring them up to West German standards (*Sachverständigenrat Jahresgutachten 1991*, p. 238).

58. Sachverständigenrat für die Konzertierte Aktion im Gesundheitswesen (1991). *Die Gesundheitswesen im vereinten Deutschland*. Baden-Baden: Nomos Verlagsgesellschaft, p. 72.

59. Glaser (1991), p. 238.

60. Glaser (1991), pp. 238-241.

61. Personal interview, March, 1991, identity withheld on request.

62. Lang, B (1992). Personal interview with director of the Baden-Württemburg Association of Company Sickness Funds, December 9, 1992.

63. Helmich, P (1991). Personal interview.

64. Kirkman-Liff (1990), p. 89.

65. Physician Payment Review Commission (1991). *Annual Report to Congress, 1991*. Washington: Physician Payment Review Commission, p. 404.

66. Bradford Kirkman-Liff (1990, p. 91) gives a higher estimate. He quotes one unnamed German physician who has served on such committees as saying that about 20 percent of all physicians appear before an economic monitoring committee in a given year, and that 2 to 6 percent of physicians a year go through the appeal process.

67. Hinz, P (1992). Personal interview with Peter Hinz of the *Kassenärztliche Vereinigung für Süd-Württemburg*, December 9, 1992.

68. Lang (1992).

69. Kirkman-Liff (1990), p. 91.

70. Kirkman-Liff (1990), p. 79.

71. Kirkman-Liff (1990), p. 80.

72. Hurst (1991), p. 82.

73. Altenstetter, C (1987). An End to a Consensus on Health Care in the Federal Republic of Germany? *Journal of Health Politics, Policy and Law*, Vol. 12, No. 3, pp. 523-524.

74. Wicks (1992), p. 47.

75. Eastaugh, SR (1992). Lessons from the First to the Latest Nation to Enact National Health Insurance. *Journal of American Health Policy*, Vol. 2, No. 6, p. 34.

76. Sachverständigenrat für die Konzertierte Aktion im Gesundheitswesen (1992), p. 232.

77. Levit et.al. (1989), p. 45.

78. Ibid.

79. Kirkman-Liff (1990), p. 89.

80. Schneider, M (1992). BASYS (Beratungsgesellschaft für angewandte Systemforschung), Augsburg. Data supplied in personal interview, December, 1992.

81. Kassenärztliche Bundesvereinigung (1993). *Schaubildsammlung zur Information und Argumentationshilfe: anlässlich der Diskussion um ein Gesundheitsstrukturgesetz 1993*. Köln: Kassenärztliche Bundesvereinigung, chart C-8.

82. Sachverständigenrat für die Konzertierte Aktion im Gesundheitswesen (1991). *Das Gesundheitswesen im vereinten Deutschland*. Baden-Baden: Nomos Verlagsgesellschaft, Table 9.

83. American Medical Association (1992). *Socioeconomic Characteristics of Medical Practice 1992*. Chicago: American Medical Association, pp. 106, 134.

84. Abel-Smith, B (1992). Cost Containment and New Priorities in the European Community. *The Milbank Quarterly*, Vol. 70, No. 3, p. 406.

85. Sandier (1989), p. 42.

86. Ibid.

87. Dale A. Rublee, PhD, a staff policy analyst at the American Medical Association, presents German physicians' earnings as a multiple of average German business-sector wages in an article in *The Internist* (May 1991, p. 17). The trend is the same, but by this index, physicians earned slightly more than 6 times the average wage in 1983, declining (after an tick up in 1986) to about 5 times the average in 1988.

88. Sandier (1989), p. 42.

89. Wicks (1992), p. 46.

90. Abel-Smith (1992), p. 406.

91. Kassenärztliche Bundesvereinigung (1993). *Schaubildsammlung zur Information und Argumentationshilfe: anlässlich der Diskussion um ein Gesundheitsstrukturgesetz 1993.* Köln: Kassenärztliche Bundesvereinigung, chart E-3.

92. Kassenärztliche Bundesvereinigung (1991). *Grunddaten zur kassenärztlichen Versorgung in der Bundesrepublik Deutschland 1991.* Köln: Kassenärztliche Bundesvereinigung, chart D-1.

93. American Medical Association (1992), pp. 106, 134.

94. Sachverständigenrat für die Konzertierte Aktion im Gesundheitswesen (1992), p. 236.

95. Personal interview, December, 1992. Identity withheld on request.

96. Schneider, M, Biene-Dietrich, P, Gabanyi, M, Huber, M, Köse, A, Scholtes, L, Sommer, JH (1993). *Gesundheitssysteme im internationalen Vergleich.* Augsburg: Beratungsgesellschaft für angewandte Systemforschung mbH, p. 50.

97. Sachverständigenrat für die Konzertierte Aktion im Gesundheistwesen (1992). *Ausbau in Deutschland und Aufbruch nach Europa.* Baden-Baden: Nomos Verlagsgesellschaft, p. 80.

98. Rodwin et.al. (1990), p. 21.

99. Kirkman-Liff (1990), p. 88.

100. Sachverständigenrat für die Konzertierte Aktion im Gesundheitswesen (1992), pp. 217, 219.

101. Kirkman-Liff (1990), p. 88.

102. Pope, GC and Schneider, JE (1992). Trends in Physician Income. *Health Affairs*, Vol. 11, No. 1, pp. 183-184.

103. Pope and Schneider (1992), p. 188.

104. Rublee, DA (1991). Trade-offs for German Physicians: A look at Income and Supply. *The Internist*, May 1991, p. 14.

105. Sachverständigenrat für die Konzertierte Aktion im Gesundheitswesen (1992), p. 233.

106. Abel-Smith, B (1992), p. 407.

107. Schulte, G (1992). Problems of Health Care in the Conflict Area between Market Economy and Government Economic Control. Address at a Goethe Institute of Boston conference on German health care, October 17, 1992.

108. Organization for Economic Cooperation & Development (1992). *The Reform of Health Care: A Comparative Analysis of Seven OECD Countries.* Paris: OECD, p. 68.

109. American Medical Association (1987). *Physician Characteristics and Distribution in the U.S.* Chicago: American Medical Association, p. 13.

110. Brenner, G (1989). Cost-Controlling Measures in Out-Patient Medical Care in the Federal Republic of Germany." Paper presented to the First European Conference on Health Economics, Barcelona, September, 1989.

111. Arnold et.al. (1982), p. 77.

112. Arnold (1991), p. 33.

113. Arnold et.al. (1982), p. 83.

114. Schroeder, S (1992). Physician Supply and the U.S. Medical Marketplace. *Health Affairs*, Vol. 11, No. 1, p. 235.

115. Certified "specialists in general medicine" make up only a fraction (less than 20 percent) of all generalists. The term "specialist" as used below includes this 8 percent of active physicians who are certified general medicine specialists.

116. Bundesministeriums für Gesundheit (1991), p. 188.

117. Ibid.

118. Sachverständigenrat für die Konzertierte Aktion im Gesundheitswesen (1992), p. 50.

119. A study conducted in 1981-83 by the U.S. National Center for Health Statistics (*Ambulatory Care: France, Federal Republic of Germany, and the U.S., 1981-83*, Washington: U.S. Dept. of Health and Human Services, June, 1989, p. 16.) came up with a somewhat different distribution of specialist encounters in Germany: 41 percent of all ambulatory encounters versus 61 percent in the U.S. In both nations, the definition of "specialists" included primary care specialists, such as internists, pediatricians, and obstetrician-gynecologists. It could not be ascertained whether this difference stems from definitional issues, sampling methods, or other factors.

120. Sachverständigenrat für die Konzertierte Aktion im Gesundheitswesen (1991), p. 65.

121. Brenner, G and Rublee, DA (1991). The 1987 Revision of Physician Fees in Germany. *Health Affairs*, Vol. 10, No. 3, p. 148.

122. Ibid, p. 155.

123. Arnold et.al. (1982), p. 60.

124. Ibid, pp. 14-15.

125. Ibid (1982), p. 121.

126. OECD (1992), p. 64.

127. Abel-Smith (1992), p. 410.

128. Kassenärztliche Bundesvereinigung (1991), Chart A-15.

129. Arnold et.al. (1982), p. 127.

130. Schröder, K (1992). *The Statutory Health Insurance System: Social Report 6*. Bonn: Inter Nationes, p. 17.

131. Schulte (1992).

132. *Die Woche*, February 18, 1993, p. 33.

133. Pfaff, M (1992). Personal interview, December 6, 1992.

134. Schulte (1992).

135. Hinz (1992).

136. Bundesverband der Pharmazeutischen Industrie e.V. (1993). The Healthcare System in Germany. Special Report, January 1, 1993, p. 6.

137. Schulte (1992).

138. *Deutsche Ärzteblatt* (February 1993), Vol. 90, No. 6.

139. *Arzneimittel Zeitung* (1992). In Focus: The Health Systems and Pharmaceutical Markets in 16 Countries. Special Report, p. 38.

140. Lang, B (1992), personal interview.

141. *Frankfurter Allgemeine Zeitung* (1992).

142. *Die Woche*, February 18, 1993, p. 33.

143. *Der Spiegel*, February 1, 1993, p. 201.

144. Stone (1980), p. 156.

A Closer Look: Doctors in Germany

Germany's Malpractice Uncrisis

Like their American colleagues, German doctors are increasingly at risk of being sued. During the 1980s, a physician's chances of encountering a malpractice claim rose by 80 percent, according to some estimates. Judge Erich Steffen of Germany's Federal Supreme Court (*Bundesgerichtshof*) reported in 1989 that intermediate appellate courts were seeing a "small explosion" of medical malpractice cases.[1]

In 1991, an estimated 15,000 malpractice claims were lodged against German physicians compared to about 6,000 a decade earlier.[2] This seems a small number compared to the approximately 46,300 claims filed against U.S. physicians in 1990.[3] But it translates to a rate of 7.7 malpractice claims for every 100 practicing physicians—the same rate reported by the American Medical Association for U.S. physicians in 1990.[4] This is surprising since Germans profess greater satisfaction with their health care than Americans,[5] and Germans still have high respect for authority, with physicians ranking higher in social esteem than any other professionals.[6] Yet the malpractice situation in Germany often has an American ring: Patients complain about arrogant and unfeeling physicians and doctors deplore patients' "whining mentality" and bemoan the good old days when patients had boundless trust in their physicians. Many German physicians even refuse to utter the term "malpractice" (*verkehrte Behandlung*), preferring the euphemism "treatment error." As in the U.S., some are urging their colleagues to attend to the problem rather than simply rail against it: "The cold wind of public opinion is blowing in our faces, and with some justification," Gert Muhr, a professor at the University of Bochum, admonished in 1989.[7]

However, the risk of malpractice claims is not the high-visibility political issue in Germany that it is in the U.S. Part of the reason is the different trajectory of the claims rate in the two nations. The 1990 U.S. rate represents a moderation from the mid-1980s, when there were 10.2 claims per 100 physicians, according to the AMA,[8] and malpractice insurance premiums were rising at a rate of 12.1 percent a year. At the same time, total practice revenues were rising at only 7.5 percent.[9] American doctors' malpractice premiums are much higher, and while they levelled off around 1990, U.S. doctors have the uneasy feeling that the malpractice cycle will repeat itself. The German rate has increased inexorably rather than in sudden jumps, and rising malpractice premiums there represent an annoyance rather than a crisis. "I worry very little. It's no problem," says Dr. Irwin Widmann, chief of surgery at a district hospital in Bad Waldsee, a town in southwestern Germany. "When I went to San Diego, all the doctors asked the same question about malpractice. They couldn't believe I have never been sued."[10]

Going to Court. Of the reported 15,000 malpractice claims filed with German physician insurers in 1990, about 4,000 end up in court. A minority are won by plaintiffs, according to the *Allgemeine Patienten Vorband*, a patient advocacy group based in Marburg, though exact figures are unavailable.[11] Other sources have estimated that plaintiffs prevail in 30 percent of civil malpractice cases.[12]

In 1990, 5,165 malpractice claims were logged by arbitration panels set up in each German state by Physician Chambers (*Ärztekammer*), "bodies of public law" controlled by physicians that conduct licensure, specialty certification, and physician disciplinary activities. The arbitration panels, founded in the late 1970s, are voluntary alternatives to the courts. The vast majority of complaints are brought by patients, and both parties must agree before a hearing ensues. In recent years the number of complaints received by state arbitration panels has risen about 10 percent per year, according to Judges Erwin Deutsch and Karl-Heinz Matthies of the Provincial High Court and Court of Appeal at Göttingen.[13] Of the panels' 5,165 claims in 1990, 4,766 were pursued to conclusion. Of those:

- □ 1,501 or 32 percent were dismissed on grounds of no jurisdiction by the Physicians Chamber;

- □ no suspicion of malpractice was found in 919 cases, or 19 percent; and

- □ the expert panel found grounds for malpractice in 2,346 cases, or 49 percent.[14]

Plaintiffs' chances of success before these physician-dominated arbitration panels have apparently risen in recent years. In 1989, 1 in 3 plaintiffs prevailed, about the same rate as in civil court proceedings.[15] The arbitration panel's decision is not legally binding. If a plaintiff wins a decision, he can go to civil court, where the panel's decision can be admitted as evidence. Court decisions typically are decided by a panel of one judge and two physicians, who rely heavily on court-appointed expert witnesses rather than on adversarial proceedings with contending

---

Table 4.9

Doctors' Views of Malpractice in the U.S. and Germany, 1991

Number/percent of physicians who ranked medical malpractice among the two most important problems with the health care system of their country:

U.S.	(Western) Germany
69/602	2/519
11%	0%

Responses to the question: "How often do you do more for your patients than you think is clinically appropriate because of the threat of being sued for malpractice?"

	U.S. N=602		(Western) Germany N=519	
Often	195	(32%)	104	(20%)
Sometimes	174	(29%)	124	(24%)
Only occasionally	168	(28%)	129	(25%)
Never	61	(10%)	122	(24%)
Not applicable	4	(1%)	32	(6%)
Not sure	—		8	(2%)

Source: Robert J. Blendon, et al., Harvard School of Public Health, April 1993.

experts. Many plaintiffs with favorable arbitration panel decisions reportedly settle out of court. However, there is no evidence that the arbitration panels have filtered out many cases from the civil court docket, nor that they have increased the rate of out-of-court settlements.[16]

Plaintiffs' lawyers may also seek criminal prosecution of physicians on battery charges arising from alleged malpractice. Almost 30 such complaints are filed against doctors every day throughout Germany, but few result in an indictment and hearing, and only 1 in 100 results in prosecution.[17] (There is considerable overlap between the civil and criminal cases.) Though a physician is rarely convicted on criminal charges, the damaging effect on reputations is greatly feared and deplored by physicians.[18]

Paying the Premiums. Malpractice premiums are not that burdensome to German doctors. In 1991 they ranged from DM 700 for a general practitioner to DM 20,000 for an obstetrician ($335 to $9,600 on a purchasing power parity basis), for a policy with a coverage limit of DM 2.5 million ($1.2 million).[19] American doctors in 1990 paid on average $4,500 (psychiatrists) to $34,300 (obstetrician-gynecologists).[20] Even allowing for the fact that U.S. physicians had gross incomes 23 percent higher in 1990,[21] American premiums still consumed a significantly greater portion of the practicing physician's practice revenues.

Many factors make up a malpractice insurance premium, including claims frequency, proportion of paid claims, the size of awards and settlements, and the costs of investigating and defending against claims. No information is available on the average size of German awards and settlements or other components of malpractice premiums. However, it is likely that premiums are lower in part because health insurance coverage is universal. This relieves malpractice insurers from the burden of paying medical costs, which comprise one-quarter of U.S. awards and settlements.[22] German plaintiffs can claim monetary damages for pain and suffering, as well as loss of income, but their medical costs are generally borne by their sickness funds. "It would be possible for sickness funds to go to the malpractice insurer and say we should not be liable for medical or rehabilitation expenses if the doctor is at fault, but it is seldom done," reports Christian Zimmermann, director of the *Allgemeine Patienten Vorband.*[23]

Doctors Disciplining Doctors. Traditionally, the Physician Chambers, which have legal jurisdiction over physician licensure and discipline much like state medical licensure boards in the U.S., have done relatively little to attack the problem underlying medical malpractice — doctors with patterns of incompetent practice. According to a 1990 international study by Timothy S. Jost of Ohio State University's Center for Socio-Legal Studies,[24] about 10 percent of all complaints against doctors are reviewed by the executive committee of the Physicians Chambers. Cases are handled privately and public hearings are rarely held. The chambers may dismiss the complaint, admonish the doctor, proceed to prosecute the case in the state "professional court" (*Berufsgericht*), or advise the state health minister to revoke the doctor's license (a power reserved for the minister).

There are no national statistics on medical discipline cases. Practically speaking, Jost reports, a German doctor loses his license "only if he is convicted of a crime or becomes disabled."[25] In some states, the health minister has revoked a physician's license on his own initiative, most commonly for conviction of fraud against sickness funds. Disciplinary actions for malpractice, or substandard quality of care, are apparently a distinct minority. The director of the Physicians Chamber in Northrhine-Westfalia, Germany's largest state with a population of 17.1 million, told Jost that about one-quarter of disciplinary cases in that jurisdiction deal with quality of care issues, including alcohol and drug abuse; another quarter address physician advertising (which is taboo), and the rest deal with various ethical and professional issues. In another state, the Physicians Chamber reported that 27 of 37 disciplinary cases in one recent year dealt with fraud against sickness funds and the others concerned "a variety of professional disciplinary matters generally not related to quality of care."[26]

Political consciousness about the quality of physician care is rising, however. A federal health care reform act of 1989 makes quality assurance programs mandatory in both the ambulatory and hospital sectors, and directs the sickness funds and regional associations of sickness fund doctors (*Kassenärztliche Vereinigungen*, or *KV*s) to develop practice [7]?

References and Notes

1. *Der Spiegel* (1989). We Must Ask Ourselves: How Is This Possible? *Der Spiegel*, Cover story. Vol. 17, pp. 86-107.

2. Christian Zimmermann, director, *Allgemeine Patienten Vorband* [General Patients Union], Marburg (1993), personal communication of March 23, 1993, based on 1991 data from leading German and Swiss malpractice insurers. Malpractice suits in Germany are not centrally registered, so there are no reliable statistics. Rainer Hess, legal adviser to the *Bundesärztekammer* (Federal Physicians Chamber) estimated in 1989 that 10,000 malpractice claims were being filed annually with West German liability insurers. (*Der Spiegel*, No. 17, 1989, pp. 86-107.)

3. Calculated from data in *Socioeconomic Characteristics of Medical Practice 1992*, Chicago: American Medical Association, p. 24; and *Health Care Financing Review* (1992), Vol. 13, No. 4, p. 45.

4. The American Medical Association rate is derived from the AMA's Socioeconomic Monitoring System, an interview-based source of information on physicians' practice, including malpractice claims experience. Other U.S. data sources suggest a higher rate, though this may represent differences in definitions regarding what is counted as a "claim." For instance, the St. Paul Fire and Marine Insurance Co., which insures about 30,000 U.S. physicians, reports a 1990 rate of 13.8 claims per 100 physicians (personal communication). For purposes of this discussion, the general point is that the malpractice claims rate gap between Germany and the U.S. appears to be closing.

5. Blendon, RJ et.al. (1990). Satisfaction with Health Systems in Ten Nations. *Health Affairs*, Vol. 9, No. 2, pp. 186-192.

6. Zimmermann (1993), personal interview.

7. *Der Spiegel* (1989).

8. The St. Paul Fire and Marine Insurance Co. reports a 1985 rate of 17.9 claims per 100 physicians (personal communication).

9. American Medical Association (1992). *Socioeconomic Characteristics of Medical Practice 1992*. Chicago: AMA, pp. 23-26.

10. Widmann, I (1992), personal interview, March 2, 1991.

11. Zimmermann (1993), personal interview.

12. *Der Spiegel* (1989).

13. Deutsch, E and Matthies, K-H (19**XX**). *Physicians Liability Law: Principles, Administration of Justice, Advisory and Arbitration Boards*. Köln: Verlag Kommunikationsforum GmbH

14. Selbmann, H-K (1992). Health Status in the Federal Republic of Germany and Approaches to Quality Assurance in Health Care. Address at a Goethe Institute symposium in Boston, October 15-18, 1992.

15. *Der Spiegel* (1989).

16. Deutsch and Matthies (19XX).

17. *Der Spiegel* (1989).

18. Zimmerman (1993), personal interview.

19. *Allgemeine Patienten Vorband* (1993), personal communication.

20. American Medical Association (1992), p. 25.

21. Sachverständigenrat für die Konzertierte Aktion im Gesundheitswesen (1991). *Gesundheitswesen im Vereinten Deutschland.* Baden-Baden: Nomos Vorlagsgesellschaft, Table 9; and American Medical Association (1992). *Socioeconomic Characteristics of Medical Practice 1992.* Chicago: AMA, pp. 106, 134.

22. General Accounting Office (1987). *Medical Malpractice: Characteristics of Claims Closed in 1984.* Washington: GAO/HRD-87-55, pp. 44, 50.

23. Zimmermann (1993), personal interview.

24. Jost, TS (1990). *Assuring the Quality of Medical Practice: An International Comparative Study.* London: King Edward's Hospital Fund, pp. 25-26.

25. Ibid.

26. Ibid.

27. Jost (1990), pp. 61-63.

CHAPTER 5

Hospitals in Germany: A Case of 'More Is Less'

T he German hospital system poses a paradox. For its population, Germany's hospital infrastructure is significantly larger than other developed nations', and it is also more highly utilized. Nevertheless, it is considerably *less* costly by all the usual indicators. Even so, German authorities, including many leaders of the hospital community, think their hospital system contains major structural inefficiencies — and are taking steps to weed them out. This conundrum is actually a prism that casts light on how the German health care system works, and on other nations' cherished assumptions about health care.

In international rankings, and especially compared to the U.S., Germany's hospital sector is among the world's largest. Germany has more than twice as many hospital beds per 1,000 residents as the U.S., 63 percent more than Canada, and 68 percent more than the United Kingdom. (See Table 5.1) Due to steady capital investment over the past three decades, German hospitals are also among the most modern and well-equipped anywhere, with excellent physical plants (in former West Germany) and a technological base second only to the U.S.

German hospitals enjoy higher occupancy rates than those of any other developed nation. More than 85 percent of Germany's acute care beds were occupied in 1989 compared to only 66 percent in the U.S. (See Table 5.2) Germans also utilize hospitals more often than Americans. One in five Germans is hospitalized each year, versus one in seven Americans. On a population-adjusted basis, Germans rack up more than two-and-one-half times the number of days in the hospital each year than Americans, due to a combination of higher admission rates and acute care stays averaging more than 12 days — five days longer than in the U.S.[1] (See Table 5.3)

At the same time, Germany spends less on hospital care than the U.S. or many other developed nations — 60 percent less per hospital stay than the United States, and 70 percent less per day.[2,3] The hospital sector in Germany also consumes less of the total health care dollar — 22 percent less than in the U.S. in 1989 — though this difference is diminishing. (See Table 5.4)

Table 5.1

1989 Hospital Bed Ratios: An International Comparison: Average Daily Census

Nation	Total beds/1000 pop.	Acute beds/1000 pop
Australia	9.8	5.3
Canada	6.6	5.2
Germany	**10.8**	**7.3**
France	9.9	5.3
Japan	15.7	NA
Netherlands	11.6	4.4
Sweden	12.9	4.1
United Kingdom	6.4	2.8
United States	**4.8**	**3.6**

Source: Health Care Financing Review, *Summer 1992.*

Table 5.2

1989 Hospital Occupancy Rates and Lengths of Stay: An International Comparison of Acute Care Hospitals

Nation	Occupancy % of available beds	Length of stay in days
Australia	71.1	5.6
Austria	80.9	10.9
Canada	82.7*	10.5
France	77.7	7.2
Germany	**85.2**	**12.4**
Netherlands	74.3	11.5
Sweden	75.5	6.8
Switzerland	79.6	14.0
United Kingdom	76.2**	7.7**
United States	**66.2**	**7.3**

*1988; **1986

Source: Health Care Financing Review, *Summer 1992.*

Table 5.3

1989 Use of Hospital Services: Germany vs U.S.

	Bed days/person		% of pop. hospitalized/yr.	
	All Hosps.	Acute Hosps.	All Hosps.	Acute Hosps.
Germany	3.4	2.3	21.5	18.7
United States	1.3	0.9	13.7	12.5

Source: Health Care Financing Review, *Summer 1992.*

Table 5.4

Hospitals' Share of Total Health Expenditures in Germany and the U.S.

Year	Hospital care as % of total health spending*		Ratio U.S.:Germany
	Germany	U.S.	
1965	18.7	33.7	1:8
1970	23.9	37.5	1:6
1975	28.7	39.4	1:4
1980	28.3	41.1	1:5
1985	30.7	39.9	1:3
1989	31.4	38.6	1:2

*Figures for Germany are hospital spending as a percent of all spending by statutory sickness funds, which cover 88 percent of the population. U.S. figures are hospital spending as a percent of total national health expenditures.

Sources: Daten des Gesundheitswesen 1991, *German Federal Ministry of Health;* Rising Health Care Costs: Causes, Implications and Strategies *(1991) Congressional Budget Office.*

Solving the Puzzle:
Partial Answers

The reasons for these striking differences in hospital infrastructure, utilization, and cost are many and complex. Some of the principal factors are:

☐ A long tradition of universal health insurance coverage, with only nominal (and recent) copayments, has eliminated financial barriers to hospital care, and helped to foster a public sense of entitlement to such care.

☐ Politics at the local, state, and federal level has favored the buildup of a strong hospital system as a symbol of equitable access to care and a source of community pride. This priority has been enshrined in federal and state legislation, which has mandated state governments and regional sickness funds to guarantee citizens access to adequate hospital care.

☐ The strict division of German medical care into ambulatory and inpatient sectors[4] results in hospitalization for many patients who would be treated as outpatients in the U.S. system. This lowers the average intensity and cost of German hospital patients, and increases the utilization of inpatient facilities.

☐ Hospital care in Germany tends to be less intensive than in the U.S. This is rooted in cultural and historical factors, but in recent years, it stems from paying hospitals for each day of care they provide, a method which gives a strong financial incentive to hospitalize patients (who in the U.S. would not be considered acute care cases) and, once in the hospital, to keep them there longer.

☐ Reflecting this lower intensity of service, staffing ratios in German hospitals are much lower than in America, a disparity that has widened over the past three decades. (Table 5.5 and Figure 5.1)

☐ Hospital staff tend to have less training and be lower-paid than their U.S. counterparts, though the difference has narrowed recently. During the 1980s, incomes of German health workers (excluding physicians) were 64 percent of the average German employee. In the U.S. health workers have incomes 88 percent of the average wage.[5]

☐ Operating costs in German hospitals do not reflect capital investment or debt service. Investment in bricks-and-mortar, major equipment and even medium-term replacement of capital assets (those with a useful life of 3 to 15 years) is almost totally financed through state governments (in the case of university teaching hospitals through state and federal funds). Operating costs include replacement costs only for physical assets with a life of less than three years.

☐ Administrative staffing and costs are far lower than in American hospitals. For instance, one 727-bed community hospital in southern Germany has a nonclinical staff of only 60. Hundreds more would be employed in a comparably sized U.S. hospital to do admissions, billing, accounts receivable, budgeting, bookkeeping, and other administrative functions.[6] This reflects Germany's streamlined all-payer reimbursement system and its simplified billing and budgeting requirements compared to the unparalleled complexity of the U.S. payment system.

Despite Germany's favorable hospital costs compared to other countries, there has been highly visible political debate since the 1970s about inefficiencies

Table 5.5

Hospital Staffing Ratios*: An International Comparison

Nation	1960	1970	1980	1989
Australia	NA	NA	3.27**	3.91
Canada	NA	NA	2.09	2.4
Germany	**0.62**	**0.80**	**1.08**	**1.31**
Japan	0.54	NA	0.75	0.78
United Kingdom	NA	NA	2.1	2.6
United States	**0.96**	**1.57**	**2.56**	**3.21**

*Personnel per occupied bed
**1987

Source: Health Care Financing Review, *Summer 1992.*

Figure 5.1

Hospital Staffing Differentials: Germany vs U.S.*

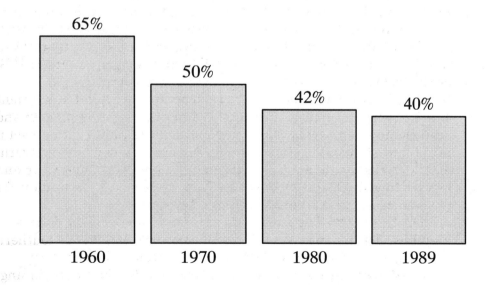

*Germany's staffing ratios (personnel per occupied bed) as a percent of U.S. ratios

Source: Health Care Financing Review, *Summer 1992.*

in the hospital sector, resulting in a series of federal laws aimed at bringing hospital costs under control. These laws have had much to do with shaping the system, but are widely regarded as having fallen short of cost-containment goals. Consequently, the Parliament in December 1992, enacted a new *Health Care Structural Reform Act* with the most stringent hospital-budgeting provisions ever designed in Germany. The background of the 1992 law and its provisions will be discussed later in this chapter.

It seems ironic to Americans that such stringencies would be imposed on a hospital system with costs so much lower than in the U.S. However, "German politicians and the German federal government...do not orient themselves [to] statistics of international comparison," notes Heinz P. Dörner, chief executive officer of the University of Tübingen Hospitals. "They are rather exclusively concerned with the fundamental stability of the premium rates paid to sickness funds."[7]

Since hospital spending is the largest component of these premium rates, the recent reform law has targeted the hospital sector for special attention. The result, German hospital officials expect, will be the most fundamental reordering of the hospital system in a generation. Some see a move away from the German tradition of *Selbstverwartung*, or "self-regulation," toward more central control. In this view, the exigencies of hospital cost-containment may be forcing a convergence of hospital finance and regulation in the U.S. and Germany, starting from very different points. Others say the important new trend is a diminishing of states' prerogatives regarding hospital policy, enabling the federal government to play a stronger role.

The Changing Face of German Hospitals

Hospitals are unique institutions in contemporary society. By any definition, they have become big businesses and major economic engines. The German auto industry employs fewer people than the German hospital industry — nearly 900,000 people, or 3.2 percent of the German workforce.[8] By comparison, the U.S. hospital sector gives work to more than 4 million people, 3.5 percent of all workers.[9] Yet no other business can lay claim to the social approbation that clings to hospitals, an advantage that is rooted in their charitable mission and immeasurably aggrandized by their modern image as "awesome citadels of science and bureaucratic order,"[10] in the phrase of sociologist Paul Starr of Princeton University. In Germany, where hospitals have not yet been transformed into the aggressive, market-driven competitors that U.S. hospitals have become, their special aura shines more brightly and influences hospital politics more strongly, inside and outside their doors.

A Heritage of Charity Care

For centuries, hospitals throughout Europe had nothing to do with medical care. They were sanctuaries founded by churches and knightly orders to shelter the sick poor and homeless. Their buildings and equipment were donated. Staff were often nuns and monks, supplemented by other volunteers. Hospitals lucky enough to be bequeathed land collected rents from tenant farmers. Hospitals did not have budgets nor did they set prices for their services until the last half of the 19th century, writes William Glaser of the New School for Social Research.[11]

The necessities of life for hospitals were also very different, and more modest, a century or so ago. In contrast to modern hospitals, which devote 70 percent of their budgets to personnel costs, at least half of hospital expenditures in the mid-19th century were for food. Wages were a small fraction of their outlays. (Table 5.6)

The seeds of the modern hospital were planted in the 18th century. The best-known and earliest German example, which still operates today on an expansive campus in former East Berlin, is the **Charité Hospital**, founded in 1727 with six departments, 200 beds and an operating room. By 1800, the Charité had expanded to 800 beds. Its main purpose was to provide bedside training and hands-on experience to army surgeons, as well as to treat military patients and the sick poor.[12] But inpatient mortality was high — 15 percent and more — and there was little medicine could offer in the way of cures. Well into the 19th century, anybody who could afford it was attended by his doctor at home.

A More "Public" Character

As charitable works, hospitals expected to run deficits that were covered each year by their sponsors. In practice, this often meant heavy public subsidies, since many German hospitals were taken over by municipalities as long ago as the late Middle Ages, a fact that helps explain why about half of all German hospitals are publicly owned, compared to 32 percent in the U.S. (Figure 5.2) Yet these publicly sponsored hospitals "were not secularized," notes sociologist George Rosen. "Essentially the hospital was a religious house in which the nursing personnel had united as a vocational community under a religious rule."[13] This vocational character has colored the development of nursing in Germany, where female nurses are still known as "sister" and are paid less than their more-professionalized American counterparts. Unsalaried religious sisters, who worked night and weekend shifts without complaint, were a common feature of German hospitals as late as the 1960s, when retirement and flagging recruitment to religious orders made secular nurses a necessity.[14]

There is another, broader sense in which German hospitals have remained more "public" than U.S. hospitals — that is, conceived as something more akin to public utilities, and less private in terms of hospitals' institutional mission, their relations with the outside world, and in individual patients' experience. Princeton University's Starr points out that American hospitals have retained a distinctly private flavor compared to those in Europe, largely because private practice American physicians won access to hospitals in the 19th century so they could admit patients and retain control over their patients' care, yet preserve their economic autonomy from hospitals. In Germany private physicians do not generally have access to hospital practice. "In Europe, and most other areas of the world," Starr writes,

> when patients enter a hospital, their doctors typically relinquish responsibility to the hospital staff, who form a separate and distinct group within the profession....American hospitals not only have private doctors; their architecture creates more private space for the treatment of patients. Hospitals in Europe...typically offer more of their care in large open wards, while American hospitals tend to be smaller in size, with more private accommodations. The economic organization of hospitals in the United States also reflects a less public conception of their function.[15]

Table 5.6

A German Hospital's Expenses in 1851

Category	Yearly Cost*	% of Budget
Food	571	57%
Wages:		
Honorarium for principal doctor	50	
Lump sum/community of Deaconesses	23	
Craftsmen	39	
Service workers	66	
TOTAL WAGES	178	18%
Supplies:		
Medications	27	
Surgical instruments	9	
Wearing apparel	9	
Bedding and linen	64	
Household/kitchen utensils	25	
Furniture	8	
Writing materials	1	
Printing and paper	8	
TOTAL SUPPLIES	151	15%
Laundry supplies and wages	41	4%
Light and heating	62	6%
Postage	1	<1%
TOTAL	1004	100%

*In Reichstalers (the form of currency being used in the 1850s).

Source: Glaser, WA in Kosten und Effizienz im Gesundheitswesen *(1985).*
München: R. Oldenbourg Verlag.

Figure 5.2

Hospital Ownership: Germany vs U.S.

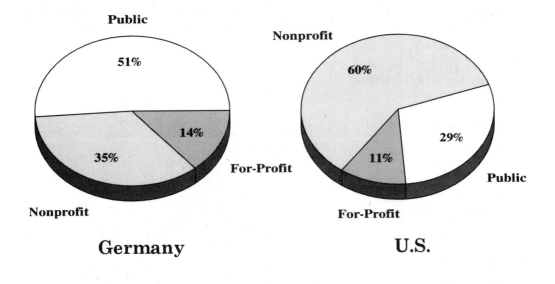

Germany

U.S.

Source: Weil, TP, Hospital & Health Services Administration, *Winter 1992.*

That German hospitals have a more public character is not to suggest they were always more egalitarian than the typical American hospital. In fact, until 1972 they were quite explicitly class-conscious. The poor and most members of statutory sickness funds, the so-called *Reichsversicherungsordnung* or *RVO* funds that make up the national health insurance system in Germany, were hospitalized in what were called "third class" wards, which typically contained up to 20 beds, where they received inferior food. Members of the largely white-collar "substitute" funds, or *Ersatzkassen,* were entitled to "second-class" care, while "first-class" was reserved for the well-off who could self-pay.[16] Today **private** patients, the 10 percent or so who are privately insured, retain privileged status in German hospitals. They may choose to be treated by a hospital department chief, and they may gain direct access to hospitals, while members of statutory sickness funds must be referred (except in emergencies) by an office-based doctor who is a certified participant in the statutory sickness fund system. In general, it is said that privately insured patients do not get better treatment in a medical sense, though they are entitled to more **comfort services,** such as more nicely furnished private rooms and more immediate attention from the staff. Statistics on inpatient mortality do not show differences between privately and statutorily insured patients.

The Modern Hospital Era

German hospitals, like those across the Atlantic, were transformed in the 1800s by the confluence of historic social, economic, and intellectual forces. Possibly because Germany became a nation later than its neighbors, 19th century German society was highly self-conscious about developing the elements of a modern, progressive state. Education and science became bourgeois virtues, recognized as indispensable for economic progress. University reform especially favored the natural sciences and medicine. The flowering of microscopic anatomy, physiology, physiologic chemistry, cellular pathology and pharmacology, which attracted the most serious medical scholars from the U.S., laid the basis for the prime of German medicine in the second half of the 1800s.

The "modern" German hospital sector — composed of institutions with departments of surgery, internal medicine, obstetrics and, after 1840, infectious disease — underwent explosive growth in this era. In 1822 Prussia had 155 public hospitals; by 1855 the number had grown to 684. The ratio of hospitals to population dropped from 1:75,000 to 1:25,000 during this period.[17] Meticulous observation, physical examination and pathological explanation of disease were the cornerstones of the "age of hospital medicine." Large numbers of patients provided illustrative material for education and research. Morton's demonstration of ether anesthesia in 1846, and Lister's 1867 demonstration of the virtues of antiseptic surgery, later followed by aseptic techniques, made hospitals far safer, less horrific, and more efficacious places.

The birth of medical disciplines in this era was often connected with the founding of small private hospitals. Famous "founders" such as Albrecht von Gräfe, credited as the father of ophthalmology, opened such establishments, which would later be integrated into public hospitals as independent departments.[18] The advent of new specialties, such as radiology, also required continuous expansion of hospital facilities.

The advent of Chancellor Bismarck's succession of social reforms — health insurance for workers in 1883, insurance for the accidentally injured in 1884, and coverage for the aged and disabled in 1889 — definitively shaped the German hospital sector from then on. The number of hospitals doubled between 1877 and 1913, the number of hospital beds tripled, the number of patients quadrupled, and the number of patient-days quintupled.[19] At one Berlin hospital, the number of patients whose hospital care was covered by statutory health insurance rose from 3.8 percent in 1884-85 to 50 percent in 1910. Not surprisingly, the growth of health insurance improved the fiscal health of hospitals; per diem hospital payments covered 75 percent of hospitals' operating costs on average during this period, leaving one-quarter to be subsidized by the hospitals' sponsors. Statutory health insurance also fostered acceptance of hospitals as useful institutions among the middle- and upper-middle classes. Partly because of this acceptance, and partly due to surgery's need for a hospital environment, increasingly fewer surgical procedures were performed at home.

Two world wars and the economic and political upheavals of the 1920s and 1930s were not conducive to hospitals' development. Nevertheless, by 1931 Germany boasted 4,951 hospitals with 595,103 beds. Of these beds, more than 60 percent were in publicly owned institutions, about a third were in nonprofit, mainly church-sponsored facilities, and the rest in privately owned hospitals.

The Nazi years brought hospitals one boon: Hitler's government, which was inimical to the interests of sickness funds, forced the funds to contract with nearly all hospitals instead of selectively directing their members to institutions offering favorable terms. But in 1936, wartime demands brought a general price freeze that included hospital per diem rates, a measure that brought hospital development to a virtual halt. The price freeze was finally lifted at the war's end in 1945, to be followed by another one in 1948.

The Postwar Years: Bust and Boom

World War II left Germany's hospitals in disastrous condition. Many buildings had been erected before World War I and poorly maintained for decades. There were severe shortages of nurses and of well-trained doctors. In East Germany, hospitals were nationalized in 1951. In the West, hospitals' capital and operating costs were both supposed to be covered by per diem rates but, even when rates were not frozen, patient revenues never covered all costs. In the early 1950s, West German hospitals' aggregate annual deficits mounted to DM 120 million. By the mid-1960s, shortfalls had reached DM 890 million — a sobering sum in those days.

This situation led to the federal government's first intervention in hospital rate-setting, the 1954 *Regulation on Per Diem Reimbursement*. This law provided for states to set hospital payment rates after consultation with hospitals and associations of statutory sickness funds. The motive was ensuring hospitals' viability, not controlling their costs, and it did improve their financial situation. But it left them with operating shortfalls, largely because the 1954 law also specified that the regulated rates had to be "socially bearable," a requirement that the sickness funds used, successfully, to keep rates low. Consequently, hospital deficits continued to rise, and states picked up the loss on an ad hoc basis to keep their hospitals afloat. But the decisions "tended to be more...random than rational," according to economist Helmuth Jung, a German health care consultant.[20] Some states began to formulate hospital plans, though these amounted to guidelines without the teeth of enforcement provisions.

Despite financial uncertainty, West German hospitals expanded at a fast clip during the 1960s, a movement driven by a booming economy and local chauvinism. Politicians pushed for funds to build the newest, biggest, and most modern hospitals, many of which would later be called "local politicians' monuments." Between 1960 and 1973, the number of West German hospital beds increased by 21 percent, the per-capita number of beds by 9 percent, hospital admissions by 36 percent, patient-days by 13 percent, per capita admissions by 22 percent.[21] Salaries of staff doctors and nurses were raised during the prosperous 1960s, and the number of physician and nursing personnel per bed increased by more than one-third. Communities ended up subsidizing the operating costs of modernized facilities as well as their capital costs because sickness funds refused to raise per diem rates fast enough. Patient care revenues in this period covered less than half of all hospital costs, and only about 40 percent of teaching hospital costs.[22] But heavy public subsidies from communities and states were not enough; the supposed shortage of hospital beds, and of nurses, became a major public preoccupation in the late 1960s.[23]

"Reform of the Century"

Growing political pressure led to a 1969 amendment to the West German constitution declaring that "it is a predominant task of federal health policy to provide the basis for economic security of hospitals...and to assure that there is a structured system of hospitals according to the [population's] needs." This constitutional commitment, which has no parallel in the U.S., laid the basis for federal subsidies to the states for hospital funding and for health planning. That came in 1972 with passage of the *Hospital Financing Act*. Ambitiously called the "reform of the century," it has been substantially revised four times but is still the cornerstone of the complex relationship between German hospitals, third-party payers, and governments at federal, state, and community levels.

The goals of the 1972 law were to
- provide hospitals with a viable economic base;
- develop a regionalized hospital system by distributing facilities, beds, general and specialty services and medical hardware in all regions and communities; and
- set reasonable hospital charges that were supportable by the statutory health insurance system.[24]

Within these broad aims, the statute made sweeping changes that shaped the German hospital system over the next two decades — and that sharply differentiate the German system from that of the U.S. One of the most important changes was the so-called "dual financing" of all hospitals, which split hospitals' sources of capital and operating funds. Under dual financing, the 11 individual West German states and the federal government shared the financial cost of acute care hospital capital investment.[25]

Operating costs would continue to be paid out of per diem payments from sickness funds and private payers. In a provision that U.S. hospitals might well envy, hospitals were legally guaranteed that their full operating costs in a given year would be covered by third-party payments as long as they operated "economically and efficiently." This feature is called *Selbstkostendeckungs-Prinzip*, or **self cost-reimbursement principle**. The law required that any cost-overruns during the year would be made up by a corresponding increase in the next year's per diem rates, and any profits would be deducted from the subsequent year's rates.

The pot was further sweetened for hospitals by a provision that automatically granted a lump sum per bed, over and above per diem reimbursements, to cover medium-term capital needs — the costs of maintenance and replacement for assets deemed to have a useful life of 3 to 15 years.[26] Assets with less than a three-year life are to be paid for out of the per diem rate.

Such statutory reimbursement guarantees may sound ideal to U.S. hospital administrators, who have been struggling in recent years to fund debt service on capital borrowing and to balance operating shortfalls from government reimbursement and discounted private payers by cost-shifting to any other payers who would tolerate it. The hitch was that German hospitals, to qualify for both capital investment grants and sickness fund reimbursement, must be included in (and met the terms of) their respective states' hospital "need plans," called *Bedarfspläne*.

About three-quarters of all hospitals were eligible to participate in dual financing and full-cost reimbursement in the mid-1970s, including most acute care hospitals. To be eligible for this program, a hospital must be nonprofit and at least 100 beds in size (or certified as geographically indispensable), a provision aimed to weed out the smallest and least efficient institutions. Also excluded were

- university teaching hospitals — a large omission, to be sure, but in Germany all such hospitals are owned by state governments, as are all medical schools, so it was presumed they were already sufficiently under state control;[27]
- rehabilitation hospitals and other long term care facilities, many of which are owned by pension funds;
- Spa hospitals, known in German as *Kurkrankenhäuser*, which are uniquely European facilities offering mud baths, massage, mineral water baths, and some conventional rehabilitation services in scenic spa settings.

Certificate of Need — With Teeth

By German standards, the 1972 federal law was unusually interventionist in the affairs of states, which in 1949 had been given broad powers over health care, and of the private institutions — hospitals and sickness funds — that deliver health services. The 1972 statute basically set up a federal framework for hospital rate-setting, though states had to ratify the per diem rates promulgated by federal civil servants. To be eligible, hospitals had to adhere to federal accounting and bookkeeping standards.[28]

The federal statute also empowered and exhorted states to create hospital **need plans**, but under the federal constitution it could not require them to do so. Consequently, German states differ considerably in their approaches to health planning. The city-states of Bremen and Hamburg and the states of Saarland and Schleswig-Holstein have never developed formal hospital need plans. Among those states with need plans, Christa Altenstetter, professor of political science at the City University of New York, points out, some, such as Bavaria, are centrally dictated by state government; others, such as the most populous state, North Rhine-Westfalia, have opted for a decentralized strategy. Practically speaking, the different approaches may not have made much difference in who finally decides. "The evidence suggests that the differences are largely those of form and political style," Altenstetter reports. In both Bavaria and North Rhine-Westfalia, for instance, "the central ministries have controlled decision-making. Hospitals were not treated as independent voices."[29] Still, the German states differ widely in the subsidies they have offered hospitals (Table 5.7) and consequently, in the size of their hospital sectors (from 9.5 beds per 1,000 population to 15.4 per 1,000 in 1988). "Such a wide range indicates there is an excessive supply of acute care beds in some areas, a view supported by the fact that German states with fewer acute care beds do not complain about hospital deficiencies," observes Markus Schneider, director of BASYS, a statistical consulting firm in Augsburg, Germany.[30]

The German hospital planning apparatus set up in the early 1970s — the same time U.S. states were enacting certificate-of-need, or CON, laws — is basically CON with teeth. By linking "need plan" compliance with the powerful

Table 5.7

Varying Hospital Subsidies* in West German States, 1972-91

State	Subsidy per inhabitant	Subsidy per "planned bed"
West Berlin	3,371	315,272
Bavaria	1,537	220,122
Rhineland-Palatinate	1,277	182,379
Baden-Württemberg	1,070	174,640
Saarland	1,255	174,480
Hamburg	1,322	173,331
West German average	**1,269**	**172,795**
Hesse	1,092	163,849
Bremen	1,756	163,619
Schleswig-Holstein	848	160,423
North Rhine-Westfalia	1,180	139,254
Lower Saxony	945	135,351

*In deutschmarks, 19-year average, including funds for both major construction and renovation and for routine maintenance/replacement costs

Source: Ernst Bruckenberger, Lower Saxony Ministry of Social Affairs, 1992.

carrots of capital funding and the guarantee of full operating cost reimbursement, West Germany would appear to have created a strong enforcement mechanism for resource, or supply-side, control in its hospital sector. There is evidence, especially by comparison with the U.S. hospital system during the same period, that German laws constrained hospital overbuilding and, especially, excess acquisition of high-technology equipment. The mechanisms are also credited with nurturing a remarkably uniform regional hospital infrastructure that guarantees citizens all over former West Germany ready access to all levels of care. At the same time, however, the 1972 *Hospital Financing Act* fell far short of the Germans' hopes and expectations. In particular, the law
   ☐ failed to reckon with the strength of local politics in driving hospital construction and equipment acquisition, and the effectiveness of state politicians in tailoring the need plans to their ambitions; and

☐ set up perverse financial incentives to perpetuate an excessively large bed complement, and unnecessary utilization of those excess beds, that even hospital administrators acknowledge as the most important flaw in the German hospital system.

Constrained...But Not Too Much

There is little academic analysis of the effects of health planning in Germany. The 1972 law's capital financing provisions, according to one hospital administrator, "have indeed contributed greatly to modernization of German hospitals during 1970s and 1980s and have ensured the maintenance of their relatively high standard of technology."[31] During this period, facilities were rebuilt, hospital wards containing five or more beds were phased out in favor of two- and three-bed rooms, and equipment was brought up to date. Between 1970 and 1977, hospital costs increased by 12.2 percent annually.[32]

At the same time, German-U.S. comparisons clearly indicate that German hospitals have significantly less high-tech equipment (such as computed tomography, CT, and magnetic resonance imaging machines, MRI) and service capacity (such as open-heart surgery and organ transplants), on a population-adjusted basis, than their American counterparts — though Germany generally has more than high-tech capacity than Canada. In 1987 Germany apparently had only

☐ 23 percent of the U.S. open-heart surgical capacity;
☐ half the cardiac catheterization capacity;
☐ about one-third the organ transplant capacity;
☐ three-quarters of the radiotherapy units;
☐ 36 percent of the lithotripsy machines; and
☐ one-quarter of the MRI machines.(Figure 5.3)

Such figures are illustrative, but they should be interpreted with caution. As Table 5.8 indicates, Germany has added substantially more medical technology since Dale Rublee's 1987 survey, in both the former West Germany and the former East Germany. For instance, it appears that the 1992 ratio for MRI is 2.59 machines per million population, nearly three times higher than the 1987 ratio calculated by Rublee. Similarly, there were about 1.4 lithotripsy units per million people in all of Germany in 1992, four times the 1987 ratio. Second, anecdotal evidence from German hospital officials suggests that utilization of high-tech services, such as open-heart surgery units, may be significantly higher than in the U.S., a factor not captured by units-per-population ratios.

No one knows the "right" ratio of high-tech capacities per million people. Whatever the precise current comparative ratios, the outlier status of the U.S. on these measures, combined with lack of evidence that morbidity and mortality measures in Germany show adverse effects from lower high-tech capacity, has led some experts to speculate that Germany has approximately "enough" and the U.S. probably has "too much." In recent interviews, German physicians, hospital administrators, and health researchers said troublesome waiting lists for high-tech services rarely occur, nor do such allegations often surface in the German media. "We don't have any rationing in technical services," asserts Peter Rosenberg, a policy analyst at the German Ministry of Labor and a veteran observer of the German health system.[33] In fact, the spectre of waiting lists for

Figure 5.3

High-Tech Units per Million Persons, 1987

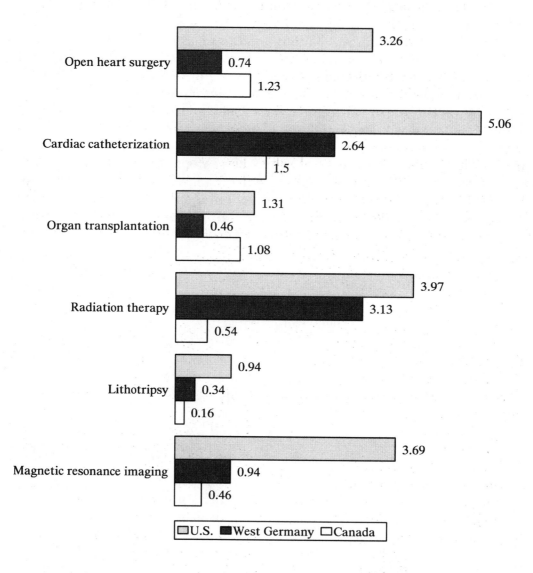

Source: Rublee, DA (1989), Health Affairs, Fall 1989.

high-visibility services has occasionally led, through political pressures, to building excess capacity. When the University of Tübingen Hospitals developed waiting lists for open-heart surgery in the late 1980s, the state of Baden-Württemberg permitted two other open-heart units to open in the region. The result was a precipitous drop in cases done at Tübingen, from 1,500 a year to only 500. "It was very painful for us," says Mark Vukovic, the chief financial officer at the Tübingen teaching hospital complex. "Heart surgery is very profitable."[34]

One effect of state health planning programs has been to concentrate high-tech services in tertiary hospitals, though not exclusively. "A university hospital is almost never refused anything it really wants to do," says Dörner, although department chiefs increasingly may be asked to make tradeoffs in their budget to add new services.[35] (Teaching hospitals must get approval from the Federal Science Board in Bonn for new equipment and facilities costing more than DM 1,500, about $900.) In addition, equipment manufacturers often donate units to teaching hospitals as a way of establishing new technologies. Health planning, by constraining what services hospitals can offer, has also driven enterprising doctors to set up high-tech machinery in outpatient facilities and contract with hospitals for such services. This is especially evident in the distribution of CTs and MRIs. MRIs are almost as plentiful outside hospitals as inside. (Table 5.8)

Table 5.8

"Big Technology" Units in Germany, Early 1992

Type	Hospital Based	Office Based	TOTAL
Cardiac catheterization	232	15	247
Computer tomography	512	328	840
MRI scanners	105	102	207
PET scanners	6	0	6
Linear accelerators	193	5	198
Cobalt Radiotherapy	154	15	169
Lithotripsy	108	4	112

Source: Bruckenberger, E, Ministry of Social Affairs, Lower Saxony.

The Era of
Cost Containment

Between 1970 and 1975, the outlays of statutory sickness funds for hospital care rose 24 percent — outpacing expenditures on outpatient physician care, dentistry, and pharmaceuticals, and rising almost 60 percent faster than they had during the previous five years.[36] But this sharp increase in hospital spending was not a cause for political concern at a time when the German economy was booming, wages were rising, and the coffers of sickness funds were full. This changed after the oil shock of 1973 and the subsequent recession. These events "brought about a rapid change of priorities in German health politics," observes Douglas Webber of the European Institute of Business Administration.[37]

By 1975, unemployment had reached 4.8 percent, the highest since 1955,[38] federal funds for hospitals' capital investment were restricted, states were feeling the economic pinch and sickness funds began pressuring hospitals and politicians for greater efficiency controls on all health providers — especially hospitals. The sickness funds argued for the ability to contract selectively with hospitals, instead of being obligated to do business with any hospital included in states' need-plans — virtually all eligible hospitals. The term *Kosten-Explosion* was born, and health analysts warned politicians that Germany could be spending half of its gross national product on health care by the year 2000 if stern measures were not taken.[39]

The jawboning led to some voluntary steps — for instance, office-based physicians agreed to restrain fee increases — that did slow the growth of health care expenditures in 1976. But the level of concern was too high to be appeased by nonbinding promises. In mid-1977 the German Parliament enacted the first *Health Insurance Cost Containment Act*, launching an era of cost-control efforts that continues to the present day. "The law marks an important watershed in German health policy development," Altenstetter wrote in 1980. "A period of expanding health services rights, coverage and benefits through legislation...may have come to an end."[40] Among the law's many provisions, it

- created a national Concerted Action in Health Care council, representing nearly all major health care stake-holders, which meets twice annually to issue influential, though nonbinding, guidelines on how fast health spending should be permitted to rise and what measures should be adopted to improve efficacy and efficiency in health care;
- introduced consumer copayments for the first time since the late 1930s, covering prescription drugs, dentures, and orthodontia;
- permitted sickness funds to reject contracts with hospitals that had not been included in a state hospital need plan, on grounds either of inferior quality or because the hospital interfered with hospital planning objectives;
- required sickness funds to pay for home nursing care under certain circumstances to reduce hospital utilization rates;
- tightened eligibility for sickness fund membership — for instance, by barring pensioners from membership if they had not paid in during their working years.

The most important of these provisions was the **Concerted Action** panel. This committee of approximately five dozen members represented virtually every important actor in health care, including federal and state governments, with one telling omission: the hospital sector.[41] Hospitals were originally included in drafts of the 1977 law. After all, hospital care consumed more than 30 percent of sickness fund total outlays in 1977,[42] more than any other category of service and twice their share only a decade earlier. Yet a fierce territorial battle between the federal and state governments resulted in hospitals' exemption from Concerted Action's cost-control purview. Hospitals historically had been the province of state governments, which jealously guarded their prerogatives of hospital regulation. States own university teaching hospitals, and have a stake in ensuring that these institutions have high reimbursement rates. In addition to their health planning powers, states also are responsible for medical education and research.[43] The federal government in Germany is constrained from passing legislation over states' objections because proposals affecting states' powers must be approved by the *Bundesrat*, the upper chamber of Parliament made up of states' representatives. Through the *Bundesrat*, the state governments were successful in having the proposals affecting the hospital sector deleted from the bill.

Even though hospitals were exempted from Concerted Action strictures, they were affected by other cost controls enacted during the late 1970s. For instance, new guidelines on the allowable number of staff per bed were partly responsible for reducing annual growth in hospital prices from 12.2 percent between 1970 and 1977 to 3.8 percent between 1977 and 1989.[44]

However, the issue of hospitals' exemption from global cost controls was not resolved by the states' 1977 victory. Physicians, pharmaceutical manufacturers, and others subject to new cost constraints complained loudly about the hospitals' exclusion, keeping the debate alive. Finally, hospitals were brought into the Concerted Action mechanism in the *Hospital Cost Containment Act* of 1981, which also

- introduced nominal cost-sharing by hospital patients;
- lowered government subsidies for hospitals' capital spending to reduce unneeded beds;
- gave sickness funds, private insurers and hospital associations a formal role in state hospital planning programs; and
- decentralized negotiations on per diem rates between sickness funds and individual hospitals, reducing the rate-setting role of state governments.[45]

The most contentious of these reforms was cost-sharing, even though it obligated patients to pay only about $2.25 per day for the first 14 days of hospitalization. The insistence on cost-sharing by the ideologically conservative Free Democratic Party, "almost sufficed to collapse" the ruling coalition, reports Webber, since the liberal Social Democratic Party has always opposed putting any burden for cost-control on patients.[46]

Despite these concessions, hospitals and state governments forced significant compromises in the 1981 and 1982 statutes. After several rounds of heated federal-state debate, a conference committee "dropped the provisions most offensive to the *Länder* [states], which represent territorial and hospital interests," Altenstetter reports.[47] Of these failed amendments, the most significant was a cap on hospitals' per diem rates tied to general wages and salaries.[48]

Figure 5.9

German Hospital Admissions, 1965-88

Year	All hospitals		Acute care hospitals		Other hospitals	
	Admissions	per 1,000 residents	Admissions	per 1,000 residents	Admissions	per 1,000 residents
1965	8,121,225	138	7,147,753	121	973,472	17
1970	9,337,705	153	8,190,454	134	1,147,251	19
1975	10,426,753	169	9,032,121	147	1,394,632	23
1980	11,595,558	188	10,033,004	163	1,562,554	25
1985	12,154,998	199	10,603,962	174	1,551,036	25
1986	12,601,063	206	10,983,090	180	1,617,973	27
1987	12,868,684	210	11,197,657	182	1,671,027	27
1988	13,226,550	214	11,482,256	186	1,744,294	28

Source: German Hospital Association.

1980s: Mounting Pressures for Cost Control

Although hospitals escaped the most onerous cost-control provisions others wanted to impose upon them in the late 1970s and early 1980s, the pressure to do something about rising hospital costs did not abate. The number of hospital admissions climbed steadily during the 1960s, 1970s, and 1980s. So did the number of admissions per 1,000 residents, which increased 56 percent between 1965 and 1989, or 6.5 percent per year on average. (Table 5.9). By contrast, the West German population was essentially static, growing an annual average of only 0.2 percent during this 24-year period. This left a 33-fold difference between average population growth and the annual increase in hospital admissions.[49] Most important politically, the outlays of sickness funds for hospital care consistently outpaced the increase in wages — the basis for calculating the sickness funds' annual revenues. Between 1980 and 1987, the funds' hospital payments rose 54 percent while base wages went up 39 percent, a difference of nearly 40 percent. (Figure 5.4)

Many of the reasons were well-recognized. The average age of German hospital patients has steadily increased (Figure 5.5). Technological progress and intensity of care increased in Germany during this period, paralleling trends in the U.S. and other industrialized nations. The number of hospital personnel in all categories increased by 50 percent between 1970 and 1985, and the number of doctors, nurses, and technicians jumped by 79 percent, 76 percent, and 92 percent, respectively. (Figure 5.6)

But many of the forces behind hospital cost inflation were clearly structural, as was (and is) also widely recognized in Germany. First and most important, a fixed per diem reimbursement rate was a powerful incentive to keep patients hospitalized beyond the dictates of medical necessity. "Because hospitals are reimbursed by the number of patient-days they tally," acknowledges Dörner of the University of Tübingen Hospitals, "they often find themselves forced to offset the high costs of the first days of treatment by increasing the number of days of low cost towards the end of treatment and thereby unnaturally lengthening the patient's time of stay."[50] (At the same time, hospitals must be careful not to exceed an occupancy target of 85 percent, since sickness funds can deny payment for "over-occupancy.")

As consultant Jung put it, a fixed hospital per diem rate

> leads to indifference to cost containment. The fixed rate thus has the exact opposite effect from the one intended: it forces hospitals to operate at full capacity. The more beds are, on the average, occupied by patients with minor illnesses, the greater the margin for diagnosis and treatment of the seriously ill....If the average length of hospitalization is reduced...the income of the hospitals must surely decline....The hospital is punished for its own cost efficiency.[51]

The full cost reimbursement principle, established in 1972 as a way of providing hospitals with a sound fiscal base, also punished hospitals for economizing by lowering subsequent-year per diem rates for any spending reductions, since hospital budgets are historically based. German hospital administrators have a descriptive word for this hazard: the *Kellertreppeneffekt*, or **cellar-stairs effect**. Full cost reimbursement also rewarded hospitals deutschmark-for-deutschmark in subsequent-year budgets for increasing their patient care expenditures.

Health planning rules provided another incentive for hospitals to keep as many beds as they could. Since hospitals received lump sum payments for each planning-certified bed, a feature intended to provide for routine medium-term maintenance and replacement costs, administrators were loathe to make reductions in their bed complement, and this put pressure on state health planners to certify more beds than were actually needed. In view of this, it is remarkable that German states were able to make significant reductions in hospital beds and in the ratio of beds to population in the early 1980s, before these incentives were substantially changed. (Table 5.10)

The split responsibility between planning and funding hospital capital (which rested mainly with state bureaucracies) and reimbursing for operating costs (a function of sickness funds, pursuant to federal guidelines and negotiations with each hospital) has also worked against hospital cost control. The

Figure 5.4

Increase in Wages and Statutory Sickness Fund Payments to Hospitals, 1980-87

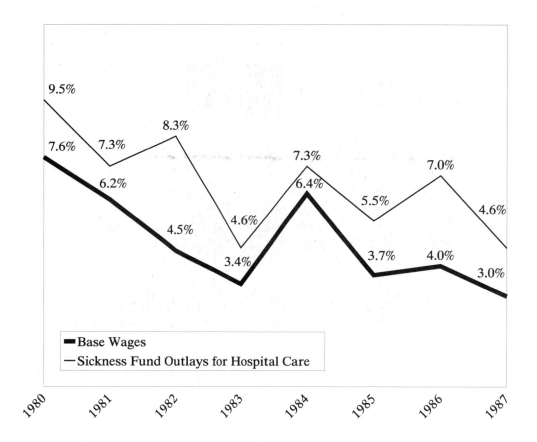

Source: *Sachverständigenrats für die Konzertierte Aktion im Gesundheitswesen , 1989.*

officials responsible for approving additional hospital capacity, new equipment, and renovation projects are a separate group of people, operating under different political constraints and with different constituencies, than those who must pay the additional operating costs connected with this capital spending.

Finally, the benefit structure of health insurance in Germany has been a barrier to shifting patients from acute care settings to long term care and home care. Though recent statutes are aimed at changing this, sickness funds historically have paid only for acute hospital care, not for long term care. This has stifled the development of alternatives to acute care; enactment of a national insurance program to cover long term care has been on Parliament's agenda of upcoming initiatives for a decade, with no action as of 1993.

Given all these incentives to overutilize, the surprising aspect of the German hospital system is that it is not more costly compared to the U.S. inpatient sector. The answer apparently lies in the low intensity of the services

Figure 5.5

German Hospital Patients Are Aging*: Proportion of Hospitalized Patients Over 60 Years Old

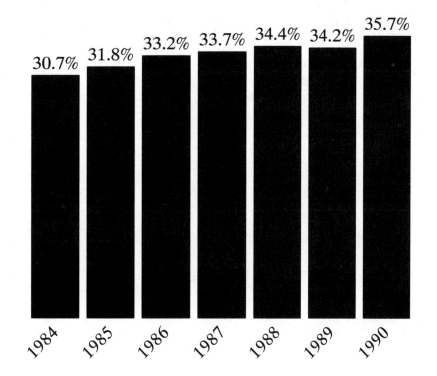

*Data are for western Germany only

Source: Sachverständigenrats für die Konzertierte Aktion im Gesundheitswesen and Deutsch Krankenhausgesellschaft, 1992.

provided, on average, in combination with the lower wage and salary structure for hospital employees — a fact all the more remarkable considering that German hospital operating costs include physicians' salaries, a component largely absent from most U.S. hospitals' budgets. Asked the secret of Germany's lower health costs, health economist Rosenberg replied: "I think the main difference is in the price level of the two countries. Doctors get less than in the U.S., and especially hospital prices are much lower than in the U.S."[52]

International comparisons bear this out. The cost of a hospitalization episode in West Germany during the 1980s averaged only 42 percent of the U.S. average cost per case. During the decade, the German cost per hospital case increased 34 percent, but the U.S. cost more than doubled. (Figure 5.7) Moreover, the price of all medical services in Germany is growing much more slowly than U.S. medical prices; between 1985 and 1990, German prices increased only 10 percent, compared to 34 percent in America.[53]

Figure 5.6

Personnel Trends in German Hospitals, 1970-89

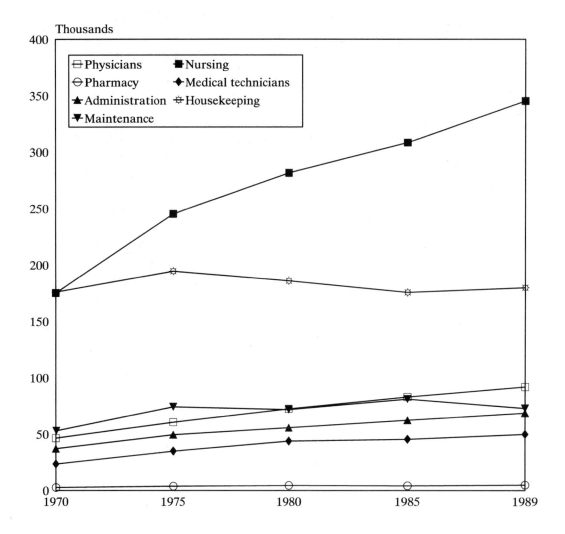

Source: Sachverständigenrat für die Konzertierte Aktion im Gesundheitswesen, 1992.

Table 5.10

Hospitals and Hospital Beds in Germany, 1960-89

Year	No. of Hospitals	No. of Beds	Beds per 1,000 pop.
1960	3,604	583,513	10.5
1965	3,639	631,447	10.7
1970	3,587	683,254	11.2
1972	3,519	701,263	11.4
1975	3,481	729,791	11.8
1980	3,234	707,710	11.5
1984	3,106	678,708	11.1
1985	3,098	674,742	11.1
1988	3,069	672,834	10.9
1989	3,046	669,750	10.8

Sources: German Federal Ministry of Health, 1991; German Hospital Association, 1990-91.

Hospitals Become a Target

Despite hospitals' rapidly rising expenses and the supposed guarantee of full cost reimbursement, hospitals were not recouping all their costs in the early 1980s, according to a study of hospital cost increases between 1979 and 1984.[54] At the same time, that widely-cited study asserted that 17 percent of hospital patients did not need care in a hospital.[55]

The growing dilemma of rising costs, revenue shortfalls and excess capacity sparked a series of federal health reforms throughout the 1980s. In 1985, a *Federal Regulation on (Hospital) Care Charges* partially withdrew from the seven-year-old principle of guaranteed full-cost reimbursement. In its place the law introduced a "flexible prospective budgeting" system, which sets a global budget in advance of a hospital's fiscal year and limits the amount the hospital can profit from increased volume, while cushioning its loss if inpatient volume drops. This feature, which U.S. hospital administrators would call a "reimbursement corridor," allows for reimbursement of only marginal costs — 25 percent of the agreed-upon per diem rate — for patient-days beyond the projected number; for every day below the projected volume, hospitals are paid 75 percent of the per diem rate, a penalty for over-projecting that still allows institutions to meet payrolls and other fixed obligations. The rationale is to blunt the incentive for hospitals to increase their volume.

Figure 5.7

Average Hospital Cost Per Case*: Germany vs U.S.

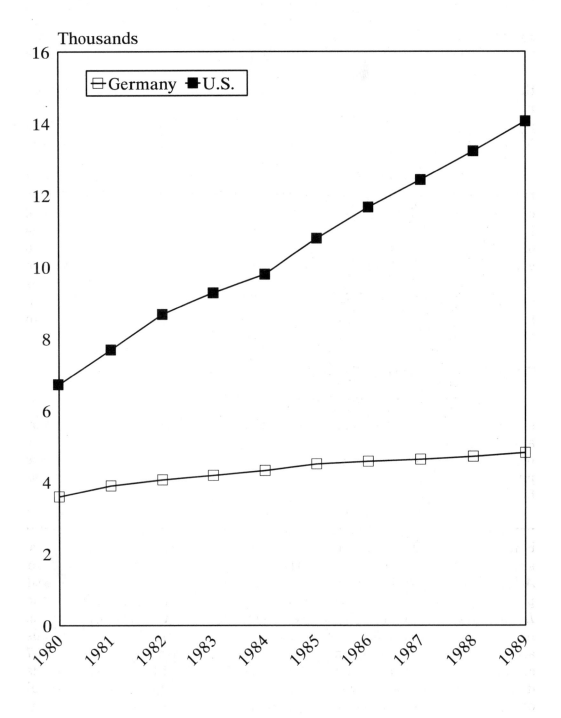

*In deutschmarks

Source: Markus Schneider, BASYS, Augsburg, 1992.

The 1985 reform also took what might be considered the first step toward a **diagnosis-based payment system** conceptually related to the U.S. Medicare program's DRG (diagnosis-related groups) payment. It introduced special, prospectively negotiated flat rates for specialized treatments, such as cancer treatment, thoracic surgery, organ transplants, joint replacements, lithotripsy, and other innovations. Rates were also negotiated for special patient groups, such as burn victims, neonates, and dialysis patients. Intended to increase "transparency" — that is, make true costs more visible — this optional system of "special payments" (*Sonderentgelte*) also relieves local sickness funds from the sole burden of subsidizing tertiary services that draw patients from a wider population area. So far only about 4 percent of all German hospital payments are rendered on this basis, or 10 percent in university teaching hospitals.[56] As hospital officials point out, whatever its virtues, it is not a cost-saving measure.

Nineteen eighty-five also saw the implementation of a separate landmark statute, the *New Hospital Regulation Law*, which ended the 13-year era of joint federal-state responsibility for hospital capital investment. The states had long objected to federal interference with their prerogatives to budget for and control hospitals in their purview. Moreover, federal subsidies had fallen far short of the originally intended one-third share, dropping to 16 percent by 1983.[57] The step was logical, Altenstetter says, because shared authority does not work well in German-style federalism: "It hampers priority-setting and thoroughly diffuses accountability."[58] The law also represented a statement by the federal government to the states, along the lines of "Prove your constant claims that you can do a better job of hospital planning by yourselves."

"Negotiations, Negotiations, Negotiations"

What is the "magic" of cost control in German health care? "The answer," says J.-Matthias Graf von der Schulenburg, director of the Institute for Insurance Economics at the University of Hannover, "is negotiations, negotiations, negotiations." Other aspects of the 1985 payment reform altered the way these pivotal budget negotiations are conducted between hospitals and sickness funds.

Unlike physicians' payments, which are negotiated by regional groups of physicians and groups of payers under binding national guidelines, hospital bargaining occurs between individual hospitals and associations of their payers, and has been open-ended until recently. The local sickness funds, called *AOK* for *Allgemeine Ortskrankenkassen*, play the lead role, since they insure the most people in any hospital's service area and the next-largest insurance funds, the *Ersatzkassen* or substitute funds, are national in scope. As in any negotiations, information is power. Under one provision of the 1985 reform, German hospitals are required by law to fill out a standardized 30-page questionnaire with 9,537 separate pieces of data. A national research institute of local sickness funds digests these data and provides the *AOK*s with information on each hospital compared to institutions of similar size, number, structure, service complement, market areas, and patient characteristics (age, sex, case mix based on primary discharge diagnosis). The *AOK*s screen for outliers on per diem rates as a bargaining chip, but there is controversy about the adequacy of case-mix data.

It is not clear these data make much difference in actual negotiations, which anecdotal evidence suggests are dominated by local economic and political circumstances. Those involved in negotiations indicate that, after introduction of more sophisticated hospital statistics, the new data were left aside during bargaining sessions. Though the 1985 law directed sickness funds to look at cost and performance data of individual hospital departments, they aren't usually doing it. In 75 percent of the cases examined in 1987, the sickness funds conceded global increases for the hospital as a whole, as in the past.[59]

The hospitals' interest in negotiating is "pretty much defined," said one hospital financial officer. "We want to expand our services in any way we can."[60] Furthermore, adds this official, hospital budgeting methods in Germany are "very primitive," based on historical cost. "The total cost is calculated based on previous year and projections of the current year, and a prospective budget is made for the following year. The negotiators for the sickness fund have a very much more difficult position than we do."

"Individual *AOK*s face a real dilemma," agrees Altenstetter. "They have to pay for the hospital care of their members out of their contributions. They also face their members who, when sick, want the best and most advanced care which commonly means technology-intensive and expensive care."[61]

Hospital negotiations include a maximum of 16 individuals, representing
- ☐ the hospital's administration, its sponsor (which can include a mayor or county executive in the case of public institutions), and its medical staff;
- ☐ sickness fund directors, technical experts, and representatives of both employers' and employees' interests, which share equally in sickness funds' contributions; and
- ☐ chairpersons of local political parties.[62]

The tenor of negotiations varies considerably from one region to another, based on local economic conditions, traditions and long-standing human relationships. German sickness fund and hospital officials explain that it is difficult to strike an agreement that will raise fund members' contributions by a half-percentage point in areas where premiums are already high, by virtue of expensive health care facilities, low wage rates (which put more burden on each wage-earner to fund sickness fund coffers), or both. "In Tübingen we have always had a very close, good relationship with the *AOK*," says Dörner of the University of Tübingen Hospitals in the southern German state of Baden-Württemberg. "My partner in Ulm has a very different relationship. They never come to an agreement, they always had to go to an arbitration."[63]

The 1985 law provided for compulsory arbitration of hospital budgets when the parties deadlock. The arbitrators are jointly appointed by the state hospital association and the state association of statutory sickness funds. A state Price Office, which had ultimate rate-setting powers, retained approval power over the arbitrated prices. The existence of compulsory arbitration reportedly is a strong incentive to agree, lest the arbitrated rate turn out to be less favorable to one side or the other. Even before the advent of compulsory arbitration, however, negotiations rarely deadlocked, for fear of the state-determined rate. Between 1974 and 1985, 97 percent of 4,500 negotiations were directly settled between the two parties, according to one study.[64] One reason, according to Altenstetter, is that state price offices — usually staffed by one or two civil servants — "acted through subtle or overt threats to manipulate each side into an agreement, hinting that if they didn't like the bargained rate they would fare worse with the arbitrated one."[65] The 1985 compulsory arbitration requirement may have increased the proportion of failed negotiations somewhat. A 1987 study indicates that 10 percent of per diem negotiations were settled by arbitration.[66]

The effectiveness of German hospital negotiations is difficult to determine, and academic studies are rare. Despite Germans' concern about rising hospital costs, comparisons with U.S. hospital inflation rates raises the question of whether the negotiating process, as Schulenburg suggests, plays a role in keeping German hospital prices low. Some German observers think so. As Uwe E. Reinhardt of Princeton University writes: "Germany has concentrated the flow of health care payments into channels "whose valves are operated through negotiation." Although there are more than 1,000 of these revenue "pipes," channelling money from sickness funds to hospitals and other providers, Reinhardt continues, the flow is coordinated "into all-payer systems which offer the payer a degree of market power similar to that enjoyed by truly single-source payers."[67]

Dörner also reports, despite generally amicable relations with his local *AOK*, that sickness fund negotiators can be tough. "We had to fight for years and years for new nursing positions," he says, adding.

> Only when political climate changed in Germany were these organizations willing [to allow more RN positions]. The opinion changed that we had shortages of nurses. Nurses had demonstrated. They began to shut down entire wards, the public became aware of these problems, and this had influence on the *AOK's* attitude....In my opinion, negotiations with sickness funds have been a very effective mechanism to hold down costs.[68]

The Problem That Wouldn't Go Away

The mid-1980s brought renewed debate over health cost containment, despite the legislation of 1984 and 1985. It was not because the governing coalition in Bonn liked health care reform for its own sake. According to Webber, the coalition which came to power in 1982, made up of the Christian Democratic Union and Free Democratic Party, "shared an antipathy to state intervention in health care as well as in other sectors."[69] However, the coalition had campaigned for *Wende* — a fundamental change in public policy — and in particular had stressed the dangers of rising health insurance contributions, which the coalition warned was undermining the international competitiveness of German exports and subverting the work ethic. Moreover, health costs continued to rise despite the earlier reforms, perhaps because they had been so "half-hearted and heavily diluted" in their approach to hospital costs, Webber says.[70] In 1986, spending in all major categories except ambulatory physician care and dentures rose more than twice as fast as wages. (See Table 5.11)

Reform was postponed until after the 1987 federal elections, but the Kohl government's reelection put the coalition on the spot for its promise to stabilize the contribution rates for statutory health insurance. The health reform debate of late 1987 and 1988 was unusually intense, with fierce opposition from an array of provider interests ranging from doctors, dentists, and drug companies to funeral directors (who opposed cutbacks in historically generous death

Table 5.11

Spending Trends* in German Statutory Health Insurance Compared to Average Salaries, 1984-87

Year	Total health spending	Hospital spending	Average wage	Average contribution per worker
1984	+8.0%	+7.3%	+4.7%	11.44%
1985	5.0	5.5	3.1	11.80
1986	4.8	6.9	3.1	12.19
1987	4.4	4.9	2.2	12.47

*Changes in percent from prior year compared to average contribution per worker (shared equally by employees and employers) for each year.

Source: Kassenärztliche Bundesvereinigung, 1988

benefits) and taxi owners (who were outraged about new limits on subsidized transportation to the doctor's office). But when the dust had settled, major cost-containment reforms had again passed hospitals by. In his analysis of the reasons, Webber describes how the state governments, through their veto power in the *Bundesrat*, once again blocked a formidable coalition made up of the labor wing of Kohl's Christian Democratic Union, the Free Democratic Party, and pro-business elements of the coalition, which were united in their determination to pass effective hospital cost-control measures.[71]

In the end, the most concrete hospital measure in the 1988 health care reform was a doubling of copayments that patients were expected to bear for the first 14 days of hospitalization, from DM 5 to DM 10 per day ($2.39 to $4.78) — hardly a great cost-saving or cost-offsetting step. "It is questionable whether the low copayment has had even a negligible effect on demand for hospital services," says statistics consultant Schneider.[72] To move more chronically ill patients out of acute care hospitals, the statute also increased sickness fund benefits for home care.[73] For instance, the funds were required to pay for four weeks of respite care so relatives who provided home care could take a holiday; family caregivers were also given a monthly allowance of DM 400 ($192) or DM 750 ($360) to hire professional nursing services, sufficient for up to 25 hours of home care per month. Evidence is sparse on the impact of these long term care benefits on the acute care burden.

Another provision of the reform permitted sickness funds to cancel contracts with hospitals (or refuse to renew) if they could demonstrate chronic inefficiency and waste. However, the *Bundesrat* amended the measure, making the standard of proof difficult, and there have been few attempts to exercise this supposedly cost-saving prerogative. In any case, the statute simultaneously gave state governments veto power over such cancellations. By 1991, four inefficient hospitals had been closed, and 20 more institutions had been targeted for closure.[74] Finally, the legislation required hospitals to publish price lists, and required ambulatory-care doctors to refer their patients to the cheapest hospitals. However, the law imposed no sanctions against hospitals or doctors who did not comply, and this provision is not believed to have made any difference in terms of either cost control or patient referral patterns.[75]

The 1992 Reform: No Escape for Hospitals

The 1988 reform, which took effect January 1, 1989, was German hospitals' last in a decade-long string of victories over major new cost-containment constraints. In December 1992, both houses of Parliament passed a sweeping new *Health Care Structural Reform Act* that aims to save a total of DM 11.4 billion annually (about $5.4 billion) in statutory health insurance spending, of which more than 20 percent (DM 2.5 billion, or $1.2 billion) is to come from hospitals. To put this in perspective, such a savings would be 66 percent of the increase in hospital spending between 1989 and 1990, the most recent available figure. The latest reform was stimulated by a projected DM 12 billion ($5.8 billion) annual deficit in the statutory sickness funds' accounts, a 10.5 percent annual inflation rate in statutory health insurance spending — more than twice as high as sickness fund income growth — and the pressures of investing vast sums in former East Germany.

The man most responsible for the reform, and for the fact that hospitals did not elude a significant impact this time, was Horst Seehofer, who became Minister of Health in May 1992. This was ironic, since Seehofer, as second-in-command to Labor Minister Norbert Blüm and as a states-rights advocate from Bavaria's conservative Christian Social Union party, had been instrumental in the successful fight to protect hospitals in the 1988 fight over health care reform. (At that time, the Labor Ministry had jurisdiction over statutory health insurance.) Seehofer has since stated publicly that it was a serious mistake to have excluded hospitals from major cost control programs in 1988.[76] Hospitals have the consolation of knowing that the 1992 law spreads considerable pain among doctors, pharmaceutical companies, dentists, pharmacists, and patients.

Perhaps the latest reform's most significant departure for hospitals is its clean break from the 20-year-old principle of full cost reimbursement. While the 1985 reform modified the full cost-reimbursement principle by allowing hospitals only their marginal costs for patient-days above or below their projected volume, the fundamental guarantee had been left intact. Now, however, the principle has been thrown out the window, "a tremendous show of political strength" over both hospitals and their traditional protectors, the states, according to Gerhard Schulte, assistant secretary in the Federal Health Ministry.[77] From 1993 through 1995, increases in hospitals will be held to fixed budgets supposedly limited to inflation in the gross wages and salaries of statutory health insurance members. "We reckon with a yearly increase of approximately 4 percent," Schulte says. "If the doctors and the hospitals do not keep within the budget, they will have to pay the surplus out of their own pockets."

Schulte also acknowledges that the 1992 reform violates the far older principle of self-regulation, which has permitted providers' budgets to be set through negotiations with payers. "This is without any doubt an act of interference, on the part of the legislature, in the right to self-government vested in the hospitals and the health care providers," he says. "However, we consider such an intervention to be justified and expedient in order to strengthen the willingness of these parties to take the necessary action."[78]

That said, it must be noted that the 1992 law has provisions to cushion the impact of a 4 percent budget ceiling. Hospital spending above this limit will be allowed for

□ increases in salaries and wages of hospital employees in excess of the German average;

□ higher costs attributable to new nursing staff regulations;

□ additional costs shown necessary to provide adequate care to the population the hospital serves; and

□ costs due to new services approved by states' hospital need plans.

Also in the hospitals' favor, the 1992 reform eliminates the much-feared "cellar-stairs effect": Hospitals will no longer be penalized in their subsequent-year's budgets if they achieve reductions in length-of-stay or other efficiencies.

In 1996, German hospitals are scheduled to begin moving away from the global per diem payment method, in effect for more than a century, in favor of a more complicated reimbursement scheme that has often been characterized as a "DRG-like" payment system. While it is true that the envisioned new German payment system is based in part on diagnosis-specific rates, there are significant departures from the DRG method that would appear to work on hospitals' favor — or at least give them room to try to win payment-enhancing exceptions. Under the new system, hospital payments are to be disaggregated into seven components:

1. basic per diem rates to cover nonclinical "hotel services," such as room and board;

2. department-specific per diem rates to cover physician and nursing services associated with particular inpatient departments;

3. lump-sum payments called *Fallpauschalen* to cover the particular costs of treatments and procedures related to certain diagnoses, such as transplants for organ failure;

4. "special payments," called *Sonderentgelte*, flat rate payments to cover particular services and material costs for procedures such as pacemaker insertion — to be charged in addition to basic and departmental per diem rates;

5. flat-rate payments for preadmission procedures;

6. flat-rate payments for postadmission follow-up care; and

7. per-case payments for outpatient surgery.

By 1996, a federal expert committee is to draw up a list of 40 diagnosis-related payment categories and at least 160 procedure-related payment categories, covering 30 to 40 percent of all hospital services. The actual payments associated with these categories will be calculated on a state level, leaving open the possibility that rates will reflect individual hospitals' special pleadings, such as an unfavorable case mix. Basic per diem rates will also be calculated at the state level, and will reflect individual hospitals' economic situations.

Breaching the Wall

Several aspects of the 1992 reform are intended to reduce unnecessary hospitalization and breach the time-honored wall between hospital and ambulatory care. Hospitals will be explicitly allowed to do ambulatory surgery (at per-case rates that match those of procedures performed in doctors' offices) and deliver pre- and post-admission care — prerogatives fiercely defended in earlier years by office-based physicians. In the end, the most important changes in the face and function of German hospitals may come about as the result of changes in the outside world rather than in their own financing. For instance, if Germany succeeds in reorienting its ambulatory physicians toward a predominance of generalists (now the ratio of specialists to generalists is 4:6), reliance on hospital care may be lessened, despite an aging population.

Even more important, the demand for acute care hospital services could be strikingly reduced if Germany succeeds in enacting a workable insurance scheme for long term care — an item that has been somewhere in the middle of the political agenda for several years, but which leading politicians say is likely to be debated in earnest in the mid-1990s. "One of the major future problems for the German health care system is the provision of adequate services for patients in need of nursing care," says consultant Schneider. These expenditures are the fastest-growing health expenses but reimbursement mechanisms are nonexistent and the organization of long term care services is "very poor," Schneider adds.[79] For instance, western Germany has approximately 2.5 nursing home beds per 1,000 population,[80] compared to 5.8 beds per 1,000 in the U.S.[81] (although the U.S. long term care bed ratio is not necessarily the "right" one).

Finally, the 1992 reform attempts to open the door to more private capital investment in hospitals by making it possible for statutory sickness funds to reimburse the costs of borrowing for planned projects that are likely to reduce costs. But some German observers think this innovation is likely to be less dramatic than it appears, for several reasons.

- ☐ The provision is designed to attract private investment for reconstruction of hospitals in former East Germany, but in the western states hospitals must still be conservative about any borrowing that would inflate their per diem rates because the rates of "comparable" hospitals must be similar.
- ☐ Most hospitals will still rely as much as possible on public subsidies for construction, renovation and replacement costs.
- ☐ Sickness funds are expected to remain resistant to payment of debt-related costs, despite new provisions that permit short-term increases in cost if they will yield savings over a seven-year period.

Most important, it remains completely unclear how sickness funds, which are under enough pressure to stabilize their premium rates as it is, could take on the burden of a substantial amount of hospital capital investment. The total burden in hospital capital investment now subsidized by states and communities is DM 7 billion ($3.4 billion). If this entire sum were to be borrowed privately, it is estimated that interest and principle repayments would push the annual total to DM 17 billion ($8.2 billion).

A Swing Toward Central Control?

What lessons can be drawn from the German hospital experience? Certainly hospital costs in Germany have been constrained by some mechanisms, or this excessively large system (by German authorities' own reckoning) would be even more expensive to operate than the U.S. hospital sector, instead of considerably less costly. However, the reasons are difficult to isolate, and it appears that specific policies targeted toward containing or lowering costs have cut both ways, at best. That is, even though the policies may have had some cost-constraining effects, they also raised costs or preserved features of the system responsible for keeping costs high, such as excessive numbers of beds and high occupancy rates.

Sometimes these contradictory effects may have cancelled each other out. For example, the federal reform that required all German hospitals to adopt global budgets in 1985 contained incentives *not* to cut spending. A 1991 study of health care spending controls in Germany, France, and Japan by the U.S. General Accounting Office (GAO) found that German policies of the late 1980s "failed to contain spending" or to slow the growth rate of hospital spending, even though it found that Germany has been demonstrably successful in recent years in constraining physician spending. One reason, the GAO researchers say, is that

> policies that limit aggregate spending may not reward individual providers for achieving economies that permit the same volume of services to be delivered for less than the budgeted amount of spending. Nor do these policies necessarily penalize providers who, despite keeping within the prescribed budget, are wasteful and inefficient....Where hospitals' global budgets are based on past spending (as in France and Germany), hospitals may sustain high spending levels so they will be allocated larger budgets in subsequent years.[82]

Although the 1986 reform law set spending targets for hospitals, the main reason this strategy failed, the GAO researchers say, is that the limits had no teeth. "The German spending targets are not reinforced by government participation in budget negotiations or by any other formal mechanism," the report concludes.

This conclusion implicitly suggests two things. First, where budget negotiations occur and the results are binding — that is, where annual hospital spending is not open-ended, as in the U.S. — there probably is a cost-constraining effect, even though it may not, in the Germans' view, constrain hospital costs *enough* over time. As Schulenburg, Reinhardt, and many other students of the German health care have stressed, the system has long been characterized by binding negotiations between hospitals and sickness funds. And while sickness funds are quite concerned about maintain high-quality, highly accessible local hospital services, they are also quite sensitive about the need to keep members' contribution rates (and their employers') in line. The overall point is that there are coordinated, all-payer negotiations, through which these pressures can be transmitted, and the annual outcomes of these bargaining sessions do have teeth. This is very different from the fragmented U.S. hospital payment system, where there are no enforceable limits and cost-shifting to the most vulnerable payers has become standard operating procedure.

The second suggestion implicit in the GAO report's conclusions is that there should be more central control if hospital budget controls are to have more impact in the future. For example, one feature of the German hospital system that has been both a blessing and a curse is the split between capital investment and operating budgets. It has been a blessing because, once again, it represents a control system, a process, that has clearly constrained certain kinds of capacity (especially high-technology equipment), although with unintended results, such as migration of some such capacity to the ambulatory sector. In addition, public financing of hospital capital investment has relieved sickness funds from the burden of financing the debt that hospitals would otherwise have incurred, and has spread these costs more broadly. (Public financing has also perpetuated a sense that hospitals are, in some concrete sense, more like public utilities than private businesses, compared to U.S. hospitals.) But the concomitant curse has been that sickness funds are saddled with the additional operating costs of capital investment over which they have no control. The GAO report notes that some experts believe that "the persistent increases in Germany's hospital care spending are the byproduct of a fragmented system of hospital financing, in which no policymaker or entity has the authority to restrain overall spending increases."[83]

As we have seen, this "fragmented system of hospital financing" is no historical accident. German hospitals and German states have fought fiercely to retain it, because it has been a bulwark against central control of a social asset of potent symbolic value — every community's hospital. However, the most recent German reform sounds a clear tocsin. For the moment at least, politicians and officials in Bonn have seen the need for more federal control over hospital spending as the only cost-control strategy likely to succeed, and to undo the structural barriers that have kept German hospital spending higher than it probably needs to be.

References and Notes

1. Schieber, GJ, Poullier J-P, Greenwald, LM (1992) *Health Care Financing Review*, Vol. 13, No. 4, pp. 24-43

2. Comparison of 10-year averages, 1980-89, average cost per hospital case, Germany vs U.S., data from Markus Schneider, Beratungsgesellschaft für angewandte Systemforschung mbH (BASYS), Augsburg, Germany, 1992.

3. Comparison using data from German Federal Ministry of Health (1991), *Datens des Gesundheitswesens*, Baden-Baden: Nomos Verlagsgellschaft, p. 230; and Newhouse, JP (1992), "Medical Care Costs: How Much Welfare Loss?" *Journal of Economic Perspectives*, Vol. 6, No. 3. p. 12.

4. As explained in Chapter Four, hospital physicians are salaried and, except for department chiefs and a few others, are not permitted to provide ambulatory care. Conversely, the vast majority of office-based physicians are not permitted to practice in hospitals.

5. Organization for Economic Cooperation and Development (OECD) software (1992). Health Profession Earnings: Health Employees/Average Employee Compensation.

6. Bonnie Blanchfield, Harvard School of Public Health, personal communication, February, 1993.

7. Dörner, H (1992a). "Hospital Financing in Germany," talk presented at the Goethe Institute of Boston, October 16, 1992.

8. *Jahresgutacthen des Sachverständigenrats für die Konzertierte Aktion im Gesundheitswesen (1991)*. Baden-Baden: Nomos Verlagsgesellschaft, pp. 57-59, 295.

9. Schieber, GJ (1992), p. 79, and *Hospital Statistics, 1992-92 Edition*, Chicago: American Hospital Association, p. 2.

10. Starr, P (1982). *The Social Transformation of American Medicine*. New York: Basic Books, Inc., p. 145.

11. Glaser WA (1985). "Krankenhauskosten im internationalen Vergleich, ein internationaler Vergleich der Krankenhausfinanzierung: Die europäischen und die amerikanischen Traditionen," in *Kosten und Effizienz im Gesundheitswesen*, München: R. Oldenbourg Verlag.

12. Murken, AH (1991). Grundzüge der Krankenhausgeschichte in den vergangenen 200 Jahren, *Krankenhaus Umschau*, Vol. 11: 837-846.

13. Rosen G (1963). The Hospital: Historical Sociology of a Community Institution, in Freidson, E. ed., *The Hospital in Modern Society*. New York: Free Press. p. 10.

14. Altenstetter, C (1989a). Federal Republic of Germany in *International Public Policy Sourcebook*, Vol. 1, ed. by DeSario, JP. New York: Greenwood Press, p. 44. Also, Sister Marie Luise Drobnik of University of Tübingen Hospitals, personal interview, December 8, 1992.

15. Starr, P (1982), p. 147.

16. Altenstetter, C (1986). Reimbursement Policy of Hospitals in the FRG. *International Journal of Health Planning and Management*, Vol. 1, 194.

17. Nipperdey, T (1991). *Deutsche Geschichte 1800-1866*, München: Beck Verlag.

18. Ackerknecht, EH (1992). *Geschichte der Medizin*, 7th edition, ed. Murken, AH. Stuttgart: Enke Verlag

19. Nipperdey, T (1990). *Deutsche Geschichte 1866-1918*, München: Beck Verlag.

20. Jung, H. (1986). Political Values and the Regulation of Hospital Care in *Political Values in Health Care*, ed. Light DW. Cambridge, MA: The MIT Press, p. 303.

21. Müller, HW (1975). *Geschäftsbericht der Deutschen Krankenhausgesellschaft 1974/75*. Düsseldorf: Deutsche Krankenhaus Verlagsgesellschaft mbH.

22. Altenstetter, C (1973), p. 47.

23. Das Image des deutschen Krankenhauses (1970). Results of a public opinion poll conducted by the Allensbach Institute for Demoscopy. Stuttgart: Studienstiftung der Fachvereinigung der Verwaltungsleiter Deutscher Krankenanstalten e.V.

24. Altenstetter, C (1989b). Hospital Planners and Medical Professionals in the Federal Republic of Germany, in *Controlling Medical Professionals: The Comparative Politics of Health Governance*. London: European Consortium for Political Research, p. 161.

25. In practice, the federal government has contributed less than one-third of hospital capital investment funds, while states and municipalities in many states contributed more than the two-thirds share specified in the 1972 law, according to various German sources.

26. Lump-sum subsidies are not negotiated, as annual per diem payment rates are, but decided by state officials. In 1993, the lump-sum subsidies varied from DM 2,850 to DM 5,130 per "planned bed" (approximately $1,370 to $2,470), depending on the hospital's size and therefore its scope and intensity of services. In addition, additional per-bed subsidies have been added, ranging in amount from DM 75 to DM 115 ($36 to $55), to buy equipment to improve nurses' working conditions, a measure intended to address a shortage of nurses. Expenditure of these additional subsidies must be supported by receipts. In addition, hospitals may apply for extra subsidies on a one-time basis if the hospital is too small for its ordinary lump-sum subsidies to permit replacement of some expensive equipment, such as a CT scanner.

27. University teaching hospitals' per diem rates are calculated in two steps. First, each hospital figures its costs for education and research and subtracts this from its total costs. The per diem rates paid by sickness funds and other payers are calculated on the remainder, while states explicitly subsidize research and training. This subsidy varies considerably from one teaching hospital to another, ranging from about 15 to 40 percent, with an average of about 30 percent. Teaching costs are not audited.

28. Altenstetter, C (1973). Planning for Health Facilities in the United States and in West Germany, in *The Milbank Memorial Fund Quarterly*, Vol. 51, No. 1, p. 47.

29. Altenstetter, C (1989b), p. 170.

30. Schneider, M (1991) Health Care Cost Containment in the Federal Republic of Germany in *Health Care Financing Review*, Vol. 12, No. 3, Spring 1991, p. 96.

31. Dörner, H (1992a)

32. Weil, TP (1992). The German Health Care System: A Model for Hospital Reform in the United States? in *Hospital & Health Services Administration*, Vol. 37, No. 4, Winter 1992, p. 537.

33. Rosenberg, P. (1991), personal interview.

34. Vukovic, M (1992), personal interview.

35. Dörner, H-P (1992b), personal interview.

36. Altenstetter, C (1985). Hospital Policy and Resource Allocation in the Federal Republic of Germany in *Public Policy Across Nations: Social Welfare in Industrial Settings*. JAI Press, Inc., p. 241.

37. Webber, D (1988). The Politics of German Health System Reform: Successful and Failed Attempts at Reform from 1930 to 1984. Unpublished paper prepared for a workshop on policy change, University of Bologna/Rimini, April, 1988.

38. Schneider, M (1991), p. 88.

39. Ibid.

40. Altenstetter, C (1980). Hospital Planning in France and the Federal Republic of Germany. *Journal of Health Politics, Policy and Law*, Vol. 5, No. 2, Summer 1980, p. 315.

41. Another stakeholder outside of the provider community that was left unrepresented in the Concerted Action panel are consumers, largely because health care consumers have never been organized into groups the way other interests in Germany are. It has apparently been assumed that consumers are adequately represented on the Concerted Action committee by representatives of government, political parties and unions.

42. Federal Association of Sickness Fund Physicians, collected health statistics, 1992.

43. Altenstetter, C (1985), p. 246.

44. Schneider, M (1991), p. 96.

45. Ibid, p. 90.

46. Webber, D (1988).

47. Altenstetter, C (1985), p. 244.

48. Webber, D (1988), p. 64.

49. Schieber, GS (1992), pp. 70-71.

50. Dörner, H-P (1992a).

51. Jung, H (1986), p. 313.

52. Rosenberg, P (1991), personal interview.

53. Schieber, GS (1992), p. 23.

54. Infratest Gesundheitsforschung (1986). Ermittlung und Analyse der Krankenhausleistungen. München: Deutschen Krankenhausgesellschaft.

55. Abel-Smith, B (1992). Cost Containment and New Priorities in the European Community, *The Milbank Quarterly*, Vol. 70, No. 3, p. 405.

56. *Sachverständigenrat für die Konzertierte Aktion im Gesundheitsweden* (1987). Baden-Baden: Nomos Verlagsgesellschaft.

57. Altenstetter, C (1986), p. 190.

58. Ibid.

59. Schwefel D, Leidl, R (1988). Bedarfsplanung und Selbstegulierung der Beteiligten im Krankenhauswesen, in Gäfgen G. (ed.), *Neokorporatismus und Gesundheitswesen*, Baden-Baden: Nomos, pp. 178-208.

60. _____(Name withheld on request), personal interview, 1992.

61. Altenstetter, C (1986), p. 204.

62. Ibid, p. 203.

63. Dörner, H-P (1992), personal interview.

64. Zimmer, CL (1985). Zur Neuen Bundespflegesatzverordnung (BPflV). *Krankenhaus-Umschau*, Vol. 10, pp. 759-765.

65. Altenstetter, C (1986), p. 200.

66. Regler, K (1988). Ergänzende Stellungnahme aus der Praxis: Erfahrungen mit dem Steurungssystem im Krankenhausbereich, in Gäfgen, G (ed.), Neokorporatismus und Gesundheitswesen. Baden-Baden: Nomos, pp. 209-218.

67. Reinhardt, UE (1990). West Germany's Health-Care and Health-Insurance System: Combining Universal Access with Cost Control. Report commissioned by the U.S. Bipartisan Commission on Comprehensive Health Care, pp. 12-13.

68. Dörner, H-P (1992b)

69. Webber, D (1992). The Politics of Regulatory Change in the German Health Sector in *The Politics of German Regulation*, (ed.) Kenneth Dyson. Aldershot: Dartmouth Books, p. 213.

70. Ibid.

71. Webber, D (1991). Health Policy and the Christian-Liberal Coalition in West Germany: The Conflicts over the Health Insurance Reform, 1987-8, in *Comparative Health Policy and the New Right: From Rhetoric to Reality*, (ed.) Altenstetter and Haywood. New York: Macmillan, pp. 53-64.

72. Schneider, M (1991), p. 98

73. Hurst, JW (1991). Reform of Health Care in Germany, *Health Care Financing Review*, Vol. 12, No. 3, p. 80.

74. Ibid, p. 82.

75. Webber, D (1992). The Politics of Regulatory Change in the German Health Sector, in *The Politics of German Regulation*, (ed.) Kenneth Dyson. Aldershot: Dartmouth Books, p. 217.

76. Pragal, P. *Berliner Zeitung*, September 9, 1992.

77. Schulte, G (1992). Problems of Health Care in the Conflict Area between Market Economy and Government Economic Control, a talk at the Goethe Institute of Boston, October 17, 1992.

78. Ibid.

79. Schneider, M (1991), p. 100.

80. Hurst, JW (1991), p. 82.

81. Prospective Payment Review Commission (1991), *Report to Congress: Medicare and the American Health Care System*, June, 1991.

82. U.S. Government Accounting Office (1991). *Health Care Spending Control: The Experience of France, Germany, and Japan*. GAO/HRD-92-9, pp. 48-50.

83. Ibid.

A Closer Look: Hospitals in Germany

A Hospital Construction Case Study: Getting It Built in Germany

Building, renovating, or expanding a hospital in Germany requires persistence, patience and, above all, plenty of public support.

For instance, a 727-bed community facility we shall call "Fortheim Hospital" decided in 1987 that it needed more room for computer tomography, ultrasound, and endoscopy equipment. Construction of a new diagnostic wing would also free up patient-care space, allowing the 20-year-old hospital to convert its four- and five-bed rooms to more spacious two-bed rooms. The project, hospital officials figured, would cost in the neighborhood of DM 150 million, or about $72 million.[1]

Fortheim Hospital faced a problem familiar to German hospitals. Unlike the U.S. system, which permits hospitals to borrow money and add the cost of repayment to its patient-care charges, German hospitals must apply to state governments for the funding to pay for construction and routine replacement of fixed assets. They may not pay for capital investment out of patient-care reimbursements from statutory health insurance funds. And although hospitals are not prohibited from borrowing, statutory sickness funds, which cover 90 percent of the population, refuse to pay the resulting interest charges if the debt is used to pay for capital investment.

The problem: In 1992 German states had an aggregate backlog of DM 3.8 billion ($1.8 billion) in approved-but-not-funded hospital projects. The entire fund for hospital construction, renovation, and routine maintenance in the state of Baden-Württemberg, where our pseudonymous Fortheim is located, amounted to DM 646 million in 1990, or about $311 million, of which 56 percent was for major construction and renovation, 33 percent for routine maintenance and replacement costs, and 11 percent for special projects, interest, and other costs.[2] Fortheim Hospital has to compete against the other 320 hospitals in the state need plan for a share of that fund, although only 10 to 20 percent of these institutions are seeking major state subsidies at any given time (Baden-Württemberg, a fairly prosperous state about the size of Maryland and Delaware combined, but with a population twice as large, is about average among the 11 states of former West Germany in the amount of state subsidy it provides hospitals.)[3] (See Figure 5a.1)

The Fortheim Hospital case illustrates there is more than one way to build a new wing. The saga of how this institution was able to finance its project is fairly representative of how German hospitals build, expand, or renovate.

Fortheim Hospital, a public facility owned by the county, is a typical community hospital located in Fortheim, a city of 100,000 that is the center of a population area of 250,000. The county owns two smaller basic-care hospitals. Fortheim Hospital is a full-service institution with 240 medical beds and 220 surgical beds, 125 obstetrics and gynecology beds, a 70-bed pediatric department, 30 urology beds, and separate smaller inpatient units for otolaryngology, ophthalmology, and neurology; 12 hemodialysis stations; departments of radiology, anesthesia, and pathology; a clinical laboratory; and a pharmacy. The staff includes 139 physicians and 406 approved nursing positions. Fifty-five people work in non-clinical areas, including administration.

The hospital's decision-making hierarchy is topped by the county council and the county executive, who are elected for five-year terms. The council has a hospital committee to oversee management. Fortheim Hospital's board of directors includes all physician department chiefs, representatives of nonsalaried community physicians who have special admitting privileges to cover certain specialist services, the director of nursing, and hospital managers. The board's executive committee consists of the chief administrator, medical director, and director of nursing.

The first step in the years-long journey toward a major construction project is a set of internal negotiations among the hospital's board of directors. In Fortheim's case, investments of up to DM 50,000 ($24,000) can be made by this board. Projects costing up to $48,000 can be cleared by the county executive without consulting the county council. The council's hospital committee can decide on projects costing up to $480,000, and costlier projects must receive approval from the full council. If the hospital reaches internal consensus on an expensive project — weighing the likelihood of state subsidies and the county's fiscal picture — the institution's officials will proceed with plans for presentation to the county council.

In drawing up the first draft of a plan, the hospital must be mindful of the state hospital "need plan," a document updated annually that sets forth the number of hospital facilities, beds, and medical equipment needed for each of the state's planning regions. It also must win the support of county council members, because they must agree to fill the inevitable gap that will remain between the state subsidy and the project's cost. Public support at the local level is not usually a problem, Fortheim Hospital officials say, since there is a reservoir of community pride in the institution.

For hospital investments costing less than DM 5 million ($2.4 million), the first step is review by a mid-level district authority, of which there are four in Baden-Württemberg. Since the Fortheim Hospital project greatly exceeded that threshold, it went directly to the state health department, which reviews plans for conformity to the hospital need plan and, if they pass muster, refers the application to the state's finance directorate. Officials there scrutinize the plans for any evidence of inflated cost estimates, and who also examine every detail down to the cost of door handles and wallpaper to sort out all expenses not legally eligible for state subsidy. For example, the state will not subsidize land acquisition, especially spacious reception areas, or retail commercial space for gift or floral shops. In addition, replacement costs of medical equipment must come out of a separate account — a fund for automatic annual lump-sum hospital subsidies determined on a per-bed basis. (Fortheim gets DM 5,100 per bed [$2,450], or $1.8 million in 1992, in this lump-sum state subsidy.)

In the case of Fortheim Hospital, this state-level review process took about five years and reduced the project's subsidizable cost by 40 percent, to about DM 90 million ($43.3 million). This was no surprise to Fortheim officials, since it is routine strategy for hospitals to inflate their requests by 30 to 50 percent.

Baden-Württemberg guidelines require a further 10 percent reduction in subsidies for renovation as opposed to new construction, leaving Fortheim with a subsidizable volume of DM 81 million ($39 million), a little more than half of the project's estimated cost. Fortheim's subsidy amounts to about 12 percent of the total estimated Baden-Württemberg budget for hospital construction in 1992 — though in fact, the state subsidy may be paid over several years.

State budgets for hospital construction are historically based, taking into account the state hospital "need plan." But it is also considered important for hospitals contemplating projects to cultivate political connections. State associations representing hospitals and sickness funds are formally consulted in these processes, although state bureaucrats are said to retain the final decision.[4] In Fortheim Hospital's case, those political connections helped, along with the recognized merits of the project, to ensure that it was one of the projects to receive state funding in 1992. Very few hospital subsidy requests are refused, although some may be delayed for several years because of budget constraints.

Thanks to the strong support Fortheim Hospital enjoys locally, the county council agreed to fund most of the remaining DM 70 million ($34 million) out of its tax revenues; the hospital will also draw on other sources of revenue, such as the "profit" it accumulates from charging privately insured patients more than actual costs.

And so it was that Fortheim Hospital broke ground for the project in 1992 and expects completion by 1996, nine years after the project was conceived. That is about par for the course, according to authorities: Due to the time needed for planning and approval at the local and state levels, major construction projects in German hospitals tend to run in 10-year cycles.

As construction equipment worked outside his window, Fortheim Hospital's director expressed satisfaction with successful completion of the process. But he said he is worried about the future. His medical staff is reducing patients' length-of-stay in response to recent cost-control initiatives, pressure to invest more in technology is unrelenting, and somehow Fortheim, like every other German hospital, must figure out how to live within an absolute budget ceiling, projected at about 4 percent annually for the next three years.

References and Notes

1. This and other dollar figures in this article are converted from deutschmarks using purchasing power parity value for 1990, as given by the Organization for Economic Cooperation and Development Data File, 1992.

2. Baden-Württemberg Ministry for Labor, Health, Families, and Social Affairs, 1993; and Baden-Würrtemberg Hospital Association, 1993.

3. Bruckenberger, E (1992), Subsidies per Inhabitant and per "Planned Bed" in DM, Hannover: Niedersächsiches Sozialministerium.

4. Bonnie Blanchfield, Harvard School of Public Health, personal communication, February, 1993.

A Closer Look: Hospitals in Germany

Long Term Care: One Reason for Long Hospital Stays

Germany's inadequate provisions for elders who can no longer live independently is a widely recognized flaw in the otherwise comprehensive system. Sickness funds, which are governed by working-age Germans and their employers, have been focused in recent years on preserving current benefits and controlling costs — not on expanding benefits to a large and growing new class of nonworking citizens. Nevertheless, the increasing numbers of old and very old Germans needing long term care is forcing the nation to pay more attention to the problem. For instance, efforts to reduce acute hospital lengths of stay will be stymied unless alternative care can be developed for hospitals' aging patient clientele.

The proportion of residents older than 65 is significantly higher in Germany than in America (15.4 percent in Germany vs 12.5 percent in the U.S. in 1988). Germany's share of residents over 75 is also higher (7.4 percent vs 5.1 percent). Not surprisingly, Germany has a correspondingly higher percentage of older people with severe incapacity. (Table 5.12) Nevertheless, the supply of residential care beds is lower than in the U.S. Germany had 5.3 beds for every 100 people over age 65 in 1990, compared to 6 per 100 in the U.S. in 1986. [1] Elder-care facilities were better staffed in the U.S., with the equivalent of 1.7 patients for every full-time worker versus 3 patients per staffer in Germany. [2] Only half the nursing home personnel in Germany have professional training as nurses.

The supply of beds in Germany's "old people's homes" and nursing homes has nearly tripled since 1960, but provisions for financing the care have remained spotty. This may arise

Table 5.12

Elders With Severe Incapacity: Germany vs U.S.

Percentage requiring intensive care or residential facilities

Country	Age Groups (years)		
	65-74	75-84*	85+
Germany	3.8%	11.1%	31.4%
U.S.**	1.2	9.6	20+

*In U.S. figures are for people aged 75 and older
**In residential care only

Source: Adapted from Jens Alber, Residential Care for the Elderly, Journal of Health Politics, Policy and Law, Winter, 1992.

from the roots of German sickness funds, which were originally intended to support workers and their families, providing medical care and rehabilitation so they could return to productive life. Jens Alber of the University of Constance notes that German sickness funds have never recognized chronic nursing care as their responsibility.

> With respect to its benefit structure for older people, the central characteristic of the German health care system is that it draws a sharp dividing line between sickness that needs medical care, on the one hand, and decrepitude or frailty, on the other....Only the former is covered by sickness insurance, while the latter continues to be largely a private risk for which there are almost no public provisions. Once older people become dependent on residential care, they frequently have to turn to a locally administered public welfare scheme to cover the cost. Therefore, a prolongation of the stay in acute hospitals is the only way to prevent older patients from having to foot the bill for delivery into nursing homes, which they can rarely afford. [3]

The cost of nursing home care in Germany varies between DM 3,000 and DM 4,000 a month ($1,435 to $1,914 on a purchasing power parity conversion), Alber reports, an amount that far exceeds pensioners' average monthly income of DM 1,914 ($916).[4] Therefore, as in the U.S., many elders must become impoverished before they qualify for public assistance with nursing home bills. Interestingly, the proportion than the U.S. of total nursing home expenditures paid for with public funds is roughly similar in the two nations — 49 percent in the U.S. vs 52 percent in Germany.[5] Private, out-of-pocket spending for such care in the two countries is virtually an identical proportion of the total.

Germany has relied more than the U.S. on family care of elders. Demographically, it can afford to, since it has a higher proportion of women between the ages of 45 and 60 — the typical caretakers for frail elders — than the U.S. (Table 5.13) Official policy has encouraged this family caregiving mode. A *Health Care Reform Law* which took effect in January 1989, reflected the policy consensus that elders should be enabled to live at home as long as possible rather than be housed in institutions. The law requires sickness funds to cover up to four weeks of professional nursing help at home each year (up to a ceiling of DM 1,800 or $861), a provision

Table 5.13

Available Caretakers for Frail Elders: Germany vs U.S.

No. of women aged 45 to 60 per 1,000 people over age 65

Germany 656

U.S. 587

Source: Adapted from Jens Alber, Residential Care for the Elderly, Journal of Health Politics, Policy and Law, *Winter, 1992.*

intended to provide respite for family caregivers. Since 1991, sickness funds have also covered 25 nursing visits at home per year (up to DM 750 or $359).

However, Germany's family care potential is "rapidly declining," as it is in the U.S., Alber observes. This means that "traditional forms of support for older people are no longer sufficient."[6] Leading members of the *Bundestag* and health policy analysts expect that some form of long term care insurance will be hotly debated in the mid-1990s, after having been put side repeatedly to deal with cost containment in the acute care system and, more recently, with the challenges of reunification.

It will be interesting to see how both Germany and the U.S. deal with elder care in the years ahead. Despite some similarity in the underlying problem and in their respective partial solutions — for instance, both nations rely heavily on "welfare" funding for nursing home care — they start from very different points in terms of the structure of their respective nursing home industries. America's is overwhelmingly private and profit-oriented, while Germany's is mainly nonprofit (sponsored by church organizations and labor unions) and publicly owned.

Nursing home care in the U.S. has the advantage of market incentives to increase supply, but the concomitant disadvantages of quality problems that require government policing. Its challenge will be to devise forms of long term care, beyond the traditional nursing home, that provide economic and flexible arrangements for its growing burden of elders. Both the U.S. and Germany will likely to explore a financing scheme for long term care that blends public and private insurance schemes.

Long term care in Germany suffers from the fact that the health system is run largely through bargaining among "corporate actors," such as employers, unions, and groups of providers totally focused on acute care. "In the collective bargaining process between corporate actors, only the interests of the groups represented at the negotiation table are considered," Alber says, adding that the situation will not change until elders are able to articulate their interests through the political system.[7] In that regard, German elder activists would be well advised to study their successful American counterparts.

References

1. Alber, J (1992). Residential Care for the Elderly. *Journal of Health Politics, Policy and Law*. Vol. 17, No. 4, pp. 950-951.

2. Ibid.

3. Ibid, p. 931.

4. Ibid, p. 938.

5. Ibid, pp. 950-951.

6. Ibid, p. 935.

7. Ibid, p. 955.

CHAPTER 6

German Drug Expenditures: The Illusion of Control

By Joe R. Neel

Many of the mechanisms to control drug spending that tantalize would-be regulators in the U.S. have already been tried in Germany's free market for pharmaceuticals. Most have failed to meet expectations, although after many decades of trial and error, Germans at last may have hit upon a successful formula for reducing drug expenditures in the 1993 reform law. Germany's experiences provide valuable insights into which types of controls might be effective and feasible to the open market of the U.S. — and which limits might prove worthless or even disastrous.

Issues Leading to Reform

One of the most persistent problems vexing German health reformers has been how to reduce the high level of spending on prescription and nonprescription drugs by the state health-insurance funds (*Gesetzliche Krankenversicherung* or *GKV*). Over the past two decades, expenditures on drugs have stayed relatively constant at about 15 to 17 percent of total health spending. (Figure 6.1) Although direct comparisons with the U.S. are difficult because of differences in definitions and data collection, the percentage of U.S. health spending on drugs has ranged from 7 to 11 percent since 1970; in 1990 drugs accounted for only 7.9 percent of spending.[1]

Most of the dozen major health reform acts in Germany since 1972 have included measures to limit expenditures on drugs. Each successive reform has called for more intervention in the drug market, though the emphasis has wavered back and forth between limits on the supply side and limits on demand.

Figure 6.1

Expenditures on Drugs as a Proportion of Total Health Spending Germany vs U.S., 1960-90

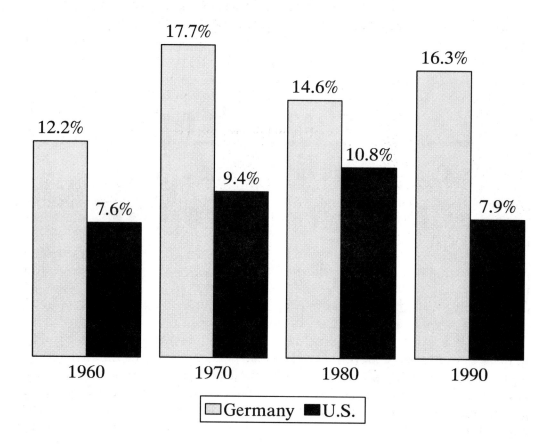

German data represent spending by *GHV* funds. U.S. data from National Health Expenditure estimates of spending by all sources.

Source: Daten des Gesundheitswesens *1991; and Levit KR, Lazenby HC, Cowan CA, and Letsche SW (1991). National Health Expenditures 1990.* Health Care Financing Review *13(1):29-54.*

Under the 1993 reforms, all sectors contribute to lower drug spending. For the first time, physicians are being held financially liable for the volume of prescriptions written. Though the penalties are generally modest, extreme outliers may face loss of income for a quarter-year or more. The reform also penalizes drug makers directly by reducing prices on selected drugs and by freezing many drug prices for a minimum of two years. This intervention may seem extreme to U.S. policymakers since drug spending in Germany has grown at a lower rate than the U.S. over the past decade. (Figure 6.2) Patients are also contributing to the savings plan by paying an increased, though still modest, copayment.

Prior to the price freeze, Germany's reference pricing system greatly inhibited drug companies' ability to set prices on certain drugs based on what the market would bear. Under the system, in place since 1989, sickness fund reimbursement limits effectively set the market price for entire classes of drugs, though manufacturers are legally able to continue charging what they like. In the U.S., such a move would have induced cost-shifting to patients who have prescription drug coverage. But all Germans have always received "free" drugs from the sickness funds and were loathe to pay even a small additional fee, forcing drug makers to lower prices on brand-name drugs. The system is another example of Germany's unique method of applying cost-containment pressure on various sectors of the health system without legislating specific prices. Germany essentially has created a situation where pharmaceuticals are still legally bought and sold on a free market—but the free market really exists only on paper.

The 1993 price freeze is the most severe intervention to date, and it effectively brings a temporary end to Germany's long-protected open market for pharmaceuticals. Drug makers will still be free to set prices on new drugs, and prices will be free to rise again once the freeze is lifted.

There is a general consensus that the relatively mild interventions before the 1993 freeze had a modest effect on limiting the *growth* of expenditures. But because the volume of prescriptions written by physicians remained very high compared with other countries, reform efforts based on limiting the price of an individual prescription have not had much success.

High prescription volume is consistently cited as the main reason for the high level of drug spending by the statutory sickness funds. German doctors write three times as many prescriptions as their American counterparts. Part of the reason lies in the higher number of patient visits and part lies with the oversupply of doctors. Cultural differences may also play a role, although the rate of consumption of ethical drugs appears to be similar in both countries.

Seeds of Change

Earlier reforms tried to filter the waste out of pharmaceutical spending, though the interventions were often half-hearted in their execution. It was only with the 1989 reform act that the upward pressure on sickness fund drug spending began to be reversed. The Act engineered a fundamental restructuring of the drug pricing system and a "negative list" of ineffective or minor drugs was expanded, making many more drugs ineligible for reimbursement. While the list may have helped improve medical care by discouraging the use of ineffective drugs, by far the most significant cost-cutting tool in the act was the creation of the **reference pricing system**.

The sickness funds, which had until then reimbursed the full price of a drug minus a small copayment, stopped reimbursing any amount above the reference price, making the patient responsible for any amount over that amount. Physicians were required to notify patients if the drug being prescribed carried an extra charge.

Figure 6.2

Annual Change in Drug Expenditures in Germany and the U.S. 1980-90

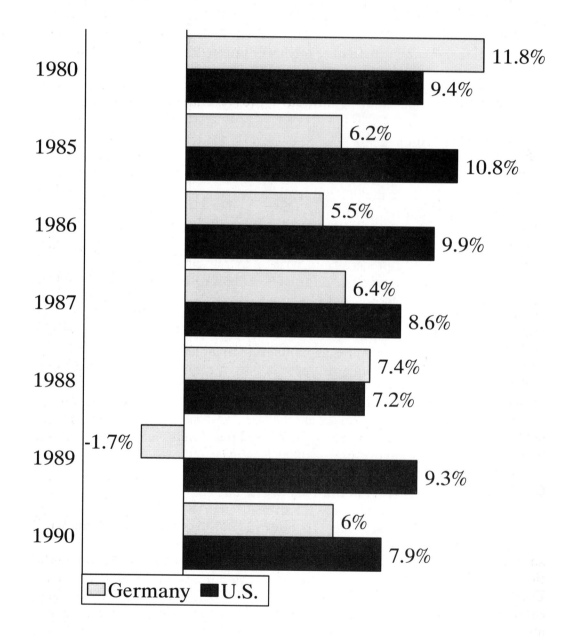

Source: Daten des Gesundheitswesens *1991; and Levit KR, Lazenby HC, Cowan CA, and Letsche SW (1991). National Health Expenditures 1990.* Health Care Financing Review *13(1):29-54.*

The reform had its intended effect: Patients and physicians abandoned higher-priced brand-name drugs that were covered by the new system. Patients were accustomed to "free" drugs and physicians were reluctant to take time to explain the financial implications of a prescribing decision with each patient. Most manufacturers instantly lowered their prices to the reference price level, although they still were permitted legally to charge any price. Companies that resisted reference pricing lost millions of DM in sales within a few weeks' time.

Yet when the dust had settled, most of the expected savings from the 1989 reform, some DM 4.3 billion (or $2.04 billion on a purchasing power parity conversion), failed to materialize. Some 80 percent of drugs were to be covered, but even after three years, less than one-third were included. While prices did fall on scores of drugs, manufacturers simply compensated for the loss by raising prices on drugs not in the reference pricing system. Actually, the most effective savings in the 1989 reform was produced by a 40 percent copayment on dentures, dental crowns, and bridges.

Because of this failure to make a dent in drug spending, backers of the 1993 reform went further. Physicians and patients were brought into the picture and made financially responsible for reducing the volume of prescriptions written. Collectively, physicians are responsible for the first DM 280 million ($134 million) in savings mandated by the reform. In addition to having more drugs placed into the reference pricing system, drug makers are responsible for the next DM 280 million in savings. Patients' DM 3 ($1.43) copayment per prescription was raised in some cases to DM 5 ($2.39) or DM 7 ($3.35).

In addition to these changes, price reductions of 5 percent were ordered on all drugs not in the reference pricing system and 2 percent cuts were ordered on over-the-counter drugs. Prices are to be frozen until 1995. The 1993 reforms also expand the so-called "negative list" of drugs that won't be reimbursed under any circumstance, even if doctor has written a prescription.

Early reaction to the "doctors' drug budget" indicates that prescribing volume has dropped precipitously in the first three months of the reform. But patients appear to be asking for larger packages of drugs to lessen the impact of the copayment. Other reforms also have produced short-lived changes in the direction desired by the government and the sickness funds, only to be subverted by clever and baroque schemes to exploit loopholes.

Germany's Drug Habit

Whether or not Germany's level of drug consumption is out of line with other countries a matter of some dispute. On the one hand, health researchers such as Michael Arnold, MD, of the University of Tübingen say drug consumption "is about average for a western industrialized nation."[2] Compared with France, with its legendary high drug consumption, this might be true. But when compared with the U.S., Germans are prescribed three times as many drugs annually (Table 6.1).

It is true that in Germany, 35 percent of prescribed drugs are over-the-counter drugs that are eligible for reimbursement simply because a doctor has written a prescription.[3] Even after over-the-counter drugs are factored out, per capita prescription drug usage in Germany still outpaces U.S. consumption (7.7 prescription-only drugs vs 6.4).

Other measures also point to higher overall drug consumption in Germany than in the U.S., though several findings complicate the picture.

- ☐ Total spending on all drugs takes up a substantially larger proportion of the German gross domestic product (GDP).
- ☐ Sickness fund spending on drugs per insured is significantly higher than comparable spending by U.S. insurers and patients.
- ☐ Prices per prescription are one-third lower in Germany, but the volume of prescribed medications ordered is three times higher.
- ☐ The U.S. has four times Germany's population and spends four times as much on drugs overall, supporting those who argue that the cultural differences between the countries aren't that great.

Spending as a part of GDP. When measured as a portion of GDP, German spending on pharmaceuticals has been consistently 30 percent higher than the U.S. for the past decade. (Figure 6.3) In 1990, prescription drugs accounted for 1.32 percent of the German GDP, but only 0.89 percent of the U.S. GDP.[4] Other sources show similar situation when over-the-counter drugs are included. The Organization for Economic Cooperation and Development (OECD) reports that combined spending on prescription and nonprescription drugs accounted for 1.8 percent of the German GDP in 1990; 1.0 percent in the U.S.[5]

In 1991, the latest year for which data are available, sickness fund spending on outpatient drugs amounted to 15.4 percent of total expenditures.[6] In the U.S., 1991 spending was estimated at 8.1 percent.[7] But the picture is more confusing when sources of drug spending are added and compared.

Table 6.1

Prescription Volume: Germany vs U.S. in 1990

	Total volume	Per capita
Germany*	751,200,000	19.8
U.S.	1,656,352,000	6.4

*Total number of prescription medications paid for by sickness funds. A single German prescription form may list more than one medication. (1990 average, 1.71). Sickness funds reimburse for all prescription-only and selected nonprescription drugs. U.S. data represent prescriptions filled at pharmacies from the National Prescription Audit conducted by IMS America Ltd., Plymouth Meeting, PA.

Source: *Kassenärztliche Bundesvereinigung, 1991, and* Pharmacy Times, *April 1992.*

Figure 6.3

Drug Spending* as a Percentage of GDP, 1980-90

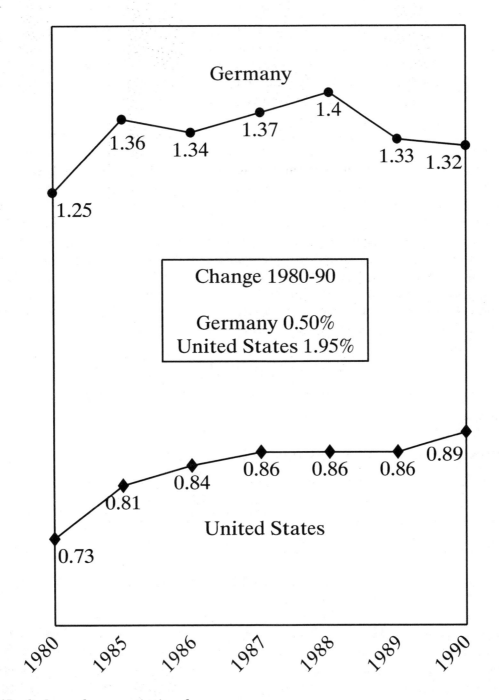

*Includes only prescription drugs.

Source: BASYS (Beratungsgesellschaft für angewandte Systemforschung mbH), Augsburg, 1992.

Total drug spending. In 1991, German spending on all types of drugs from all sources except hospitals amounted to more than DM 32.6 billion ($15.6 billion).[8] Of this, total sickness fund spending on prescription pharmaceuticals in 1991 amounted to DM 24.4 billion ($11.7 billion), up from DM 22 billion ($10.5 billion) in 1990.[9] Private insurers spent another DM 1.1 billion ($526.3 million) on drugs in 1990.[10] And approximately DM 5 billion ($2.4 billion) is spent annually by consumers on over-the-counter drugs not reimbursed by the sickness funds or private insurers.[11] The hospital drug market accounts for no more than DM 1 billion ($478 million) because of heavy discounting, though some estimates run as high as DM 2 billion ($957 million).[12] Patient copayments amounted to DM 1.14 billion ($545.5 million) in 1991.[13]

In the U.S., with four times Germany's population, prescription drug sales are four times higher. In 1990, the latest year for which data were available, U.S. retail sales of prescription drugs totalled $32.3 billion, while over-the-counter drugs and medical nondurables accounted for another $22.3 billion in sales, all of it out-of-pocket.[14] In 1990, Germany's estimated total drug spending was $13.9 billion.

It must be noted that this comparison may be misleading since some drugs that require a prescription in the U.S. don't require one in Germany, and vice versa. The German practice of reimbursing for over-the-counter drugs if prescribed by a physician further complicates international comparisons. Formal international comparative studies are not done on a regular basis. Also, U.S. data on drug spending exclude medications provided in hospitals. Subsequent discussions will refer to total drug spending by sickness funds for outpatient care.

Spending Per Insured. When sickness fund spending is examined on a per-insured basis, spending on prescription and selected nonprescription drugs in 1990 was 31 percent higher than U.S. spending per capita—in line with the GDP numbers. In 1990, this amounted to DM 576 ($275.60) per person insured by the statutory sickness funds. In the U.S. the 1990 per-capita figure was $210.35, based on total spending on prescription and over-the-counter drugs of $54.6 billion.

Other sources provide estimates at variance with these. For example, the OECD reports that the *per capita* figure for Germany was $257 in 1990. OECD estimates for other countries include: United Kingdom, $93; Japan, $179; Italy, $220; and France, $230.[15]

Though they have remained a relatively stable part of sickness fund spending, drugs have become a target for reformers because of pressure from other, more vocal sectors. Since 1970, the share of sickness fund spending on physicians has dropped from 22.9 percent to 17.7 percent, while hospital spending rose from 25.2 percent to 32.5 percent.[16] As Rainer Hess, JD, chief legal counsel of the German Physicians Chamber (*Bundesärztekammer*), observed: "The expenditure for medication prescribed by [sickness fund-] authorized physicians has almost matched the expenditure for the entire ambulatory treatment sector."[17] Pressures to cut costs were intensified in 1991, when the sickness funds ran a deficit of DM 5.5 billion ($2.6 billion), the sickness fund system's first deficit ever.

Prescription Volume. A look at differences in prices between the U.S. and Germany shows how volume can play a big role in overall drug expenditures. Though German drug prices are the highest in the European Economic Community (EC), they are one-third cheaper than the U.S. on average. In 1991, the average cost of a sickness fund-reimbursed prescription medicine in Ger-

Table 6.2

Average Drug Prices in Germany and the U.S.

	Germany	U.S.
1990	$13.87	$20.39
1991	15.15	22.44

In PPP dollars per prescription

Source: Kassenärztliche Bundesvereinigung *1992, Grunddaten zur kassenärztlichen Versorgung in der Bundesrepublik Deutschland 1991; and Hargis JR, editor (1992).* Lilly Digest. *Indianapolis: Eli Lilly and Company, p.3.*

many (either prescription-required or over-the-counter; brand-name or generic) was DM 31.66 ($15.15),[18] up from DM 28.99 ($13.87) in 1990.[19] The average U.S. prescription (generic or brand-name) cost $22.44 at retail in 1991, a rise of 10.1 percent over 1990's $20.39.[20] (Table 6.2)

Doctors Drive Drug Spending

Physicians' prescribing volume—particularly that of general practitioners (Table 6.3)—appears to be one of the main drivers of Germany's high rate of drug spending, along with patient expectations of a prescription at each visit. The volume of prescribed drugs ordered by all sickness-fund physicians rose 3.8 percent to 770 million per year in 1991.[21] (Figure 6.4)

One reason for Germany's high prescription volume is the high number of physician visits per year. This is compounded by the doctor glut described in Chapter Four. As in the U.S., there is a direct relationship between an office visit and a prescription: Each visit usually results in at least one prescription in both countries. But in Germany, patients see physicians 11.2 times a year; each insured member in the statutory health insurance funds averaged 11.6 prescriptions in 1991.[22] (Table 6.4) This situation has barely changed since 1962, when Germans averaged 10.2 physician contacts per year, resulting in 11 prescriptions.[23] In 1990, 30 percent of all prescriptions in Germany were classified as "patient desires."[24] Even when the volume of drugs prescribed by class is examined, this phenomenon of one visit-one prescription is supported; drugs for aches and pains, coughs, and stomach aches lead the list. (Table 6.5)

In the U.S., patients visit physicians only 5.5 times per year,[25] resulting in an corresponding average of 6.4 prescriptions annually, according to the Na-

Table 6.3

German Physicians' Prescribing Patterns 1988-90

	Proportion of prescriptions		Specialty distribution
	1988	**1990**	**in 1988 and 1990**
General practitioners	58.5%	49.9%	38%
Internists	17.2	16.3	16
Pediatricians	5.6	7.2	5
Ob-gyns	2.4	2.6	9
Dermatologists	2.0	3.0	2*
Other specialists	14.3	21.0	30*

* 1988 figures: Dermatologists, 3%; other specialists, 29%

Source: Sachverständigenrat für die Konzertierte Aktion im Gesundheitswesen (1990 and 1992).

tional Prescription Audit conducted by IMS America.[26] This is slightly higher than the case 30 years ago, when the average annual number of patient visits was 4.4 and the number of prescriptions was 4.7.[27]

Given these data, it should not be surprising that physicians have gradually become the focus of drug expenditure controls.

Private Insurance and Drugs

Per capita drug spending by Germany's private insurers is far lower than the statutory sickness funds. In 1990, private insurers paid out just DM 165 ($79) per insured, compared with the sickness funds' per-insured reimbursement of DM 576 ($276). Drug spending accounted for a mere 7.2 percent of private insurers' outlays, compared with 16.3 percent for the statutory sickness funds.

It's not that privately insured patients are three times healthier, although there is some evidence that because of their socioeconomic status they do enjoy somewhat better health. Instead, incentives to pay for costs out-of-pocket are strong in the private insurance sector.

Many privately insured patients don't claim small drug amounts because there is a large deductible. But more importantly, if privately insured patients do not submit any claims at all for a certain period (typically several years) they get a rebate of the premium they've paid in over the period—plus the employer's

Figure 6.4

Sickness Fund Drug Spending and Prescription Volume From 1981 to 1991

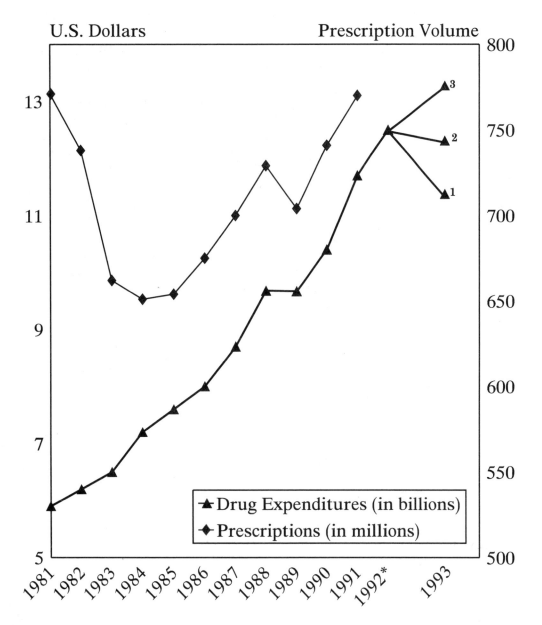

* Projected; [1] without 1993 reform law; [2] with 1993 price reductions and freezes; [3] with 1993 physicians' drug budget. DM converted to U.S. dollars using purchasing power parity conversion.

Source: Kassenärztliche Bundesvereinigung (1993). Schaubildsammlung zur Information und Argumentationshilfe, chart D6 and Sachverständigenrat für die Konzertierte Aktion im Gesundheitswesen (1992).

Table 6.4

Physician Contacts and Drugs Prescribed in 1990

	Physician Contacts/Person/Year	Prescriptions/ Person/Year
Germany	11.2	11.6
United States	5.5	6.4

German prescription forms may list more than one drug (average in 1990, 1.71), while U.S. prescription forms list only one drug.

Source: Health United States *(1991). Washington: Department of Health and Human Services, p. 219; Simonsen, LLP (1992). What are Pharmacies Dispensing Most Often?* Pharmacy Times, *Vol. 4, p. 47; and Kassenärztliche Bundesvereinigung (1992). Grunddaten zur kassenärztlichen Versorgung in der Bundesrepublik Deutschland 1991, chart E4.*

share. However, some private insurers have begun dropping their rebate program at the same time as they are increasing premiums faster than the sickness funds.

Needless to say, privately insured patients aren't happy. But because there are strict rules prohibiting a return to the sickness fund system, where rates are lower, these people appear to be stuck where they are.

Generics Arise

The development with the greatest impact on drug spending in Germany over the past decade has been the rapid rise of generic alternatives to brand-name drugs. In the late 1960s and early 1970s, generics were erroneously viewed by drug makers and the sickness funds as a disappearing market that would ultimately be replaced by the latest and greatest innovative brand-name drugs. As R.K. Schicke, of the University of Hannover's department of epidemiology and social medicine, wrote in 1973: "Attempts to alter this pattern may become increasingly futile as more sophisticated drugs become abundantly available in proprietary form and displace the generic type."[28]

In the years following World War II, proprietary drugs had made significant inroads in all western countries. The market share of generics in the U.K., for example, fell from 93 percent in 1947 to 22 percent by 1968.[29] By 1970, generics made up only 9 percent of the market in the U.S., with similarly low proportions in France, West Germany, and Italy.[30]

By 1988, this trend had been reversed in Germany. In that year, generics accounted for 20.4 percent of total prescription drug sales and for 50.4 percent of prescription sales volume in markets with generic products.[31] In the U.S., generics made up 13 percent of new prescriptions written in 1991.[32] Counting refilled prescriptions, the number of generic prescriptions written annually in the U.S. may be as high as 40 percent.[33] U.S. generic sales amount to about $4 billion, or approximately 7.3 percent of total drug spending in the U.S.[34] A U.S. Office of Technology Assessment study found that six years after patent expiration, brand-name drugs still hold over 50 percent of the market in the U.S.[35]

One of the major reasons for the shift to generics in Germany is the economic monitoring system that provides feedback to physicians on a wide range of practice patterns, including drug prescribing. These practice profiles include a comparison of costs generated by the doctor's prescribing habits and show what the cost would have been had generics been prescribed in all possible cases.[36]

More Me-Too Drugs

Because of Germany's liberal drug-approval policies, there have always been a greater number of brand-name "me-too" drugs available in Germany relative to the U.S. Drug makers say that this has facilitated lower market prices through competition, though others say the high cost of developing copy-cat drugs negates the savings.

Until 1986, winning approval for a generic version was exceedingly easy in Germany: All that a generic manufacturer had to do was to prove that its machines could duplicate the drug.[37] Safety data weren't required. On top of that, the generic maker could legally get all files regarding manufacturing processes from the patent holder and proceed with production on the day the patent expired. Generic makers suffered a major setback in 1986, when the federal drug act was amended to add a copyright-like protection to manufacturing processes. A drug must now be on the market for at least 10 years before generic makers are allowed to have access to manufacturing information.

The Patients Are Guilty Too

Some have ascribed Germany's high drug consumption to the strong tradition of romantic medicine that has existed in Germany since the early nineteenth century. In her 1988 book, *Medicine & Culture*, Lynn Payer quotes anthropologist Felix Moos, PhD:

> While Americans often do things simply because they are practical, "in Germany nothing is done without Geist [spirituality]. Medically this means...that while Americans see the body as mechanical, Germans see health and the body as going hand in hand with Geist and nature. Part of the focus on balance that can be seen in German society, he believes, comes from the constant effort Germans have to make to balance that side of them that is efficient with their romantic side.

Payer observes that the German health care system tries to accommodate both the efficient and the romantic aspects of the German character by allowing reimbursement for high-tech medicine as well as herbal, homeopathic, and anthroposophic remedies. To achieve internal balance between competing systems, says Payer, drugs are often prescribed in combination; some 70 percent of drugs in Germany are combination products.[3] And because more attention is paid to a patient's resistance to infection than to the infection itself, antibiotic sales are proportionately lower in Germany than in the U.S.

Alternative medicine plays a big role in the German health system. Homeopathic and anthroposophic drugs account for thousands of the 8,250 preparations listed in the *Rote Liste*, the German equivalent of the *Physicians' Desk Reference*. There are even 1,400 herbal preparations. According to Payer, about one-fifth of German physicians practice either homeopathy, anthroposophic medicine, or plant therapy, all of which are recognized as valid therapeutic options by the sickness funds.

The romantic features of German medicine and the substantial role alternative medicine plays in the German system are confirmed in drug statistics. The German pharmacopoeia contains some 130,000 formulations of drugs.

A study of drugs for coronary diseases (coronary insufficiency, arrhythmia), done by Greiser in the early 1980s, suggested just how big the problem of ineffective drugs is in Germany: He found that one-quarter of 231 single-purpose drugs to be inadequate, while nearly all of 336 multipurpose drugs study were considered ineffective.

For decades, cardiac drugs have dominated Germany's top 10 list of drugs prescribed, due in part to the widespread labelling of unexplainable ills as *Herzinsuffienz*, or heart insufficiency. German doctors also favor diagnoses related to poor circulation, including low blood pressure, circulatory collapse, and vasovegatative dystonia, when patients complain of tiredness and fatigue. The latter two diagnoses are seldom considered in the U.S. Payer links these diagnostic patterns and Germans' strong romantic streak:

> The belief in America that the heart is just a pump is so strong that we became the first nation to seriously think that a machine could in fact replace it.... For Germans the heart is not just a pump, but an organ that has a life of its own, one that pulsates in response to a number of different stimuli including the emotions.... The German heart, as opposed to the American heart, retains some of the metaphorical associations with love and the emotions. At first such a concept seems silly, but upon further reflection it offers certain advantages over a purely mechanical model. This way of thinking about the heart probably led Europeans to recognize, long before Americans, that angina pectoris ... can be cause not just by a clogging, but also by a spasm of the coronary artery, a concept hard to integrate into the mechanical model.

Given Germany's romantic obsession with the heart and their devotion to improving circulation, it is not surprising that heart drugs are so frequently prescribed. Heart drugs were the most frequently prescribed drugs in the early 1980s, and they remain second only to nonsteroidal antiinflammatories and other arthritis and musculoskeletal drugs. Some 11.9 percent of prescriptions written in 1990 were for arthritis and rheumatic-pain drugs. Heart drugs accounted for 9.3 percent.

Recent worldwide attention to the risk of elevated cholesterol levels has not gone unnoticed in Germany, although German physicians and patients are not as obsessed with cholesterol lowering and healthy diets as Americans are. But Germans are beginning to pay more attention to their cholesterol levels, which are substantially higher than average U.S. levels (see Chapter Seven). And as new cholesterol-lowering drugs become available and studies showing their benefit continue to accumulate, it is not unreasonable to presume that heart drugs may once take over the number-one spot before the end of the decade.

History of Drug Cost Controls

German efforts to control drug expenditures date back decades. In recent years, each sector of the health system has contributed to drug expenditure controls, but until the mid-1970s, these efforts focused mainly on limiting the margins for wholesalers and retailers. These controls remain in place today.

Table 6.5

Prescription Volume by Drug Class, 1990

	Volume (in millions of prescriptions)	Percent change from 1989
Nonsteroidal antiinflammatories	88.4	7.2
Cough preparations	58.9	7.4
Stomach preparations	43.3	7.2
Skin preparations	35.8	5.4
Psychiatric drugs	35.3	1.1
Coronary artery drugs	29.9	8.0
Ophthalmologic products	26.6	6.6
Antibiotics and chemotherapeutics	25.5	9.9
Bronchial/asthma drugs	20.4	1.5
Congestive heart failure drugs	20.1	1.5
Circulatory enhancing drugs	18.6	-1.1

Source: Scientific Institute of Local Sickness Funds (WiDO), 1992.

(Table 6.5) Depending on the manufacturer's price, the wholesaler may tack on only 12 to 21 percent (average, 15 percent) to the price, while a retail pharmacist is allowed to add only 30 to 68 percent (average, 35 percent).[38] On a hypothetical drug with a retail price of DM 10 (Figure 6.5), the manufacturer's price would be DM 4.67 ($2.23), the wholesaler's markup, DM 0.94 ($0.45), the retailer's markup DM 3.16 ($1.51), and the value-added tax, DM 1.23 ($0.59).

Patients have also borne some of the brunt of cost controls, though these charges have always been modest. On August 1, 1969, for example, Germany introduced a sliding-scale drug copayment, replacing an earlier per-prescription form charge of DM 1.00 ($0.33). This copayment charged patients 20 percent of the prescription price, to a maximum of DM 2.50 ($0.83). But because a large number of patients were exempt from any charges—for instance, because they were low-income, pregnant, or under age 18—some 54.8 percent of prescriptions were dispensed free of charge in 1970.[39] Overall, copayments accounted for just

Figure 6.5

The Price Components of a Hypothetical DM 10 Drug

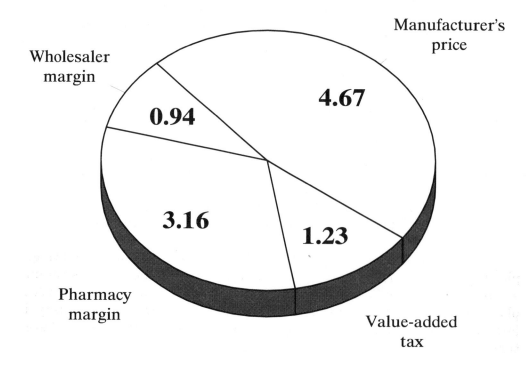

Source: *Kassenärztliche Bundesvereinigung (1993). Schaubildsammlung zur Information und Argumentationshilfe, chart D1.*

6.1 percent of German drug sales that year.[40] In contrast, only 9 percent of drugs in the U.S. were distributed at no cost to patients in 1964-65.[41]

German physicians have long been required to conform to "economical prescribing" rules, under threat of liability for monetary restitution (*Regresspflicht*).[42] But these rules were often vague and information about prices was not readily available to physicians. As Schicke wrote in 1973: "Needless to say, the available volume of preparations and the lack of accessibility to instant price information place rather heavy demands upon the physician's prescribing skills." In less polite terms, the rules were generally ignored.

Unlike today, the sickness funds in the 1970s weren't very concerned about drug prices and did not pressure retail pharmacies to compete on price. Indeed, they seemed more concerned with avoiding the bureaucratic complexity that competition might entail. As Schicke tells it:

> Surprisingly, it seems that in the Federal Republic competition at the retail level reflected in price differentials is thought to be "not quite desirable" for the Local Sick Funds... according to the director of the Funds' Federal Association this would make auditing more difficult and "impair" the comparability of drug statistics. Moreover, it is argued that the financial interests of the insured are not affected by possible price differentials. The desirability of more agile and competitive forces may well be doubtful to a system characterized by a very modest price-competitive mechanism at the industrial level, combined with adherence to recommended wholesale prices set by the manufacturers, and reinforced by expectations of retail price uniformity promulgated by the statutory insurance structure.[43]

Schicke concluded:

> In the Federal Republic the sellers' market is buttressed by a relatively insignificant degree of price competition both at the wholesale and retail levels. It is interesting to note that comprehensive drug benefit insurance schemes as existing in the Federal Republic may favor cost uniformity or condone minimal price competition, whereas in countries with pluralistically conceived, voluntary health and drug schemes, organizational diversification and experimentation seem to foster cost sensitivity and vigilance.[44]

The reform act of 1975 made the first meaningful efforts at bringing physicians into the loop of price-consciousness. The act called for publication of a **transparency list**, which would list the price of a drug, along with its pharmacokinetic data, active-agent content, identity, purity, and stability. By law, physicians were required to consider each of these factors each and every time a drug was prescribed. But because enforcement was lax, few did.

Voluntary Limits

During the 1970s, the German Pharmaceutical Manufacturers Association (*Bundesverband der Pharmazeutischen Industrie e.V.* or *BPI*) repeatedly negotiated voluntary self-restriction agreements between its members. The self-restrictions ran the gamut of perceived drug industry ills, from promotion to prices. Unlike the federal association of sickness funds and the sickness fund physicians' association, the pharmaceutical association is not a public corporation. Therefore, it cannot draw up binding contracts on prices and sales volumes between its constituent members. But it was more than happy to make broad, if often meaningless, pronouncements on behalf of members.

Prices were the focus of voluntary price controls recommended by the German pharmaceutical association to members in 1976, 1981, 1982, 1985, and 1987. Some of these came after federal investigations of "excessive" pricing. Under the various agreements, the association requested that members refrain from increasing prices and stabilize existing prices.[45] But these controls had little effect on the overall level of prices and did not appreciably slow the rate of sickness fund spending on drugs. (Figure 6.4)

In 1975, the association negotiated a self-restriction agreement on advertising practices, limiting the size and frequency of drug advertisements in medical journals. The agreement also established maximum expenditure figures for professional education about products and continuing medical education, and it set limits on the type and costs of presents that may be given to physicians.[46] U.S. drug companies' promotional practices also came under scrutiny in the 1970s and 1980s, but the first voluntary limits were not put into place until 1992, after intensive pressure from the U.S. FDA Commissioner, David Kessler, MD.

Government Weighs In

The German government was also actively involved in indirectly manipulating drug prices in the mid-1970s. The most significant effort came in the *Health Insurance Cost Containment Act* (HICCA) of 1977, which required that a drug-expenditure ceiling be established, in an attempt to alter physicians' prescribing practices. The limit was placed only on the sickness funds; providers were not directly responsible for any overages.[47]

This ceiling was considered to be an **orientational parameter** or voluntary global budget—the ceiling could not be enforced because it set no limits on the liability of the sickness funds for drug utilization by insureds. The ceiling also had little effect because drug makers are not contractually bound to abide by sickness fund rules.

The 1977 law also set targets for physicians' prescribing patterns for the first time, establishing thresholds above which physicians would receive a call from sickness funds to discuss budget overruns. But the law required proof that an individual physician had been intentionally "uneconomical" before financial penalties could be invoked. In an interpretation of the 1977 law, the University of Tübingen's Arnold wrote:

> Should an impermissible prescription practice be detected, the [sickness fund] physicians who are substantially responsible for the overexpenditure on drugs must be individually informed or counseled where necessary. Only after information or counseling has been unsuccessful should additional selected individual checks be carried out.... It must be proved that a physician has prescribed drugs uneconomically before regression of drug costs can be granted; regression of drug costs merely because the maximum level of drug expenditure has been exceeded would be illegal.[48]

In practice, most physicians ignored the ceiling, though they became more sensitized to the price of drugs. Writes Arnold:

> The contractual parties to medical care...agree that the drug expenditure ceiling which must be negotiated between the parties has primarily an advisory value.... When the maximum is exceeded, the severity of the overexpenditure must be determined. In general, the contractual parties have agreed to view a 10 percent cost overrun beyond the planned rate of growth in drug expenditures as *slight* [*emphasis added*].[49]

Price List. A more effective part of the 1977 reform act was the creation of a comparative list of single-agent drugs and their prices (*Preisvergleichsliste*) as an appendix to earlier drug guidelines.[50] The list divided products into three categories: products that are appropriate for relevant indications; products that are appropriate for relevant indications in some cases; and products which require careful consideration.[51] Products are then listed according to their average daily cost.

The 1977 Act also called for creation of a **negative list** or "blacklist" of drugs shown to have no value and those for minor ailments such as coughs and colds. But the federal health minister at the time did not immediately approve this list, and implementation of a negative list did not come until 1983.[52]

But the negative list proposed in 1977 laid the groundwork for the list enacted in 1983 and expansion of the list in later reforms. Drugs on the list were to be excluded from the rules requiring reimbursement of all prescribed drugs whether prescription-only or over-the-counter. Some drugs were to be ruled out altogether, while others could be prescribed if the physician justified the medical need. According to a publication by Arnold in 1981,[53] the list would have prohibited.

- ☐ weight-reducing drugs/preparations,
- ☐ cellular therapeutics,
- ☐ tonics,
- ☐ ablactation drugs (unless medically indicated),
- ☐ geriatrics (when they are intended to influence physiologic effects of aging), and
- ☐ vitamin preparations (except in vitamin deficiency).

Also to be prohibited from reimbursement were drugs for minor health ailments such as coughs and colds. Dressings and bandages were also *verboten*.

Drug Industry Structure

The German pharmaceutical industry is made up of some 1,000 manufacturers, which employ 122,200 people.[54] There is a huge number of preparations sold in Germany with 8,262 substances currently licensed for sale.[55] The industry is characterized by a large number of small companies with very low market share. (Table 6.7) About half of Germany's domestic market is dominated by foreign companies, compared with 31 percent penetration by foreign companies in the U.S., and 20 percent in Japan. Non-European community manufacturers have 30 percent of the total EC market.[56] Viewed another way, the five leading pharmaceutical companies hold just 12 percent of the market in Germany, while the 10 leading companies hold 21.6 percent.[57]

Table 6.6

Maximum Allowable Retail Drug Markup

Retail price in DM	Maximum markup in percent
0 to 2.40	68.0
2.64 to 7.60 (between 7.61 and 8.26, a fixed price of DM 4.71)	62.0
8.27 to 14.28 (between 14.29 and 16.96, a fixed price of DM 8.14)	57.0
16.97 to 23.75 (between 23.76 and 26.51, a fixed price of DM 11.40)	48.0
26.52 to 38.00 (between 38.01 and 44.16, a fixed price of DM 16.34)	43.0
44.17 to 57.00 (between 57.01 and 70.30, a fixed price of DM 21.09)	37.0
above 70.30	23.1

Source: German pharmacists' handbook.

Table 6.7

Germany's Pharmaceutical Industry 1990

Sales (in million of DM and $U.S.)	Number of firms	Percent distribution
to 7.5 ($3.6)	23	15.6
7.5 to 15 ($7.2)	11	7.4
15 to 45 ($21.5)	34	23.0
45 to 150 ($71.8)	36	24.3
over 150	37	25.0
Eastern states	7	4.7
TOTAL	**148**	

Soruce: Bundesverband der Pharmazeutischen Industrie e.V. (1992). Pharma Daten '92. *Hofheim: Gutenberg-Druck und Verlag.*

The leading 10 products in Germany account for 10 percent of the market; the leading 1,000, 77.4 percent; the leading 2,000, 95 percent. As Dietrich Nord, PhD, assistant professor of sociology at the University of Constance, observed in 1986:

> The special drugs contained in the remaining 5 percent are, however, hardly superfluous. Many can be kept on the market only through manufacturers' balancing their business calculations since there is usually little demand for them and in numerous instances they fail to meet their costs. This applies to almost all drugs against tropical diseases (which must be available in the FRG if they are to be administered appropriately) and to drugs against very rare diseases and organic disorders (such as the drug "Androcur," which treats sexual deviations and hypersexuality. It also applies to vaccines stockpiled in case of epidemics.[58]

Nord also observed that West Germany's 2,000 leading drugs were roughly equivalent to the number decreed as essential by the more financially strapped East German government. Deborah Stone, professor of law and social policy at Brandeis University, made a similar observation in 1991:

An East German surgeon who now practices in the West showed me her catalogues of available pharmaceuticals for the two countries, the equivalent of the *Physicians' Desk Reference*. The East German book was about one and a half inches thick, the West German one, about four inches. She felt the pharmaceutical armamentarium of the East was fully adequate. There seems to be general agreement that East Germany had some supply problems with certain classes of drugs, such as antibiotics and chemotherapeutic agents for cancer. But West German health experts have conclude that almost a third of prescription drugs on the West German market have not been proven effective, and drugs are overused in a variety of ways.[59]

Exports Start To Slip

The German pharmaceutical industry is one of the world's leading exporters, though it falls far behind Japan and the U.S. Germany's premier position as the world's leading drug exporter during the 1970s has been diminishing steadily over the past two decades. Between 1968 and 1973, Germany held the top rank in world drug exports, while it remained third in total drug output.[60] Now the U.S. leads exports with 31 percent of world pharmaceutical market, followed by the EC as a whole (30 percent), Japan (18 percent), and Germany (7 percent).

In 1990, West German companies exported pharmaceuticals with a value of 10.6 billion DM ($5.1 billion) or 41.3 percent of the total production. Companies in eastern Germany produced pharmaceuticals valued at DM 5 billion in 1989 and exported about 50 percent.[61] By 1991, German pharmaceutical exports after reunification had risen to DM 12.1 billion ($5.8 billion). The total production value of the German pharmaceutical industry is estimated to be DM 30.9 billion ($14.8 billion), of which the new eastern German states account for DM 1.7 billion ($813.4 million). In contrast, U.S. exports of pharmaceutical products to all countries by members the PMA were $22.2 billion in 1991, or 33 percent of production.[62]

East Germany: A Drug Industry Evaporates

Within a year of reunification, the new eastern states' drug industry had shrunk dramatically. Before the Wall fell, the East German drug industry supplied not only that country's entire drug needs — more or less — it was also a major exporter to other nations in the Communist Bloc. But by the end of 1991, the companies that remained in the east held only 40 percent of the eastern states' pharmaceutical market.[64]

The demise of the eastern drug industry is blamed on two things: the "solidarity rebate" and the costs of modernizing often-decrepit manufacturing plants. Immediately after the Wall fell, all western companies were ordered to discount prices by 55 percent to eastern German pharmacies. On April 1, 1991, this discount was modified: All German companies—including those in the east—were required to grant a 25 percent discount on all deliveries to eastern Germany. A solidarity rebate was also required to be carried by wholesalers (24 percent) and retailers (22 percent). The hope was to ease the economic integration of the two countries—at the time, marks from the east were officially exchanged at a 3:1 rate and unofficially exchanged at much lower rates.

In 1989, East German companies produced pharmaceuticals valued at DM 5 billion ($2.4 billion) and exported about 50 percent of total production. By 1991, however, total production had fallen to DM 1.7 billion ($813 million) and exports had essentially stopped. A campaign among western physicians to increase prescribing of eastern-produced drugs to bolster employment there failed to have much effect. In 1992, pharmaceutical sales in the eastern states amounted to DM 4.1 billion ($2 billion); DM 28.5 billion ($13.6 billion) in the west. Spending in the eastern states rose at an annual rate of 27.3 percent between January and September 1992, according to *Deutsches Ärzteblatt* in January of 1993.

When the wall fell, numerous discrepancies between pharmacotherapy in the east and west appeared. Easterners didn't have cimetidine or angiotensin-converting enzyme inhibitors, two of the most frequently prescribed drugs in the west. Eastern manufacturers tried to invade the western market, especially with birth control pills, but they were ill-equipped to challenge the more advanced western companies.

When the sickness funds took over health care in the eastern states, there was much confusion. Many citizens, unaccustomed to western ways, didn't understand why toothpaste was no a longer covered expense. After all, it had been a long tradition under the Communists.

European Community

A major external factor influencing Germany's drug industry was the removal of trade barriers between the 12 European Community trading partners at the end of 1992. Though this was not expected to have an immediate impact on individual countries, it did affect some $34 billion worth of pharmaceutical products throughout Europe. According to the PMA, U.S. manufacturers account for one-quarter of the European drug market.

Major issues regarding patent protection, product registration, pricing, reimbursement, and approval standards have been the subject of negotiations for years, but relatively little has been resolved. The EC Parliament and Council are now considering a proposal that would establish a system transferring authority for approval of pharmaceutical products from member states to the EC.

Patent issues are furthest along. The EC legislature has approved rules that extend patent protection through a supplementary protection certificate. According to PMA, these rules provide compensation during the period devoted to product development and testing when the patent protection has a small financial value. The certificate will have a maximum of five years' duration, and it will provide up to 15 years' effective coverage. Similar legislation has recently been enacted in the U.S. and Japan, according to PMA.

On pricing, the EC adopted in 1989 a **pricing transparency directive** that requires each EC member to disclose pricing policies and reimbursement decisions, and that such decisions be made on the basis of objective and verifiable criteria. The EC has officially certified that all member states have complied with this directive, but the PMA says that it hasn't significantly changed pricing and reimbursement. Yet the PMA complains that these measures are taking the EC away from the free market it so cherishes. The PMA warns that as trade barriers are lowered, lower prices will result, "which will make it increasingly difficult for industry to fund essential research and development."[63] It also warns that product trade will flow from low-price EC member states such as Greece and Spain to members with higher prices, such as Germany. PMA has lobbied the EC for an U.S.-like open market in pharmaceuticals, but given the nature of members' socialized health care economies, that is unlikely.

Developing and Selling Drugs

Though they make up a relatively small proportion of the market, Germany's largest drug firms proportionately allocate far more of their budget to research and development than do smaller companies. (Table 6.8) According to the German pharmaceutical association, approximately DM 5.1 billion ($2.4 billion) was invested in 1990 by pharmaceutical companies in research and development in Germany. The association reports that only about 15 of 1,000 manufacturers carry out fundamental research.[64]

Overall, research and development accounts for 19.4 percent of manufacturers' costs in Germany; according to the PMA, U.S. companies invested 15.9 percent of U.S. sales plus exports in R&D in 1990. Because U.S. R&D expenditures have been rising by about 10 percent annually since 1980, U.S. firms had increased the percentage of sales plus exports devoted to R&D to 16.7 percent by 1993. The U.S. Office of Technology Assessment estimates that U.S. pharmaceutical firms spent $8.13 billion worldwide on R&D in 1990.[65]

Drug Approval in Germany

The large number of drugs available in Germany can be tied to its drug approval process, which until 1978 required only proof of safety, not efficacy. It has been estimated that 31 percent of drugs currently available in Germany are ineffective,[66] amounting to approximately DM 6.1 billion ($2.9 billion).[67] Many are homeopathic or anthroposophic remedies of questionable value. Both of these movements have deep roots in German history and politicians are loathe to limit reimbursement for these remedies.

Compared with the U.S. Food and Drug Administration's stringent, years-long process for approving new brand-name drugs, the German Federal Health Agency, appears casual. Before 1978, all a German manufacturer had to prove was that a drug did no harm before being granted a license to market a new chemical entity. This law dated back to the early 1960s, when all industrialized nations restructured their drug approval process in the wake of the thalidomide tragedies.

In 1968, several years after drug laws had been revamped, the German Federal Health Agency approved 1,739 preparations—versus 11 by the U.S. FDA. Between 1978 and 1990, the German agency approved approximately 9,750 drugs.[68] During this period approximately 10,000 unprocessed applications accumulated, along with 30,683 applications for drugs approved before 1978. By 1987, the average time between patenting a new entity and its approval was 12.3 years, leaving only 7.7 years for marketing under patent.[69]

Because of increasing data showing that many of the drugs available in Germany were of little or no value, the 1978 health reform law required the Federal Health Agency to include efficacy studies as part of the approval process. This measure, the *Second Medication Law*, required efficacy studies for

Table 6.8

German Pharmaceutical Manufacturers' Distribution of Costs, 1990

Size of firm	<$3.6	3.6-7	7-21	21-72	>72	East	All
Production	49.9%	39.9%	45.4%	37.9%	38.8%	37.1%	39.0%
Research & development	3.9	4.5	5.5	8.2	21.8	4.5	19.4
Licensing	1.1	2.5	1.8	0.8	1.9	0.0	1.7
Professional education	17.3	9.8	15.0	17.3	10.5	0.8	11.2
Advertising	4.2	8.0	6.8	7.8	3.3	1.2	3.9
Marketing	8.3	19.9	7.5	12.7	8.8	6.5	9.2
Administration	17.7	10.8	12.0	8.9	8.0	19.0	8.4
Interest	1.9	1.9	1.2	1.2	1.9	0.4	1.8
Taxes	2.4	1.4	1.4	1.7	2.6	0.1	2.4
Other expenditures	6.7	1.3	3.4	3.5	2.4	30.4	3.0

Size of firm in millions of dollars in sales. Converted to U.S. dollars using a purchasing power parity conversion.

Source: *Bundesverband der Pharmazeutischen Industrie e.V. (1992)*. Pharma Daten '92. *Hofheim: Gutenberg-Druck und Verlag.*

pre-1978 drugs also, but as the backlog indicates, very few drugs have been formally approved, though they remain on the market.[70]

With the new rules have come delays in approval times and increased research and development costs. By 1988 the costs of developing a new chemical entity and submitting it for review before the Federal Health Agency were estimated at DM 250 million ($116.8 million). The U.S. Office of Technology Assessment, which advises Congress, estimated that the average cost of bringing a new chemical entity to market in the U.S. in the 1980s was $194 million.[71] Observers attribute the higher U.S. costs to stricter FDA rules, which necessitate larger numbers of subjects in clinical trials, and longer FDA backlogs. The average time for FDA approval of new drugs in the U.S. in 1990 was 27.7 months; 1991, 30.3 months; and 1992, 29.9 months.

In 1992, innovative drugs accounted for 35 percent of the total prescription volume in Germany, and they are responsible for about two-thirds of the increase in spending.[72] By contrast, brand-name drugs in the U.S. accounted for 86.3 percent of prescription volume in 1991. As noted earlier, U.S. sales of generics amount to about $4 billion, or approximately 7.3 percent of total drug spending. That share of the U.S. market is expected to change dramatically during the mid-1990s as more than 60 major drugs lose patent protection or other exclusive rights between 1992 and 1995.[73]

According to pharmaceutical industry officials, German authorities are far less restrictive than the U.S. when considering innovative new drugs.[74] Companies do not have to prove that a product is better than other existing drugs, as is often required by the U.S. FDA. According to Hans Hapke of Gödecke, a medium-size drug firm, the German approach translates into "far less" innovative competition to establish a new drug, meaning that delays are shorter for me-too products. "Within three to four years of marketing a new drug, a slightly similar drug will appear on the market," Hapke says.[75]

Promotion

As in the U.S., German drug companies spend more on "professional education," advertising, and marketing than on research and development, but they spend even more on this sort of promotion than U.S. companies do. Combined, these three areas accounted for 24.3 percent of German drug costs in 1990, according to the German pharmaceutical association,[76] although some estimates run as high as 30 percent[77] or 40 percent.[78] In contrast, U.S. companies spent about 22 percent of their budgets on marketing in 1991.[79]

High promotional expenses have existed in Germany for more than two decades. In the late 1960s, promotional costs accounted for 18.8 percent of drug sales in the U.S., while at the same time in Germany, a federal commission estimated that promotional costs made up 25 to 40 percent of total drug sales.[80] In contrast, promotional costs were 12.2 percent in the U.K., 17.6 percent in Canada, and 16 percent in Belgium.[81]

In noting Germany's large number of **detailers**—salespeople who visit doctors to provide scientific "information" and patient samples, Arnold chides the companies for their insistence that such "consultants" are needed for physician education about their products: "Given the infrequency with which new drugs representing real breakthroughs are launched onto the market, it is evident that the essential function of pharmaceutical consultants is not to provide physicians with information on new products and substances, but to promote the sale of pharmaceutical products."[82]

Anecdotes about lavish promotional spending by drug companies are as legendary in Germany as they are in the U.S. One physician interviewed for this book noted that oversized leather chairs in his office came from a drug company seeking to "educate" him about its product. Another related an unconfirmed story that a large drug maker bought television sets for every room in a hospital in order to get its drugs on the hospital's formulary.

There is no question that German physicians are bombarded by as much promotional literature and publications in the mail as their U.S. counterparts, and perhaps even more. There are even *daily* medical newspapers filled with advertisements that are sent free to physicians. Such aggressiveness by drug promoters is made possible only because of Germany's highly efficient postal system, which guarantees next day delivery of common mail nationwide.

Drug makers' largesse has not gone unnoticed by federal regulators. In 1986, federal limits were passed restricting the number of free drug samples to two per physician per year. But physicians report that this has had little effect on the practice—an eastern German physician says she liberally supplies free samples to her patients as a marketing ploy of her own.[83]

Pharmacies

Over the years, drug spending in Germany has been largely a factor of its noncompetitive retail structure. Prices in retail pharmacies are strictly regulated and are uniform.[84] In 1970, the maximum allowed markup at the retail pharmacy before tax was 33.5 percent.[85] During the same period, markup in the U.S. averaged 44.3 percent.[86] The average prescription cost in the U.S. in 1970 was $4.02, as reported by the *Lilly Digest* that year, while the average cost in West Germany was $1.57. As quoted by Schicke, the *Digest* concluded that "more than 50 percent is attributable to the acquisition cost of the drug product dispensed.... [The report suggests] that drug product costs are generally artificially inflated due to lack of meaningful price competition among manufacturers of prescription drug products." Schicke adds that a similar statement could be made about the German drug-price situation, particularly because Germany also regulated the wholesale price set by manufacturers,[87] a practice that continues to this day.

Drug prices in the U.S. have always been moderated to some extent by the growth of chain-store drug outlets and discount pharmacies—two phenomena without analogies in Germany. Between 1964 and 1970, chain and discount pharmacies grew from 11 percent to 32 percent of the U.S. market.[88] The National Association of Chain Drug Stores says that chain drug stores filled 40.5 percent of all outpatient prescriptions in 1991, up from 39.5 percent in 1990.[89] Total sales of prescription drugs through chain stores was $17 million in 1991.[90]

In contrast, proprietary drugs are sold almost exclusively through licensed independent pharmacies in Germany. (Table 6.9) Pharmacies in Germany are mom-and-pop affairs, on the whole, and are tied culturally into the country's long tradition of skilled craftspeople who are trained in a particular field beginning in their mid-teens. These stores sell only prescription and nonprescription drugs and related sundries; pharmacies in supermarkets or large discount stores are more or less unknown.

Table 6.9

Pharmacies in Germany, 1985-90

	Retail		Hospital		Pharmacists	
	Total	Change from prev. year in %	Total	Change from prev. year in %	Total	Change from prev. year in %
1985	17,705	--	518	--	32,234	--
1986	17,960	1.4	521	0.6	33,025	2.5
1987	18,161	1.2	524	0.6	33,903	2.7
1988	18,301	7.7	520	-0.7	34,498	1.8
1989	18,432	0.7	522	0.4	35,181	2.0
1990	18,549	0.6	520	-0.4	36,474	3.7

Source: Sachverständigenrat für die Konzertierte Aktion im Gesundheitswesen (1992). Jahresgutachten 1991. *p. 256.*

German pharmacies do have one advantage over American pharmacies when it comes to nonprescription drugs. Most over-the-counter drugs can be sold only in pharmacies. Aspirin, ibuprofen, and even some vitamins and mineral supplements are restricted to sale only in government-licensed pharmacies.

Hospital Market

In 1973, hospital pharmacies were found in barely 9 percent of the 3,494 hospitals in West Germany.[91] The purchase of drugs by hospitals is conducted mainly via retail stores. These costs are not reflected in sickness fund totals for drug expenditures, though they are occasionally calculated for comparison purposes.

Only larger hospitals tend to have in-house pharmacies.[92] Even so, hospital pharmacies accounted for 14 percent of total drug costs incurred by the statutory sickness funds in 1973, according to Schicke. In the U.S. in 1970, 75 percent of hospitals had a pharmacy, but these commanded only 11 percent of all medications sold in the U.S.[93] By 1991, drug sales through U.S. hospitals accounted for 23 percent of all drug sales, or $11.4 billion.[94]

Today in Germany, manufacturers sell brand-name drugs to hospitals at markedly reduced rates in the hopes of stimulating demand in the outpatient market. The 1989 reform tried to restrict this practice by requiring hospitals to release only the name of the active ingredient—not the brand name—when a patient is given a continuing prescription at discharge.[95]

Undercurrents for Reform

By the mid-1970s, the funds had come under increasing pressure to control costs. Premiums to individuals and employers were rising steadily. And Germany's drug prices were becoming legendary as the highest in Europe. Prescription volume and physician prescribing patterns were increasingly the focus of concern. As Arnold noted in 1982:

> In 1979, a general practitioner wrote an average of about 2,300 prescriptions per quarter, with the average prescription comprising two drugs. The average cost of drugs per general practitioner prescription in 1979 was DM 24.00 [$9.30]. Thus the GP causes more costs to the [sickness] funds through drug prescription for his patients than he receives in fees for [sickness fund] practice. General practitioners accounted for 66.4 percent of total prescriptions of [sickness fund] physicians in 1979, internists accounted for 15.8 percent.[96]

The first meaningful laws on physician prescribing took effect in 1977, with the enactment of the HICCA. This Act for the first time placed full responsibility on physicians for prescription volume. Average prescribing patterns for each specialty were added to the profiles already in use and adjusted for practice demographics. Doctors who fell outside the acceptable limits forfeited income. As a result, prescription volume fell precipitously during the early 1980s, reaching a nadir of 651 million prescriptions in 1985. But the reform failed to make a dent in sickness fund spending on drugs, which continued its sharp upward curve. And by 1988, prescription volume had risen again to 729 million, just under the 1982 level.

During the early 1980s, it became attractive to doctors to prescribe parallel-imported drugs as a way to lower costs. German companies typically exported their drugs to another country then reimported them at a lower price. Most drugs were routed through France, where drugs were much cheaper.[97] Parallel-imports' share was 10 to 15 percent of the original brand, accounting for 2 to 3 percent of the total pharmaceutical market, a figure that has not changed appreciably today.[98]

The other major reform that laid the foundation for the 1989 and 1993 reforms was the negative list, first proposed in 1977, as described above, and enacted in 1983. The 1983 list, for the first time, prohibited reimbursement for drugs for coughs and colds; mouth, nose, and throat conditions (other than fungal infections); travel sickness; and laxatives. There were no relevant savings from this attempt to reduce prescriptions for minor ailments, as Figure 6.4 demonstrates. According to several observers, doctors simply changed the diagnosis and prescribed drugs that were reimbursable.

Planting the Seeds of Structural Reform

While the 1993 reform officially ordered a structural overhaul of Germany's health system, the seeds for structural change were planted in the 1989 reform. The most significant provisions of the 1989 reform called for sweeping changes in pharmaceutical pricing and physician prescribing patterns. Like earlier reform laws, the 1989 reform didn't tear down existing structures. Rather, it built new layers of regulation utilizing the successful strategy of negotiations between providers.

The pharmaceutical provisions of the 1989 reform act set out four cost-containment measures, of which "reference pricing" has garnered the most attention internationally. The Act (known as the *Gesundheitsreform Gesetz* or *GRG*) also increased the number of nonreimbursable drugs on the negative list, and it introduced **prescription volume controls** (*Richtgrössen*), which put individual doctors at direct financial risk for the volume of drugs they were prescribing, rather than penalizing them for the somewhat vague sin of "uneconomical prescribing." The Act also raised patients' copayments from DM 2 ($0.95) to DM 3 ($1.42). The average copayment was DM 24 ($11) in 1990 (DM 48 for pensioners and DM 17 for others).[99]

The stated goal of the 1989 pharmaceutical measures was to induce more price competition among pharmaceutical suppliers and to instill a more cost-conscious attitude in physicians. It called for total health care savings of DM 13.9 billion ($6.6 billion), of which pharmaceuticals were to provide DM 4.3 billion ($2 billion), or about 30 percent of the total savings. Many drug industry officials expressed outrage at the time, complaining bitterly that the drug industry was being asked to contribute far more than its fair share to savings. At the time, drugs accounted for "only" 15 percent of sickness funds' spending, as the German pharmaceutical association frequently noted. Even liberal members of Germany's Parliament (*Bundestag*) agreed that the reform was uneven, although they were less sensitive to drug makers' concerns. As Martin Pfaff, a professor of economics at the University of Augsburg and a Social Democrat in the *Bundestag*, recalls:

> I remember stating to the *Süddeutsche Zeitung* [newspaper] that we knew very well that the package as it existed, to be quite blunt, would not suffice to guarantee medium or long-term stability to expenditure growth.... First, the distribution of burdens between the insurer and the providers was not equitable. Of course that's a normative judgment and somebody else may come to a different conclusion. But the sacrifices expected were largely on the side of the insured, and to be more specific, on the side of sick persons. About 7 billion deutschmarks of coinsurance payments were expected.... [Federal health minister] Blüm expanded this to the extent of about 7 billion and I felt at that time and still feel today that this was not equitably distributed.[100]

As it turned out, the drug industry's worst fears didn't materialize, though some smaller firms with only a few products did take a beating. The reference price system did lead to a "perceptible intensification" in drug-price competition, according to Gerhard Schulte, a federal health official. But in the end, economy-wide spending on all drugs (reimbursed and nonreimbursed) dropped just one one-hundredth of a percentage point of GDP between 1989 and 1990. (Figure 6.3) After a run up in the final quarter of 1988 by patients seeking to beat the copayment increase, sickness-fund expenditures on drugs dipped slightly in the first quarter of 1989 (Table 6.10), but then began a steady rise in the following quarter. Similarly, prescription volume dropped by 25 million prescriptions for 1989 as a whole, but jumped back to the high 1982 levels in the following year. Other data also point to the measure's limited effect: Total sickness fund

Table 6.10

Impact of 1989 Reform Law on Sickness Funds' Expenditures for Prescription Drugs

Quarter	Payments (millions)	Change over previous year, same quarter (in percent)
I/1988	$ 2,229.6	
II/1988	2,336.4	
III/1988	2,348.3	
IV/1988	2,663.5	
I/1989	2,236.6	-1.1
II/1989	2,447.0	+3.3
III/1989	2,437.0	+2.3
IV/1989	2,467.0	+8.7
I/1990	2,472.1	+9.5
II/1990	2,622.2	+6.1
III/1990	2,587.6	+5.2

Source: Sachverständigenrat für die Konzertierte Aktion im Gesundheitswesen (1992). Jahresgutachten 1991. *pp. 107.*

spending on drugs fell just DM 218 million ($104 million). The pharmaceutical price index remained unchanged between 1989 and 1990, at 126.3, but it rose again in 1991 to 127.9. (Table 6.11) And per-insured sickness fund spending on drugs was only one dollar lower in 1989 than 1988. (Table 6.12)

Schulte believes that the increasingly intense competition among doctors in private practice promotes a willingness to prescribe generously and thus uneconomically. He notes that expenditures rose by 10.2 percent in 1991, while drug prices rose only 2 percent. Additionally, innovative drugs accounted for only 2.5 percent of the cost increase. The rise in the amount of drugs prescribed per insured person was consequently responsible for 5.7 percent of the increase. "There is no medical explanation for this development," Schulte says. "However, it is a fact that, over the same period, the number of doctors had risen by 3.5 percent, and it would seem that more physicians prescribe more drugs."[101] (Interpretations of what drove up prices in 1991 vary, see Figure 6.7.)

Dental Copayment Takes a Bite

The impact of the 1989 law on other sectors has been discussed in other chapters. As the per-insured data show, most of the savings from the reform was gained from reduced spending on dentures, dental crowns, and bridges. (Table

6.12) The GRG raised the copayment on dentures and dental materials such as crowns and bridges from zero to 40 percent, effective January 1, 1989.[102] But even the decreased spending on dental appliances did not last long. As drug industry analyst Heinz Redwood wrote in 1992:

> By 1990, the sickness funds' net dental costs, after deducting copayment receipts, began to rise substantially, as patients became accustomed to paying for part of the cost of their crowns and bridges when there was no free alternative, and as dentists found ways and means of raising the volume of materials anchored in patients' mouths. In other words, behavioral patterns developed not as officials had planned, but apparently "perversely." There are lessons in this for pharmaceutical cost containment.[103]

Table 6.11

Trends in Cost of Living Compared with Pharmaceutical Prices, 1980-91

	Living costs all private households		Pharmaceutical prices	
	Index 1980 = 100	Change in percent	Index 1980 = 100	Change in percent
1980	100.0	5.4	100.0	4.8
1981	106.3	6.3	105.6	5.6
1982	111.9	5.3	108.2	2.5
1983	115.6	3.3	113.5	4.9
1984	118.4	2.4	116.9	3.0
1985	121.0	2.2	120.3	2.9
1986	120.7	-0.2	121.8	1.2
1987	121.0	0.2	122.8	0.8
1988	122.4	1.2	124.1	1.1
1989	125.8	2.8	126.3	1.7
1990	129.2	2.7	126.3	0.0
1991	133.9	3.5	127.9	1.3

Source: Sachverständigenrat für die Konzertierte Aktion im Gesundheitswesen (1992). Jahresgutachten 1991. p. 108, and Bundesverband der Pharmazeutischen Industrie e.V. (1992). Pharma Daten '92. Hofheim: Gutenberg-Druck und Verlag.

Negative List Grows

Indeed, the widespread and often baroque manipulation of loopholes by patients, physicians, and drug makers is one of the main lessons of the 1989 reform. Reaction to the expansion of the 1983 negative list is a case in point. The 1989 reform broadened the list beyond drugs for minor ailments, to include all uneconomical drugs. A committee made up of appointees from the federal doctors' panel and the sickness funds plus three independent members was to oversee and approve all additions to the list. The reform law called for an end to reimbursement for drugs that

☐ contain active ingredients not needed to fulfill their therapeutic purpose or to reduce risks;

☐ contain more than three medically active ingredients (does not apply to natural remedies); and

☐ are therapeutically unproved.

The Health Ministry printed and distributed its version of the new negative list, even though the private-sector committee had refused to agree to it. But because of the health minister's reserve powers, a court ruled that the health minister's list was legal and enforceable.[104]

The original aim of the expansion was to create a new negative list of 6,000 products with sales of about DM 4.5 billion ($2.1 billion). Redwood says the threat of delisting persuaded the affected companies to withdraw 3,500 products voluntarily. But these products were often reformulated and relaunched as products acceptable for reimbursement. The remaining 2,500 accounted for about DM 1.5 billion ($711 million) in sales.[105]

Table 6.12

Impact of 1989 Reform Law, Selected *GKV* Spending Classes Per Insured

	Total services	Physician services	Dental appliances	Dental	Drugs from pharmacy	Durable equipment	Misc.
1987	$1,554	261	92	78	235	98	88
1988	1,697	273	97	122	258	113	54
1989	1,654	288	98	62	257	100	50
1990	1,787	307	103	61	276	106	67

Does not include hospital care, disability payments, prevention, or maternity care, all of which demonstrated modest rises after the 1989 reform law (when converted to a PPP basis).

Source: Daten des Gesundheitswesens *(1991). Page 175.*

Figure 6.6

Value-Added Taxes, 1992

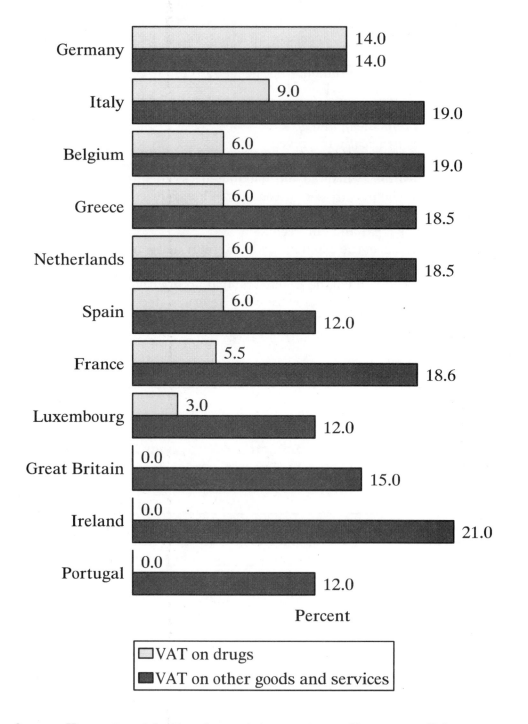

Source: Kassenärztztiche Bundesvereinigung, 1992, Kassenärztztliche Bundesvereinigung (1993). Schaubildsammlung zur Information und Argumetationshilfe, chart D3.

At the time, federal health officials asserted that savings were not the primary goal of the list; rather the list was intended to promote "more rational" prescribing practices and to discourage the use of Germany's long list of ineffective medications. The total negative impact on drug companies sales was estimated at only DM 200 million ($95 million). Larger declines did not occur because the drugs were still available for purchase by patients with their own money.[106] Indeed, by 1990 the sales of self-medication products had reached DM 4.8 billion ($2.3 billion), an increase of 12 percent over the previous year.[107] Physicians also reacted by substituting medicines not on the negative list so that patients would get a reimbursable—and probably more costly—drug.[108]

Reference Prices (*Festbeträge*)

The cornerstone of the 1989 reform law was the creation of an elaborate new pricing system designed to force the price of brand-name drugs down to generic levels. Some 80 percent of drugs reimbursed by the sickness funds were to be covered by the reference pricing system within three years of the law's enactment. Initially, reference pricing had the intended effect on drugs that were covered, but gaping loopholes in the system subverted its overall savings goals. As noted above, reforms in the pharmaceutical sector were supposed to produce DM 4.5 billion in savings for the sickness funds, but didn't. The reference price system did, however, lower prices on affected drugs by 7.3 percent overall. (Table 6.14)

Figure 6.7

Components of Drug Price Increases* Between 1990 and 1991

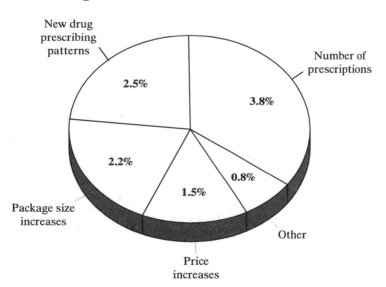

*Drug spending by sickness funds rose a total of 10.8 percent during this time.

Source: Kassenärztliche Bundesvereinigung (1993). Schaubildsammlung zur Information und Argumentationshilfe, chart D3.

Table 6.13

Annual Change in Spending on Dental Materials, *GKV** Funds, 1960-90

	GKV spending (in millions)	Dentures' portion of *GKV* outlays (in %)	Change in total spending over previous years (in %)	Per capita *GKV* spending on dental materials
1970	$ 273.3	3.5	--	$ 9
1980	2,964.1	8.6	--	83
1985	3,468.8	7.1	+ 4.5	96
1986	3,106.8	6.0	-10.0	85
1987	2,868.9	5.3	- 8.9	78
1988	4,509.8	7.5	+53.6	122
1989**	2,325.8	3.9	-49.6	62
1990	2,315.8	3.6	- 0.4	61

*Statutory health insurance funds
**Forty percent copayment introduced January 1

Includes dentures, crowns, and other dental materials.

Source: Sachverständigenrat für die Konzertierte Aktion im Gesundheitswesen (1992). Jahresgutachten 1991. *p. 225; and* Daten des Gesundheitswesens *(1991), p. 175.*

First, a definition: **Reference prices** in Germany are not prices per se, but allowable reimbursement levels. Manufacturers are allowed to set prices at any level, though the reference price system effectively controls prices by setting sickness funds' maximum reimbursement levels for listed drugs. And while "reference price" systems in other countries fix prices on the basis of prices in the country of origin or other countries, Germany's reference price system is completely internal.

Under the 1989 reform, a reference price level was established for groups of related therapeutics. The drugs chosen for reference pricing are selected by a federal committee made up of equal numbers of doctors from the sickness funds physicians' associations and the funds, themselves. The funds alone are responsible for setting the actual reference price, contingent on the committee's recommendation. The price that is set falls somewhere between the highest and the lowest priced drug in a product group. The price chosen is not necessarily the median price, but the "functioning market price." Often this price is very near the price of the generic drug in the category, if one exists. If the committee fails

Table 6.14

Effect of the 1989 Drug Price Reform Law

	Number	Baseline sickness fund market (in millions)	Savings		Percent savings	
			Gross	Net	Gross	Net
Level I	83 substances	$2,967.6	$529.0	$262.2	17.8	8.8
Level II	9 groups	957.9	61.2	25.7	6.4	2.7
Level III	2 groups	44.9	8.5	3.8	18.9	8.5
Total		**$3,970.3**	**$598.8**	**$291.7**	**15.1**	**7.3**

Annual savings through July 1, 1992
Converted from DM to dollars on a purchasing power parity basis.

Source: Schwabe, U and Paffrath, D (1992). Arzneiverordnungs-Report '92. (Pharmaceutical Industry Report '92.) Stuttgart: Gustav Fischer Verlag. p.446.

to come to an agreement on a reference price or delays in setting the price, the federal health minister has the power to set the reference price.

The sickness funds reimburse pharmacists for the reference price. Drugs priced at or below this benchmark do not carry a copayment. (Patients under age 18 and low-income patients with certificates from a sickness fund were exempted from all copayments.) The 1989 law also included plans to raise the copayment for medications not covered by reference prices to 15 percent (maximum DM 10) by July 1, 1993. But for reasons described below, the increased copayment was abandoned until a revised form appeared in the 1993 reform law. The law also requires doctors to disclose to patients if the drug being prescribed carries a price tag higher than the reference price level and if a copayment is necessary.

The 1989 law called for a three-phase approach to setting reference prices. Beginning in September 1989 (level I), reference prices were set for groups of products with identical ingredients—proprietary drugs and their generic offspring—that had been on the market for more than three years. For drugs on the market less than three years, the reference price is to be established at the end of the three-year period. But by December 1991, prices had been established for only 150 active ingredients in 7,000 package sizes—only half the number that had been expected for this category.

In the second phase (level II), effective July 1991, reference prices were to be set for products with pharmacologically and therapeutically "comparable" active ingredients. But after much controversy over what constitutes a comparable active ingredient, only benzodiazepines were considered. In the third phase (level III), reference prices were to be established for pharmacologically 'comparable' effects, particularly combination products. These prices have not been established yet, but will be under the 1993 reform law.

Reference Price Reaction

When pressed to choose between identical drugs—either a brand-name drug or its generic equivalent—German physicians and patients abandoned the higher-priced drug in almost all cases. The market share for drugs whose makers resisted reference prices fell dramatically overnight.[109] According to drug analyst Redwood, reference prices resulted in an uneven level of price cuts, ranging from 20 percent to 70 percent below the previous price. Among the first 15 agents, cuts averaged 30 percent. Redwood says that an uneven effect emerged in a company-by-company analysis—some companies were not able to make up for the losses, particularly if their leading brand was on the reference price list, he says. Citing a 1990 Nord study of 38 companies, Redwood reports that 23 lost more in reference price cuts than they gained in raising prices outside the reference area; 14 gained more than they lost; and one broke even. The extent of reference pricings' impact depended not only on the company's pricing strategy but also on the degree to which its product range was hit by reference prices.[110]

Despite these large fluctuations in prices, the sickness funds' savings from the reference pricing amounted to DM 1.3 billion ($616 million) in 1989, on expenditures of DM 8.3 billion ($3.9 billion) for the covered drugs. When the copayment is subtracted, there was a net savings of about 8.4 percent, or DM 698 million ($331 million), according to Rudiger Vogel of the German pharmaceutical association.[111] Pharmaceutical companies tried to anticipate reference pricing by raising prices, but the average price increase during the run-up was never more than 4 percent because nearly all the drugs had generic competition.[112]

Generic companies initially experienced increased sales, but felt the competitive heat as brand-name prices were lowered. If the price was the same, physicians reasoned, why not prescribe the brand-name drug? Generic makers reacted by lowering their prices further. Ratiopharm, Germany's largest generic maker, even lowered all its prices to 10 percent below the reference price level.[113]

One of the major reasons that overall spending decreases fell short of the projected DM 4.5 billion savings was unpredicted compensatory price rises by drug makers. Faced with the loss in profits, companies boosted prices on products outside the reference price list. For the period February 1, 1989 to June 30, 1991, one study estimated that prices for products in the reference areas were cut at an annual rate of DM 824 million ($391 million), whereas prices outside the reference area were increased at an annual rate of DM 935 million ($443 million).[114] There is little doubt that price increases would also have occurred on drugs within the reference-price system, making a direct link problematic. But clearly, most of the gross revenues lost to the government's price "persuasion" was recouped in other areas.

Finding the Loopholes

Behavior was also a major factor in the missed goals of reference pricing. As Redwood observed:

> First and foremost, [the system foundered] because its theoretical and conceptual foundations failed to take into account the quirks and psychological reactions of those who have to operate under the system: doctors, patients, and industrialists. All have "played games," as people do with all systems. Some of their games might have been foreseen. Others are as novel as the system itself.[115]

Drug makers were able exploit the slowness of the switch to reference prices. In the first year, less than 15 percent were covered by reference prices—far short of the 80 percent called for by the 1989 reform law. Even after three years, reference prices covered only 40 percent of the German drug market.[116] As noted above, much of the delay centered on definitions of therapeutic and pharmacologic equivalency.

In theory, 306 active drug substances were eligible for inclusion in the phase I list in 1991, though less than half (130) were regarded as suitable for reference pricing. To be considered suitable, a drug must have relatively large sales and a sufficiently wide gap between the price of the original brand and its generic copies, Redwood says. By July 1992, 79 suitable drugs had been given reference prices, accounting for more than 90 percent of sales of these chemical entities. Except to the extent that reference prices can be lowered still by legislative fiat, most of the savings to be extracted from multisource drugs has been accomplished.[117]

Many observers cite the physician disclosure requirements in the law as the reason the drug companies rushed to match the reference price in each group. They say that German doctors—already perpetually rushed—were unwilling to spend additional moments (and potential income) discussing with patients the financial implications of prescribing an identical drug priced above the reference level. "It is easier to avoid the issue by prescribing at or below the reference price," says Redwood. Hapke agrees: "Since 1989, doctors have been less sensitive to price than before. Because of reference pricing, they feel they don't have to worry."[118]

Innovation was another significant factor in the small savings that were realized: Since 1987, German companies have focused intensively on developing new drugs, producing a number of new angiotensin-converting enzyme (ACE) inhibitors, antiemetics for cancer patients, and cholesterol inhibitors. Innovative drugs account for about 35 percent of the total prescription volume, and that they are responsible for about two-thirds of the increase in spending.[119] For example, ACE inhibitors are three times more expensive than other hypertensives. The -statin series of cholesterol lowering drugs are also about three times more expensive than earlier generation drugs.

The limited effect of reference prices on drug spending was demonstrated in 1991, when drug expenditures increased by about 10 percent over 1990. Some 1.5 percent of the increase was due to the structural effect of introducing new cardiovascular drugs outside the reference pricing system. And a new requirement as of January 1, 1993, will add 1 percent to baseline drug spending: Birth control pills will now be provided free to all women up to age 21 years.

Despite the losses at some companies, including his own, Hapke says the 1989 reforms produced no negative effects on innovation. The principal reason for this, he says, is that most of the drugs entering the market now were developed in the years before the reform took effect. "What is in the pipeline now will be on the market in 10 years, perhaps, with or without further reforms."

Slumbering Giants. Just as some manufacturers were quick to maneuver into loopholes, others were inept when it came to judging the implications of the reference price system. According to Hapke: "Some consultants to pharmaceutical industry said: 'Do not lower your prices. The patient will pay. There is remarkable brand loyalty.' A number of major manufacturers took the gamble and kept their prices up." He cites as prominent examples CIBA's Diclofenac, Roche's Bromezapin, Beyersdorf's Beta-acetyldigoxin; and Procter & Gamble's Diazide, which at the time was the best-selling diuretic in Germany. "Some drugs that lost 50 percent of market share from one week to the next, even if the copayment was small," Hapke says.[120]

Redwood echoes this:

> Industrially, the most ominous result of the implementation of phase I has been the "capitulation" of brand manufacturers. Whether they anticipated the instant annihilation of brand loyalty in the face of a skewed "pay something/pay nothing" choice, or waited until they saw it happen, within weeks nearly every manufacturer had reduce the price of nearly every original brand in a reference group to the reference level. Two companies that attempted to resist were hit so hard by losses of market share that they felt compelled to reverse their decisions within weeks.... Companies that had done so from the start generally held their market share but did not materially increase it. Accordingly price cuts became lost profits on the affected products.[121]

Bayer reportedly lost some DM 90 million ($42.6 million) after the reference prices were introduced. While this amount may sound relatively small for a multibillion dollar company, even a 10 percent reduction in sales can lead to an 80 percent reduction in profits, when margins are in the 12 to 15 percent range. A smaller company dependent on a single product may be devastated by such a loss, whereas pharmaceuticals at giants Bayer, Höchst, and BASF account for only 10 to 20 percent of their total revenues. Still, pharmaceuticals often carry the highest margins of any product line.

The impact on profits has been severe in some cases. Gödecke AG, which once spent DM 40 million ($7.6 million) per year on research and development and employed 300 people in the effort, discontinued all domestic R&D after the 1989 reform, Hapke says. The company now relies on its American parent Parke-Davis for R&D. The company has also scaled back its budget for promotion to 1982 levels, he says.[122] It is difficult to determine how many German companies have cost-shifted their R&D operations to foreign soils or have reduced domestic R&D expenditures.

Definitional Deadlock

In the summer of 1990, the federal committee on reference pricing deadlocked over definitions of drug "comparability" when they tried to group nonidentical drugs under phase II of reference pricing. Phase I had included only proprietary drugs and their identical generic equivalents; phase II was to set a reference price for related, but not identical, compounds in the same therapeutic class. Drugs were to have "comparable" therapeutic activity at available doses.

Under the 1989 reform, the *Betriebskrankenkassen* (company-based sickness funds) take the lead in determining equivalence, making recommendations to the federal committee of sickness funds and sickness fund physicians. When considering the phase II recommendations, however, all nine doctors' representatives on the committee voted no, while all nine representatives from the sickness funds voted yes. The three independent members abstained. According to Redwood, when the discussion turned to benzodiazepines, the doctors demanded narrowly defined groups in order to allay doubts about "comparability," while the sickness-fund representatives wanted to lump nearly all benzodiazepine tranquilizers and sedatives together, with only the most glaring anomalies excluded. The benzodiazepine battle was eventually resolved by splitting the 17 benzodiazepines into a 10-member group of those with predominately anxiolytic effect and a seven-member sedative group.

Reference prices' effect on the benzodiazepine drug market, estimated in 1991 to be DM 187 million ($89 million), was almost negligible, however, says Redwood. Gross savings to the sickness funds were estimated at DM 12 million ($5.7 million), or DM 700,000 ($334,000) per substance. But the elimination of the copayment for this class of drugs triggered a shift from other classes, increasing benzodiazepine prescribing. This caused the sickness funds to pay out an additional DM 14 million ($6.7 million) for benzodiazepines in 1991.[123]

By 1992, two more level II groups had been added—beta-blockers and nonsteroidal antiinflammatories. Gross savings for level II (including benzodiazepines) were estimated at DM 127.9 million ($61.2 million) in July 1992; net savings were DM 53.7 million ($25.7 million), or 2.7 percent, on total sales of DM 2 billion ($957 million).

Still controversial is the issue of what constitutes an innovative drug under level II. If a drug is deemed noninnovative, although patented, and enters level II, this could undermine the value of patent protection by effectively forcing a patented brand to meet the reference price for an unpatented (generic) group of chemically different drug substances, Redwood says. He adds:

> These, in reality, are the kind of problems which countries with formal price control tackle day-in-day-out: Allowing a price premium for innovation whilst enforcing lower prices for copies or noninnovative products is normal in price-controlled markets. The fact that such questions are now arising in Germany illustrates how far the Reference Price System has strayed from the "market economy" principle to which the country officially adheres.[124]

Copayment Chaos

Patient contributions are universally seen as a panacea for inhibiting system utilization, though it is sometimes difficult to link cause and effect, particularly in an environment where there are other volume drivers such as new technologies and innovative new drugs that replace other forms of therapy. Yet policymakers grasp at copayments in the hope that they will do something to solve the problem at hand.

Copayments on health services in Germany have been slower to evolve than in the U.S., although token copayments on drugs have existed for decades. As noted earlier, Germany raised its copayment from DM 1 ($0.33) in 1969 to a sliding-scale fee with a maximum of DM 2.50 ($0.83). But nearly 60 percent of drugs were free of copayment, diluting much of its desired effect.

The 1989 reform made another swipe at making patients more cost-conscious. Copayments were raised from DM 2 per prescribed drug to DM 3 initially. Doctors are now required by law to tell the patient if the drug they are prescribing exceeds the reference price level. They must also tell the patient if the drug carries a copayment. The copayment was scheduled rise to 15 percent by 1993, to a maximum of DM 10 ($3.35). But public outcry over copayments during the debate over the 1993 reforms caused the copayment structure to be changed and the maximum to be watered down to DM 7 ($3.35). During the debate over the law, drug makers and physicians proposed that the patient contribution be graduated on the basis of income and be linked to indication. Both proposals were rejected.[125]

But as in earlier years, many drugs and certain classes of patients are exempted from the copayment: at least 40 percent of drugs are reference priced and are free from copayment; pregnant women, insureds under age 18, and low-income insureds are also exempted. Even so, patient resistance to copayments runs high and German politicians are often forced to retreat, sometimes to the extent of repealing copayment increases or delaying implementation.

In the debate over copayments to the 1989 law, for example, complained so loudly that the maximum amounts were never implemented. And the abandonment of drugs priced higher than the reference price was based in large measure on patients' reluctance to pay the copayment and the requirement that the patient pay the difference in price. Noting a "natural human failing," Redwood comments: "The message was crystal clear: Patients in one of the most prosperous countries in the world were not prepared to pay even DM 3 [$1.42] WHEN THE ALTERNATIVE WAS TO PAY NOTHING. Well, dear reader, what would *you* do if you were a bit short of cash?"

But the failure of the increased copayment to have a significant negative impact on sickness-fund drug spending is quite clear. After a temporary pause in spending increases in 1989, drug spending continued its upward climb. Retailers confirm that the copayment had little effect. As Tübingen pharmacist Claus-Peter Ullbricht observed: "To pay extra is not so hard for patients. Most accepted it after grumbling. Just after the 1989 reform passed, pharmacies' revenue went down for awhile, but after a half-year or so, they went up, and at more than the inflation rate. Copayments, and the limitation on total amount a doctor can prescribe only made people annoyed—it didn't have much effect [on total sales]."

Schulte estimates that the drug copayment would have to be as high as 30 percent to have any controlling effect on drug demand. "The result of this would be that pensioners and the long term sick would have to be excluded from any copayment scheme. On the other hand, since this group consumes more than half of all the drugs prescribed, the aim of cost-effectiveness would be thwarted again."

Copayment Foes. Drug makers naturally have opposed copayments, but their sophistical arguments usually emphasize the harm others will suffer, obscuring their own (profit) motives. In the current debates, drug makers painted copayments as the primary source of the system's ills. In a press release issued in early 1993, the German pharmaceutical association even blamed the 1991's DM 5.5 billion deficit on the 1989 reform law itself:

The release of the "fixed amount on medicaments" from the "prescription fee" has contributed to this large expansion [in sickness-fund drug spending] — because it is all for free — as well as the "prescription fee" of three marks itself — when three marks are paid, then for a larger package. The abolishment of the "additional payment freedom" for "fixed amount-medicaments" is an admission of this misdirection. On the contrary, the Ministry plays down the consequences of increasing life expectations and the costs of medical-technical progress, which give an uncontrollable dynamism to the development of costs of each health system.[126]

In other words, the industry group asserts, in effect, that exempting reference-priced drugs from the copayment and discouraging use of more expensive drugs will lower life-expectancy and inhibit technologic innovation because the free market is no longer free and profits are no longer easy. The German pharmaceutical association also seems to be complaining that patients seeking to maximize their DM 3 copayment by purchasing larger packages are also a threat to the integrity of the system, which may be true, but this argument inadvertently runs counter to drug makers' interest. Drug analyst Redwood also takes a dim view of copayments. The copayment system in Germany has not worked, he says,

because it unintentionally created a split market by applying a prescription charge to some drugs and not to others, instead of staying with the tried and tested principle of applying it to some patients and not to others. The intention was to induce responsible consumption; the actual result is a distorted market with as yet unforeseeable medical repercussions as a result of the perverse decision patterns which such a split market induces.

Solidarity arguments—always powerful in Germany—also enter into the debate with regularity: "It has been suggested that, whereas a patient with a painful knee stands an excellent chance of receiving a "free" drug, a cancer patient may not be so lucky," Redwood notes.[127] Others, including economics professor Pfaff, complain that people with illnesses bear a greater burden for the cost savings than healthy people.

Copayments seem likely to stay, however. All 12 European communities have some form of copayment for pharmaceuticals.

Turning Down the Volume

To slow prescribing volume and to prevent physicians and patients from shifting to more expensive drugs outside the reference pricing system, the 1989 reform act drew the outlines of a physicians' drug budget and shifted the focus to physician prescription patterns — a focus that was sharpened in the 1993 reforms. It called on the National Association of Sickness Fund Physicians to establish budgetary norms for prescription drugs as part of the extensive practice profiling system that tracks physicians' use of diagnostic tests and other procedures. The doctors' association was instructed to set norms on a regional basis for each type of generalist and specialist practice. A 2 percent sample in each region would set the standards for all physicians; each prescription written each quarter would be tracked and analyzed according to the practice's case-mix, the age of patients, and other factors. Physicians whose prescribing fell significantly outside the standard deviation were to receive personal counseling from the local panel of doctors. Recalcitrants or egregious violators were to be subject to loss of all income for a quarter or longer.

When the physicians' drug budget was proposed, and later enacted, doctors flew into a public outrage. They succeeded in delaying implementation three years, until the reforms of 1993. Experiments were allowed, however, to begin in early 1992 on a limited basis in the white-collar sickness funds (*Ersatzkassen*).[128]

Profiling prescribing habits was not new, but the link to overall spending was. In 1985 in north Germany, for example, up to 25 percent of all doctors were counseled on prescribing behavior. By 1989, however, this practice had decreased to 0.3 to 0.5 percent.[129]

Physician Gaming

Germany's profiling system has permitted sickness funds to alter physician behavior by showing them how they stack up against their peers. Sophisticated statistical analyses are presented quarterly comparing a physician's test ordering, prescribing, and referral patterns with other doctors in the same field. These analyses are corrected for case-mix, age of patients, and other factors. Physicians face an automatic reduction in reimbursement if they are more than 40 percent over the averages. Physicians whose averages are lower but consistently violate norms are asked to explain the variation. Those with an elderly practice or too many industrial workers with an occupational illness have yearly meetings with local sickness fund panels to justify the overages. There is little question that the meetings and the monitoring modify physician prescribing patterns.

But the analyses may be triggering another kind of behavior modification—gaming. Many computer software packages have been developed that show a doctor how many more tests or procedures he or she can order during the current quarter without increasing the risk of audit. The long-term pernicious effect of this practice, critics say, is to fuel unnecessary care.

"As long as auditing is based on comparing a specific practice pattern with the statistical average it is likely that this will stimulate physicians to approach, or stay slightly above, this average," observes Dominic Stillfried, a health services researcher at the University of Tübingen. "If it is possible for physicians to communicate their prescription habits among each other, it will be possible to raise the average collectively without any threat for the individual physician."

Indeed computer software already exists that tells a physician how to prescribe drugs at 108 percent of his budget, so as to stay below the dreaded 110 percent threshold where counselors from the sickness funds begin calling.

1993 Reform

It was only when the 1993 "structural" reform law was enacted that a true drug budget became effective for doctors, expanding a barely-initiated experiment to countrywide implementation. The law, known as the *Gesundheitsstruktur Gesetz* or *GSG*, reform is scheduled to produce savings of DM 11 billion ($5.3 billion) in sickness-fund spending per year: the "suppliers of productivity"—the pharmaceutical industry, hospitals, pharmacists, physicians, and dentists—are to ante up a total of DM 8 billion ($3.8 billion); sickness funds will be held liable for the remaining DM 3 billion ($1.4 billion) in savings. Physicians are collectively responsible for the first DM 280 million ($134 million) of any amount over the global drug budget which was set at DM 24.1 billion ($11.5 billion). Pharmaceutical companies as a group are responsible for the next DM 280 million. "The reason for putting a ceiling on expenditure is that, with almost 25 billion D-Marks in the western part of the FRG alone in 1991, we have reached the absolute limit on drug-related expenditure," says Schulte.[130] "In many areas, excessive expenditure on drugs not only brings no benefits; instead it even damages the patient's health."

If physicians' national prescribing on drugs exceeds DM 24.1 billion, they will be held collectively liable through the sickness fund physician associations, with the overage to be taken out of future fee reimbursements.

Should spending go beyond a DM 280 million overrun, the pharmaceutical industry will pay for the overage by having the price moratorium extended beyond 1995. Wholesalers and retail pharmacists will be compensated retroactively by drug makers through the use of discounts for any extension of the moratorium. The overall 1993 budget was set at the 1991 levels (minus 1.6 percent for the anticipated effect of expanding the reference pricing system to more drugs) so that drug makers and physicians couldn't artificially affect subsequent budgets by raising expenditures in 1992. The drug budget for 1994 will be set on the basis of expenditures for 1993. From 1994 onward, physicians alone are responsible for any overages in the drug budget, which will be determined by negotiations between the national physicians' group and the sickness funds.

Some reactions were predictable. The German pharmaceutical association couched its concern in terms of the doctors' and patients' plight:

> The Association of the German Pharmaceutical Industry rejects these budgets firmly. They endanger the trust between doctor and patient. Since the individual doctor cannot know how much of the total budget has already been used, and on the other hand when exceeding he must expect retrogressive losses in fees, he tends to be reserved about prescribing.[131]

But the association didn't hesitate to run up the well-worn flags of the threat budgetary limits pose to the vitality of pharmaceutical research and development (and profits).

> The considerable financial limitation leads to the fact that the doctor is more hesitant about using innovative, expensive drugs. The desirable change in therapy slows down and with it, the introduction of new medicines. The economic risks of research continue to increase. The basic year budget for budgets will be the year 1991. The Association of the German Pharmaceutical Industry estimates the loss of [sales] as a consequence of the budgeting (if the average market growth of past years is taken for 1992 and 1993) in billions.[132]

Others expressed skepticism about the feasibility of achieving multibillion mark savings on drugs, particularly because so many patients are being switched to newly released innovative drugs. Data from 1991 indicate that sales rose significantly on innovative drugs in that year. (Table 6.14) But lawmakers agreed with Schulte's assessment that DM 24 billion marks is the upper limit for sickness fund spending. To insure that the goal is met, legislators also mandated that prices be reduced and frozen in place until 1995.

Price Freeze

The prices of prescription drugs for which there is no reference rate are to be reduced by 5 percent in 1993. Over-the-counter drugs are to be reduced by 2 percent. The basis for the price reduction is the price on May 1, 1992. Not included are all preparations which are on the negative list, which were previously excluded from reimbursement under the 1989 reform. For drugs that enter the market between May 2, 1992, and December 31, 1992, the benchmark for the reduction is the introductory market price. Those drugs entering the market after January 1, 1993, will not be affected by the price reduction, but their price will be frozen until 1995. Drugs with an established reference price on or before January 1, 1993, are automatically excluded from the price moratorium as soon as the set rate is effective.

Not surprisingly, the German pharmaceutical association was outraged by the passage of the price reductions and the 1993-95 freeze. In an English-version press release they railed:

> The legally regulated price reduction is a previously unknown state interference in the freedom of enterprise and is highly questionable from the point of view of order and politics. The autonomous decision about one of the important instruments of competition is taken from the hands of the entrepreneur and his economic position is influenced from outside. Since the German prices have a reference function for foreign price formation, the price reduction also burdens [drug makers'] foreign business. The price reduction in the case of medicines which are not prescribed is of no use to the health insurances but at the same time reduces the [sales] of the companies involved unjustly. Such medicines as the patient buys on his own account have always relieved the national health insurances.... The price freeze hinders until the end of 1994 a pharmaceutical [enterprise's ability to] pass on cost increases (e.g., salary increases, higher raw material costs). In the case of a lost of purchasing power of about 4 percent per year, the resulting burden accumulated from this alone on industry is about 10 percent, which would correspond to an additional savings potential of 2 billion marks.[133]

But as Schulte notes, the influence of the pharmaceutical manufacturers in Germany is very strong and drug makers prevailed on many issues in the debate over the 1993 reform. Whereas the 1989 reforms were intended to control 80 percent of the market with reference prices, only 40 percent had been covered by 1993. Reformers tried to reestablish the 80 percent goal, but were only able to achieve a 70 percent target. Schulte says that the drug makers, with the help of the right-of-center Free Democratic Party, were able to enlarge the list of innovative products that are exempt from the reference pricing system.

Copayments Rise Slowly

Beginning in 1993, the copayment was calculated on the basis of package size. Patients pay DM 3 for small packages, DM 5 for medium packages, and DM

7 for large packages. (Table 6.15) Those over 70 are expected to pay about DM 60 ($29) per year; those aged 60 to 70 would pay about DM 45 ($22); ages 40 to 60, about DM 30 ($14); and ages 18 to 40, about DM 20 ($10). Patients under 18 are exempted from the drug copayment.[134]

The German pharmaceutical association argues that these broad copayments will lead to increased demand for the most expensive drug in the largest package, and instead wants a uniform 10 percent copayment. A percentage additional payment, it argues, would sensitize patients to even small differences in price and would curb the demand for larger packages.

Reference Price Tug-of-War

The 1993 reform requires reference prices for 70 percent of all drugs reimbursable by the statutory sickness funds, much the same goal as the 1989 reform. Drug makers fought against this goal and ultimately lost, but they made inroads by extending the protected period for newly launched drugs. Drugs had been exempted from reference prices for three years after introduction under the 1989 law, but the 1993 reform abolishes that waiting period. Products are now protected from reference prices until the patent expires—typically seven to eight years after the drug is introduced.

According to the Eckart Fiedler, manager of the white collar sickness funds, savings on new and revised reference prices in 1993 are expected to amount to DM 365 million ($175 million).[135]

Negative Turns Positive

The 1993 law also builds on the negative list that was most recently expanded in 1989. But the list will now be a **positive list** of approved drugs, rather than a negative list of unapproved drugs. The decision to exclude drugs from reimbursement will be made by a new Institute of Drugs to be established in association with the National Association of Sickness Fund Physicians and the sickness funds. The Institute is actually a council of 11 members and will be independent of the Federal Health Agency, which licenses new drugs and approves them for marketing. The council will be made up of three clinical pharmacologists, three practicing physicians, three physicians from the "minor" medical schools of thought (anthroposophy, homeopathy, and herbals), one medical statistician, and one pharmaceutical scientist.[136] The Institute's scope is limited to reimbursement issues.

Under the 1993 reform law, it will draw up a list of approved drugs that contains none

☐ to which are attributed only minor therapeutic benefit or of which the therapeutic effectiveness is doubtful according to the present state of knowledge;

☐ which are used for minor health defects;

☐ which are uneconomical.

The physician can deviate from this list in individual cases, but he or she must justify this decision in each case. The law also created special regulations for herbal, homeopathic, and anthroposophical drugs, facilitating their inclusion on the list, much to the chagrin of allopathic physicians.

Table 6.15

Sales Trends for Newly Approved Drugs in Germany

Therapeutic category	Sales rise from 1990 to 1991, in millions of PPP dollars
ACE-inhibitors*	$112.5
Cholesterol inhibitors	81.3
Antiasthmatics	79.4
Antibiotics/chemotherapeutics	67.5
Analgesics/antirheumatics	65.4
Beta-blocker/calcium antagonists	44.8
Sexual hormones (mainly estrogen)	38.4
Antidiabetics	38.1
Mineral supplements	36.2
Expectorants	27.9
Antiallergics	20.4
Antifungals	15.2
Total	**637.1**

*Angiotensin-converting enzyme inhibitors are used to lower high blood pressure.

Source: Kassenärztliche Bundesvereinigung (1993). Schaubildsammlung zur Information und Argumentationshilfe, chart D5.

Table 6.16

1993 Drug Copayments

Price of drug	Copayment
to DM 30 ($14.35)	DM 3.00 ($1.43)
DM 30 to DM 50 ($23.92)	DM 5.00 ($2.39)
above DM 50	DM 7.00 ($3.35)

Dollar conversion on a purchasing power parity basis.

Source: German Ministry of Health, 1993.

Newly registered drugs will be added or excluded from the list within three months under the new law. If a decision is not made during this period, the new drug will be temporarily placed under prescription, as long as it falls within one of the approved indication groups.

The drug industry has challenged the legality of creating a second panel to review drugs.[137] The German pharmaceutical association also argues that "an Institute or Federal Committee cannot decide about the therapeutical use from the conference table.... It is only the doctor who can decide about the therapeutic usefulness of a medicine in a concrete individual case." The association also "firmly rejects" the creation of another list of excludable drugs, saying that the negative list created by the 1989 reforms should be expanded instead. Again, the R&D bogeyman is raised.

> In the medium term even internationally active enterprises are affected, who have a large potential for research. In the future, they would have to invest up to a three-digit million figure in research and development without knowing whether, in the end, the penstroke of a health bureaucrat in the Institute for Drugs will eliminate any chance of economic success in Germany. With this economic risk in research is increasing and the capability for innovation is declining. This uncertainty does not speak for Germany as a pharmaceutical base.[138]

A Taxing Debate

German drug makers are also aggrieved by the 1993 reform law's ambivalence toward the effects of adjusting to the European Economic Community's uniform 15 percent **value-added tax**, as of March 1, 1993. This raised Germany's VAT one percentage point. Unlike other European countries, Germany applies the whole VAT to the retail price of drugs. EC-wide, the average VAT on retail drugs is only 5 percent. (Figure 6.7)

The 1993 reform law does not require that the VAT be added to the reference price, so sickness funds are not obligated to pay for the increase. Patients are thus held liable for the additional amount on reference priced drugs, confusing the 3-5-7 copayment system with an additional tax surcharge. (Retail prices in Germany always include the VAT; there is no additional markup at the register as in the U.S.)

The German pharmaceutical association estimates that 1,038 medicines in different formulations and package sizes will be affected by this ruling. An example from the association illustrates the confusion, which seems quaint by American standards, where poor patients often must pay for the entire cost of a drug and where applicability of state and local sales taxes is much more Byzantine.

> A manufacturer offers 100 tablets of an expectorant at the price of DM 78.31, which is exactly the set rate. The increase of VAT makes the product 68 pfennigs more expensive. Thus the new price is DM 78.99, 68 pfennigs above the set rate. In this price category, the insured party must pay the seven marks copayment plus 68 pfennigs additional payment, which makes in total, DM 7.68. The additional payment of 68 pfennigs is also payable, if the insured party otherwise is released wholly or partly from additional payments through regulations concerning the case of hardship or provision for excessive demand.[138]

Doctors are also peeved about the VAT. The Health Ministry has told doctors that it has considered the effects of the VAT increase in setting the drug budget, but the National Association of Sickness Fund Physicians claims that the increase isn't adequately accounted for and may have thrown the budget off by DM 2 billion or more.

Protest

The debates over the 1993 reforms were among the most raucous in Germany history. Prior reforms had touched only one or two sectors at a time. But the 1993 reforms aimed to spread the pain among all parties.

Among the most vocal were physicians. As noted in Chapter Four, the German Society of General Medicine called the drug budget proposal an "ugly instrument of torture."[139] The National Association of Local Sickness Funds threatened to expel any doctors from sickness fund practice if they were found to be denying patients needed medication. The doctors were mainly upset at the prospect of prescribing in the dark until the end of the year, when it would be revealed whether they had collectively exceeded the budget or not.

Pharmacists joined in the protest against the proposed 1993 reforms. Many felt the reforms posed the biggest crisis in their careers. Tübingen pharmacist Ullbricht observed: "Already many pharmacies are below the minimum to survive. They survive on their savings. They still earn what a worker would earn, but they have no profit."[140]

A brochure distributed by the pharmacy associations in Baden-Württemberg and Lower Saxony warned that the new reforms would cause 30 percent of pharmacies to close, costing 20,000 pharmacy jobs. Emergency service, such as all-night hours, would have to be curtailed. Patients were told that their pharmacists would no longer be able to give them advice, due to the staff shortages. With so many closed pharmacies, the sick and elderly would be made to travel much greater distances to get their medicines, pharmacists claimed.[141]

The pharmacy association also cautioned that cheap sundries would be a thing of the past, implying that steep price hikes were inevitable if the reform passed. Most fearsome of all was a warning that under the physicians' budget: "Imagine the time when your doctor can't prescribe the high-value medicine you need because he's over his prescribing budget."[142]

Meanwhile, the drug manufacturers were sending out all-points bulletins trying to cover all bases. The German pharmaceutical association began by insisting that the drug industry has been totally cooperative in previous cost control efforts, and emphasized its call for voluntary price freezes among members. It also trumpeted its (reluctant) backing of the reference price system, its support for reduced regulatory burdens in the new eastern states, and its achievement of "price stability" over the past few years. "The financial sacrifice has until now in total accumulated to almost 2 billion marks annually," the association noted.[143]

Stumbling Giants

But the German pharmaceutical association's public relations campaign was not always smooth. Several very public fumbles weakened support for the drug industry's point of view at critical points in the reform debate, paralleling the stupendous errors made by physicians at the same time. Two examples illustrate the magnitude and emotions of the debate.

When the January 1991 reunification law went into effect, for example, it mandated a 55 percent price reduction for drugs to be sold in the eastern states. Rather than help out the eastern states, where incomes were half those in the west, many western drug manufacturers simply boycotted the eastern states. But television cameras captured easterners queuing at pharmacists who could not supply drugs abundant only a few kilometers to the west. The public outrage that ensued is widely viewed as leaving the drug makers in a weakened position when the 1993 reforms were debated during 1992. "They simply hadn't prepared a public relations strategy to counter this," Hapke says.[144]

Doctors were hardly smarter. A television campaign against global budgeting showed doctors telling elderly patients that they could no longer prescribe needed medication and fliers in waiting rooms reinforced the message. By most accounts the campaign failed because it was spectacularly overplayed. Michael Arnold of the University of Tübingen says the campaign sunk under the weight of its own untruths.[145] And the *Frankfurter Allgemeine* editorialized against the tactics of the physicians, pharmacists, and drug makers.

> Whatever protest actions farmers might come up with to combat subsidy cuts, or miners devise to rescue their now unprofitable coal-pits, nothing can surpass the apocalyptic and drastic quality of the horror scenarios conjured up by the suppliers of services on the health care market. At the merest inkling, anywhere, that the massive sums flowing into their coffers threaten to decrease in the slightest, the lobby paints a picture of the ruin of prosperous industries, the withering of the research landscape, the impoverishment of the healing arts, and the agonizing wasting away of the population, in the grayest and blackest of tones.[146]

Initial Reaction

The early reaction to the 1993 reform was dramatic. In January 1993, there was a substantial reduction in prescription volume. Newspapers and other media reported massive outcries from patients who complained that they were being denied vital drugs and were being advised to buy reimbursable drugs themselves so as not to raise the doctors' drug budget. Pharmaceutical manufacturers reported that they lost 40 to 50 percent of their sales.[147] And pharmacies reported losses between 20 and 60 percent—losses that were at least partially due to the fact that patients asked their doctors for three months' prescriptions in December to avoid higher copayments in the new year.[148] The largest sickness fund, the *AOK*, was reportedly threatening to discharge doctors who refuse to prescribe vital drugs. Hundreds of such cases were allegedly reported.[149]

Much like the public relations campaigns conducted during the debate over reform, these events seem overblown. Taking into account price cuts and patients' contributions, the demand on doctors to lower their prescribing amounts to a mere 2.3 percent per doctor. The average doctor prescribes DM 480,000 ($229,665). Seeming not to have learned their lesson earlier, however, doctors are justifying their actions by claiming that the actual cut from their budget is DM 4 billion ($1.9 billion) when three things are considered: the VAT increase, the advent of more expensive innovative drugs, and the addition of 10,000 new doctors this year. (As discussed in Chapter Four, the German constitution forbids any limits on career choice, virtually guaranteeing an oversupply of highly paid professionals. This is being challenged by the 1993 reform.)[150]

Long Term Outlook

One of the biggest problems that may arise from the 1993 reforms could be the role sickness funds will play in determining drug makers' outlays for R&D. The sickness funds may well delve into drug company budgets and set future reimbursement levels according to what they interpret as adequate for insuring innovation. There is precedence: Austria already negotiates sickness fund expenditures on innovation.

What Would Real Reform Consist Of?

Tübingen pharmacist Ullbricht perhaps summed it up best when asked what shape real reform should take:

> Real reform would be for patients to learn that the [sickness funds] can't pay for all drugs. All the population has to change its mind about drugs. People who come to the pharmacy for self-medication drug and see it costs DM 10 say, "Oh, that is too much." Then they go to the doctor and get him to prescribe it. They have to learn that health insurance is for emergencies, for high costs, and is not meant to pay for everything.[151]

What Americans Can Learn

Germany's pharmaceutical reforms over the past two decades mainly can be characterized as reactive and patchwork. Though several of the reforms were carefully planned to deliver long term results, these voluntary plans usually failed within months of implementation, often because no enforcement was attempted. New reforms were then rushed into place in an ever-futile attempt to restrain drug spending. Only when faced with the real threat of enforced global budgets did the situation begin to change.

Given the American addiction to the quick-fix, it is tempting to speculate that a similar course would have evolved in the U.S. over the past two decades, had efforts to provide universal coverage been successful. The preference for voluntary restraints that is evidenced in Germany's many reforms would likely have been tried repeatedly in the U.S. Moreover, voluntary measures probably would have been the only possible intervention in the U.S. pharmaceutical market after the wage-and-price control debacle of the Nixon Administration. Indeed, that experience greatly colored the internal debates over drug price controls in the nascent Clinton Administration. The mere mention of price controls—in a government no longer controlled by Republicans—caused many major U.S. drug firms to rush out voluntary pledges to keep price rises in line with general inflation. As the German experience shows, such vows are worth approximately the value of the paper they are written on.

Some contend that Germany's modest interventions—physician profiling and negative drug lists—have been effective in keeping a lid on German pharmaceutical spending, holding it at a constant 15 to 17 percent of sickness fund expenditures. But drug spending in the U.S, where there are virtually no controls on drug expenditures (except those in state and federal Medicaid budgets), has remained constant, too—at about 8 percent of national health expenditures.

The underlying force driving Germany's high level drug spending is surely the high volume of prescriptions being written—a situation without direct parallel in the U.S. There is a strong belief among policymakers in Germany that the 1993 reform's attack on prescription-writing volume by physicians is the magic net by which spending can be reeled in. Earlier efforts at lowering prescription volume were quite effective, but only for a relatively brief period of time. Part of the reason lies in the oversupply of physicians. Prescription volume inevitably has risen as too many doctors compete to make too few patients happy. If Germany were to ever lower drug spending, it would seem, the only effective solution was to implement a strict global budget on drug spending and make it enforceable by financially penalizing physicians for overprescribing. Early returns from the reform indicated that physicians were overreacting to the budget, drastically cutting back on prescribing. The long term clinical implications for patients were unknown.

In the U.S., prescription volume is not a major concern, even though each patient visit results in a prescription, on average—just like in Germany. (Germans visit physicians three times more frequently than Americans, however.) Rather, rapidly rising prices have captured U.S. policymakers' attention, and with good reason. Increasing drug prices have been outpacing general inflation in the U.S. for many years now. Prices are now 30 percent higher in the U.S. than in Germany, where prices are the highest in Europe.

Mixed Results

Germany's attempts at curbing drug price rises have had mixed results. Some are directly applicable to the U.S., while others are not, due to cultural differences and variations in reimbursement methods. A brief cross-national review follows.

Price Controls. Germany's reference pricing system has dramatically lowered prices on covered drugs. But clever maneuverings by drug firms has kept many brand name drugs out of the reference price system, subverting the original goal of having 80 percent of drugs covered by 1993. Yet for the 40 percent that are now covered, prices are substantially lower than they were before the system was implemented. In the U.S., reference pricing could be implemented if drug reimbursement levels were determined by a central source. One could imagine a drug-fee schedule similar to the reimbursement schedules that have been developed for physicians and hospitals in the Medicare system. Politically, such a list might made be palatable to drug firms if health reform provided universal coverage for drugs.

Price Freezes and Reductions. The deep market interventions made in the 1993 reform have no parallel in earlier German reforms. Based on past experience, however, it is likely that German drug makers will find loopholes and exploit them to their fullest. Manufacturers will likely raise prices on drugs and related goods that are not covered by the price controls. The clinical impact of these reforms could not be predicted when the reform was enacted, though with Germany's high proportion of ineffective drugs, it is possible that the effect will be minimal. The U.S. experience with wage-and-price controls and health cost-shifting suggests that restraints imposed on one sector will trigger higher prices in other sectors.

Generics. Early attempts to encourage greater use of generics have resulted in significantly higher generic usage in Germany than in the U.S., which has helped keep sickness fund drug spending from exploding as prescription volume has risen. Regulatory approval of generics has always been simpler and faster in Germany than in the U.S., though recent changes in rules have made it somewhat more difficult to bring a generic to market in Germany. Me-too drugs also have been approved faster in Germany than in the U.S., which has fostered competition among brand-name drugs with similar indications. Faster drug approvals seem likely in the U.S. under institutional reforms put in place by the FDA in 1992. But because they involve overhauling an entrenched bureaucracy, the speed of such change is uncertain.

Copayments. Even minor changes in drug copayments have had a dramatic impact on patient behavior in Germany but little effect on overall spending. Patients, long accustomed to "free" drug coverage, have resisted increased copayments and have caused politicians who support them much grief. Indeed, the present copayment structure is actually distorting the market further by heightening demand for larger packages. Increased copayments in the U.S., where insurance coverage for drugs is already spotty, would have little effect on drug spending or drug prices.

Formularies. Germany's negative drug lists have had little impact on overall spending, but they have removed many minor and ineffective drugs from reimbursement, providing structural savings in future drug budgets. In the U.S., drug formularies are common in individual hospitals, and are viewed as essential in controlling hospital drug costs. Formularies have not been tried on a larger scale, except in Medicaid, where they have been judged a cost-containment failure. Formularies were adopted by 47 states in the late 1980s, but by 1993 only 19 states still had such list.

Markups. Germany's fixed markups at the retail and wholesale levels, in place for decades, eliminate two major price factors that are uncontrollable in U.S. These controls have helped to limit price volatility in Germany, but they also have preempted two potential levels of competition. It is hard to envision such limits on markups in the U.S., where competitive pressures are largely viewed as beneficial to consumers—whether or not they actually are.

The overriding concern in many minds when controls on pharmaceutical expenditures are discussed is the possible effect on the improvement of health and the technologic advance of medical science. There is little question that drugs have had an enormous impact on public health in the 20th century, perhaps only secondary to the improvement in public sanitation. And although it has not been proved directly, it would seem that there is some merit in the argument that drugs have helped lower health costs by obviating surgery in many cases.

Regulatory Risks

Like their counterparts in the U.S., German drug makers regularly use these arguments to counter claims that drug prices and spending are too high. German drug firms complain that lower drug prices will devastate the industry, which remains one of Germany's premier—though diminished—export industries. They warn that price freezes and controls will emasculate research and development operations, and anecdotal evidence suggests that German firms have shifted R&D to U.S. parents and subsidiaries, no doubt fueling higher U.S. drug costs. U.S. firms, if faced with price cuts, could shift R&D to other countries where costs are lower, though access to the latest technology would become a problem.

However, reduced profits may have the opposite effect. Faced with lower earnings, companies may find it advantageous to develop more products to maintain sales levels over the long term. But with each drug costing more than $200 million to develop, drug firms' ability to increase drug development is severely restricted. And as the German evidence shows, price rollbacks do not affect promotion budgets, the most likely source of funds for greater R&D. Whether price controls or freezes on U.S. drugs will have similar effects remains to be seen.

References

1. Rublee, DA and Schneider, M (1991). International Health Spending: Comparisons with the OECD. *Health Affairs* Vol. 10, No. 3.

2. Arnold, M (1991). *Health Care in the Federal Republic of Germany* Koln: Deutscher Ärzte-Verlag, p.45.

3. Scrip *World Pharmaceutical News.* June 3, 1992, No. 1,723, p. 9.

4. BASYS (Beratungsgesellschaft für angewandte Systemforschung mbH), Augsburg, 1992.

5. Organization for Economic Cooperation and Development (1991).

6. Bundesverband der Pharmazeutischen Industrie e.V. (1992). *Pharma Daten '92.* Hofheim: Gutenberg-Druck und Verlag.

7. Levit, KR, Lazenby, HC, Cowan, CA, and Letsche, SW (1991). National Health Expenditures 1990. *Health Care Financing Review* Vol. 13, No. 1,pp.29-54.

8. Scrip *World Pharmaceutical News* (1992). German Pharmaceutical Market in 1991. June 3, 1992, No. 1,723, p. 9.

9. Bundesverband der Pharmazeutischen Industrie e.V. (1993). The Healthcare System in Germany. Special Report. January 25, 1993. p.1.

10. Sachverständigenrat für die Konzertierte Aktion im Gesundheitswesen (1991). *Jahresgutachten 1991: Herausforderungen und Perspektiven der Gesundheitsversorgung.* Baden-Baden: Nomos Verlagsgesellschaft; p.267.

11. Schwabe, U and Paffrath, D (eds.) (1992). *Arzneiverordnungs-Report '92.* Stuttgart/Jena: Gustav Fischer Verlag.

12. Stillfried, D (1993), personal communication.

13. Ibid.

14. Levit, KR, Lazenby, HC, Cowan, CA, and Letsche, SW (1991).

15. Organization for Economic Cooperation and Development (1992).

16. Vogel, R (1992). Presentation at Goethe Institute Conference on German Health Care, Boston, October 17, 1992.

17. Hess, R (1992). Presentation at Goethe Institute Conference on German Health Care, Boston, October 16-17, 1992.

18. Schwabe, U and Paffrath, D (eds.) (1992).

19. Kassenärztliche Bundesvereinigung (1992). Grunddaten zur kassenärztlichen Bersorgung in der Bundesrepublik Deutschland 1991.

20. Hargis, JR, editor (1992). *Lilly Digest.* Indianapolis: Eli Lilly and Company, p.3.

21. Kassenärztliche Bundesvereinigung (1992). Grunddaten zur kassenärztlichen Bersorgung in der Bundesrepublik Deutschland 1991.

22. Ibid (1992). Chart E4.

23. Schicke, RK (1973). The Pharmaceutical Market and Prescription Drugs in the Federal Republic of Germany: Cross-national Comparisons. *International Journal of Health Services*, Vol. 3, No. 2, pp. 223-236.

24. Geursen, R (1993). *Medizin nach Listen.* Köln: Deutscher Ärzte-Verlag.

25. *Health United States* (1991). Washington: Department of Health and Human Services, p. 219.

26. Simonsen, LLP (1992). What are Pharmacists Dispensing Most Often? *Pharmacy Times* Vol. 4, p.47.

27. Schicke, RK (1973), pp. 223-236.

28. Ibid.

29. Ibid.

30. Ibid.

31. Arnold, M (1991), p.46.

32. Simonsen, LLP (1992), p.47.

33. Freudenheim, M (1992). All About: Generic Pharmaceuticals. Now the Big Drug Makers are Imitating Their Imitators. *New York Times* Sept. 20, 1992; Sect. 3, p.5.

34. Ibid.

35. U.S. Congress Office of Technology Assessment (1993). *Pharmaceutical R&D: Costs, Risks and Rewards.* OTA-H-522. Washington, DC: U.S. Government Printing Office. p. 30.

36. Kirkman-Liff, B (1990). Physician Payment Cost-containment. *Journal of Health Policy Law* Vol. 15, No. 1, Spring 1990, p.90.

37. Hapke, H (1992). Interview with R.A. Knox, December 1992.

38. Ibid.

39. Schicke, RK (1973), p.233.

40. Ibid.

41. Ibid.

42. Ibid, p.229.

43. Ibid, pp. 227-8.

44. Ibid, pp. 228-9.

45. Oberender, P (1988). Marktzugang und Tendenzen der Bedarfssteuerung auf dem Arzneimittelmarkt. In: Gérard Gäfgen (ed.) *Neokorporatismus und Gesundheitswesen.* Baden-Baden, Nomos Verlagsgesellschaft, pp. 217-226.

46. Oberender, P (1984). Pharmazeutische Inudstrie. In: Peter Oberender (ed.) *Marketstruktur und Wettbewerb in der Bundesrepublik Deutschland, Brachenstudien zur deutschen Wirtschaft.* München: Verlag Vahlen, pp. 243-310.

47. Arnold, M, et al. (1982). *The Medical Profession in the Federal Republic of Germany.* Köln-Lövenich: Deutscher Ärzte-Verlag. At 5.5.8.3.

48. Ibid.

49. Ibid.

50. Arnold, M (1991).

51. Wertheimer, A (1993). Testimony before the U.S. House Committee on Energy and Commerce Subcommittee on Health and the Environment. February 22, 1993.

52. Hapke, H (1992).

53. Arnold, M et al. (1982), at 5.5.8.3.

54. Bundesverband der Pharmazeutischen Industrie e.V. (1992).

55. Ibid.

56. Vogel, R (1992).

57. Ibid.

58. Nord, D (1986). State Control and Drug Supply. In: *Political Values and Health Care: The German Experience.* Cambridge, MA: MIT Press. pp. 360-361.

59. Stone, D (1991). German Unification: East Meets West in the Doctor's Office. *Journal of Health Politics, Policy, and Law*, Vol. 16, No. 2, p.408.

60. Schicke, RK (1973), p. 225.

61. Arzneimittel Zeitung (1992). *In Focus: The Health Systems and Pharmaceutical Markets in 16 Countries. Special Report.* pp. 31-38.

62. Pharmaceutical Manufacturers Association (1993). *New Drug Approvals in 1992.* January 1993.

63. Pharmaceutical Manufacturers Association (1992). Industry Issue Brief: Europe 1992.

64. Arzneimittel Zeitung (1992).

65. U.S. Congress Office of Technology Assessment (1993), p.24.

66. Kassenärztliche Bundesvereinigung (1993).

67. Scientific Institute of Local Sickness Funds (1992).

68. Bundesverband der Pharmazeutischen Industrie e.V. (1992).

69. Arnold, M (1991). p. 48.

70. Hapke, H (1992).

71. U.S. Congress Office of Technology Assessment (1993), p.1.

72. Hapke, H (1992).

73. Freudenheim, M (1992).

74. Hapke, H (1992).

75. Ibid.

76. Bundesverband der Pharmazeutischen Industrie e.V. (1993). *The Healthcare System in Germany. Special Report.* January 25, 1993.

77. Sachverständigenrat für die Konzertierte Aktion im Gesundheitswesen (1991). p. 92.

78. Schwabe, U and Paffrath, D (1992).

79. Rep. Henry Waxman (D-CA) press conference, February 25, 1993. Based on an Office of Technology Assessment study.

80. Schicke, RK (1973), p.225.

81. Ibid.

82. Arnold, M (1991), p.46.

83. Personal communication to R.A. Knox.

84. Schicke, RK (1973), p. 223.

85. Ibid.

86. Ibid, p. 227.

87. Ibid.

88. Ibid.

89. *The Pink Sheet*. Chain Stores Must Take Leadership Role in Health Care Reform Now That Debate Has Turned to Drug Costs, New NACDS Chairman Urges at Annual Meeting. May 4, 1992, p. 15.

90. Ibid.

91. Ibid.

92. Schicke, RK (1973), p. 228.

93. Ibid.

94. *The Pink Sheet* (1992). Mail Order Grew 37 Percent to $2.9 Billion in 1991; IMS Survey Growth May Slow Soon. March 16, 1992, p. 11.

95. Enquete Kommission (1990). Report, p. 511.

96. Arnold, M et al (1982).

97. Hapke, H (1992).

98. Ibid.

99. Sachverständigenrat für die Konzertierte Aktion im Gesundheitswesen (1992). p. 64.

100. Pfaff, M (1992). Interview with R.A. Knox in Tübingen, December 1992.

101. Schulte, G (1992). "Problems of Health Care in the Conflict Area between Market Economy and Governmental Economic Control." Speech to Goethe Institute, Boston, October 16, 1992.

102. Ibid.

103. Redwood, H (1992). *The Dynamics of Drug Pricing and Reimbursement in the European Community: Where are Control Systems Leading Suppliers, Prescribers and Patients? Assessment and Prognosis.* New York: PharmaBooks Ltd, p. 106.

104. Redwood, H (1992), p. 108.

105. Ibid.

106. Ibid.

107. Arzneimittel Zeitung (1992).

108. Geursen, R (1993).

109. Sachverständigenrat für die Konzertierte Aktion im Gesundheitswesen (1991), p. 68.

110. Redwood, H (1992), p. 112.

111. Vogel, R (1992).

112. Hapke, H (1992).

113. Redwood, H (1992). p. 110.

114. Ibid, p. 112.

115. Ibid.

116. Bundesverband der Pharmazeutischen Industrie e.V. (1993).

117. Ibid.

118. Hapke, H (1992).

119. Ibid.

120. Ibid.

121. Redwood, H (1992), p. 110.

122. Hapke, H (1992).

123. Redwood, H (1992), p. 118.

124. Ibid.

125. Arzneimittel Zeitung (1992).

126. Bundesverband der Pharmazeutischen Industrie e.V. (1993). p. 1.

127. Redwood, H (1992), p. 113.

128. Ibid, p. 109.

129. Hapke H (1992).

130. Schulte, G (1992).

131. Bundesverband der Pharmazeutischen Industrie e.V. (1993). p. 1.

132. Ibid.

133. Ibid.

134. Schwabe, U and Paffrath, D (1992).

135. Fiedler, E (1993). *Handelsblatt* No. 23, p.6. Issue date: 3 February 1993.

136. Scrip *World Pharmaceutical News* (1992). Issue 1762, p. 5.

137. Bundesverband der Pharmazeutischen Industrie e.V. (1993). p. 7.

138. Ibid.

139. Arzneimittel Zeitung (1992), p. 38.

140. Ullbricht, PC (1992). Interview with R.A. Knox, December 1992.

141. Brochure published by the Aktionsgemeinschaft Baden-Württembergischer Apotheker, ca. December 1992.

142. Ibid.

143. Bundesverband der Pharmazeutischen Industrie e.V. (1993), p. 9.

144. Hapke, H (1992).

145. Personal communication by R.A. Knox with Michael Arnold, December 1992.

146. As quoted by Schulte, G (1992). *Frankfurter Allgemeine* ca. Oct. 1992.

147. *Die Woche*, February 18, 1993, p.33.

148. *Der Spiegel*, February 1, 1993, pp. 200-201.

149. *Die Woche* (1993).

150. *Der Spiegel* (1993).

151. Ullbricht, PC (1992).

CHAPTER 7

Reunifying German Health Care: The Grand Experiment

With the signing of the historic *Treaty of Reunification* on August 31, 1990, Germany entered phase II of a grand and unprecedented natural experiment in health care delivery. Phase I formally began 41 years earlier, on October 7, 1949, with the creation of the German Democratic Republic. By then occupying Soviet forces had already dismantled what was left of the war-torn German health care system founded 66 years before by Chancellor Otto von Bismarck. Decision-making in the new East German health care system was centralized and state-controlled — a 180-degree departure from the decentralized and thoroughly private structures in the West, which carefully observes what is called a "subsidiary" role for government. In the 1950s and 1960s the East Germans achieved some public health successes impressive by any standards, but the 1970s began a long period of decline due to pinched resources and ossifying bureaucracy.[1] By the time the Iron Curtain collapsed in a heap of ideological rust, East Germany's socialist health care experiment was judged by the world — and certainly by West Germans — to be an abject disaster, a conspicuous failure in a social sphere in which socialist ideologues claimed special superiority over capitalists. "The whole system is discredited," observes Jeremy W. Hurst of Great Britain's Department of Health, "by its association with the former German Democratic Republic."[2] Without looking back, West Germany launched **Phase II**, a reconstruction of the health care financing and delivery forms that had evolved over 107 unbroken years in the west. Equally heroic, the "*Wessies*" have begun a determined effort to transform both the decrepit physical infrastructure and the *Weltanschauung* of health care personnel in former East Germany to match those in the west.

Reunifying German health care has taken place at a breathless pace. The new system, complete with West German-style sickness funds and payment mechanisms, took effect on schedule only four months after the reunification treaty's signing. A system that was, for all practical purposes, entirely socialist, with government-salaried doctors, nurses, technicians, social workers, and support personnel, was mostly privatized within two years. Dark and shabby government clinics have been transformed into bright, carpeted, computer-equipped private doctors' offices. Sophisticated new machines have quickly supplanted equipment straight out of a Norman Rockwell sepia-toned painting of a 1940s-era country doctor's office. Physicians scrambled for private office space and learned how to be hard-driving entrepreneurs, coping with sizable mortgages, fee-for-service billing systems, ruthless competition with their colleagues, and a steady influx of drug company salesmen. Even though their fees were set as much as 60 percent below prevailing western levels during a five-year transition period, doctors in the east have become financially well-off beyond their dreams.

Compared to other aspects of reunification — 15 percent unemployment rates in the east, neo-Nazism and xenophobia, widespread resentment among struggling "*Ossies*" toward the affluent and arrogant "*Wessies*," flagging industrial productivity — the transformation of health care in former East Germany has appeared to an outsider remarkably smooth and successful. That impression, while not entirely invalid, conceals fierce debates that flared over the shape of the new system. Many on both sides of the fallen Berlin Wall argued that Germany should seize a priceless opportunity to mount a different sort of experiment, preserving some of the eastern health care values and institutions that had worked well in order to point the way toward needed reforms in the west. That was not to be. There was some flirtation with the idea of experimenting with other options in Germany's new eastern states — even with adopting a British, Swedish, Finnish, or even American-style health system.[3] But in the end, the government of Chancellor Helmut Kohl decided to impose the West German system *in toto,* an outcome that resulted from adroit political maneuvering by organized medicine in West Germany and, some participants argue, from the necessity to erect a new system quickly to avoid social chaos. This chapter will examine some of the successes and failures of the East German health care experiment, the politics of health care reunification, and the challenge that lies ahead for Germany as it struggles simultaneously to bootstrap its eastern states up to the western standard and to correct emerging problems in the health structure of the "old federal states."

East German Health Care: German Ideas, Soviet Ideology

The postwar period in Germany's eastern sector presented the Soviet Union with a crisis and an opportunity. Millions of people had been killed in the war, millions more were uprooted refugees with no means of livelihood. While this was true throughout Germany, living conditions were worse in the east. Malnutrition was rampant, undermining people's health. Living conditions in the bombed-out cities were unhygienic in the extreme, setting the stage for epidemic disease. The health care infrastructure had been shattered; many physicians had fled to the west as the Soviet Army approached.[4] Strong, immediate, and centrally determined action was vital; this kind of intervention was entirely consistent with Soviet socialist ideology. The Soviets saw their sector of Germany as an ideal laboratory in which to prove the superiority of socialist health care over corrupt capitalist models. "The Soviet Union obviously attached eminent political importance to the German health system and its reorganization from the first," stresses Stefan Kirchberger, Dr.Phil., professor of medical sociology at Münster University.[5]

A National System of Local Health Clinics

One of the Soviets' first actions in the months immediately following the war was to abolish the traditional German separation between hospital and ambulatory care doctors, a decision dictated by dire necessity since there were insufficient numbers of physicians outside hospitals.[6] In 1946, they established a **Central Health Administration**, the first central authority in German history responsible for the entire health system.[7] In 1947, they proceeded to suppress private health care services and construct a hierarchical system of national, state, and district health agencies. A "pivotal point," notes Aloys Henning, MD, of the Free University of Berlin, was the Soviet authorities' decree in 1947 establishing a network of **ambulatories** (primary care centers) and **polyclinics** (multispecialty outpatient care centers)[8] — a step taken over the vehement but futile objections of German physicians in the Soviet sector.[9] However, free choice of physician was preserved, a concept unknown in the Soviet Union.[10]

Ironically, the system imposed by the Soviets on East Germany was German in conception. The Social Hygiene Movement pioneered by Johann Peter Frank, Alfred Grotjahn, and other Germans in the late 19th and early 20th centuries stressed prevention over curative medicine. Championed by German socialists in the 1920s, social medicine was emulated by Lenin "to refocus the centralized system he had inherited from the tsars toward public and occupational health," notes sociologist Donald W. Light, PhD, professor of comparative health systems at the University of Medicine and Dentistry of New Jersey. "Faced with mass starvation and epidemics, Lenin established a national system of local health stations."[11] However, Henning points out that the highly centralized bureaucracy that characterized East German health care "is neither particularly socialist — Marx seems to have considered voluntary associations — nor particularly appropriate. It is simply Russian....Its absolutist semi-military administrative structures were created by the reforms of Tsar Peter I."[12]

The Sickness Funds Persist

In contrast to the more than 1,300 sickness funds in West Germany, 89 percent of East Germans were insured through the Free German Trade Union and the other 11 percent (the self-employed, members of cooperatives, state employees, and their dependents) were covered by the state. But unlike the Soviet system, a semblance of Germany's sickness funds persisted: Most of the population paid contributions into their health insurance fund, employers contributed a portion of the premium, and higher-income workers could buy extra benefits for "voluntary surcharges."[13] Virtually all health care workers, including many doctors practicing in single-doctor settings, were employees of the state and subject to its rigid hierarchy. The East German health care delivery system was a "planner's fantasy," says Deborah Stone, PhD, Brandeis University professor of law and social policy. "A system of increasingly sophisticated treatment facilities is laid out to cover increasingly large population bases."[14] The principal aim, which was reportedly achieved in the main, was to make primary care accessible in every community and every sizable workplace. The Soviets moved quickly to establish a network of company-based clinics and health stations, which the East Germans maintained until the regime collapsed. (Figure 7.1) In fact, most East German encounters with the health system occurred in the workplace. In 1987, 7.2 million workers and their dependents were treated in company-based clinics versus 3.2 million people in the system of community-based clinics.[15] In addition, there was an extensive system of almost 10,000 maternal health centers to deliver prenatal, postnatal, and well-baby care. The far-flung network of day-care centers had its own health stations to carry out vaccinations, preventive care, and primary care, as did kindergartens and schools.

East Germany's Distorted Demographics

While concepts of Social Hygiene and the desire for a socialist showcase shaped the philosophy of East Germany's health care system, its priorities were largely determined by a less abstract factor: the new nation's skewed age and sex structure. Two world wars had "depleted the ranks of working men, resulting in

Figure 7.1

Workplace-based Health Care Centers in East Germany, 1950-89

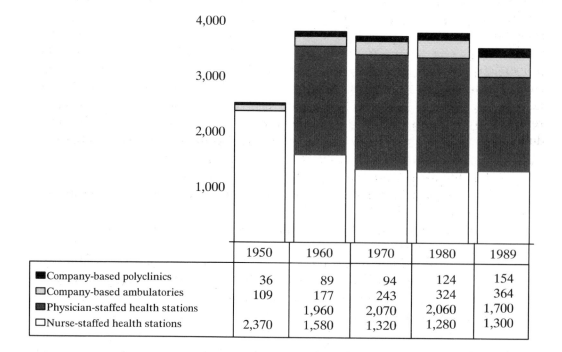

	1950	1960	1970	1980	1989
■ Company-based polyclinics	36	89	94	124	154
□ Company-based ambulatories	109	177	243	324	364
■ Physician-staffed health stations		1,960	2,070	2,060	1,700
□ Nurse-staffed health stations	2,370	1,580	1,320	1,280	1,300

Source: Sachverständigenrat für die Konzertierte Aktion im Gesundheitswesen, 1991.

a preponderance of women over men and a worsening dependency ratio of working-age people to children and older people," notes Hans-Joachim von Kondratowitz, Dr.Phil., of the German Center for Gerontology in Munich.[16] (Figure 7.2) This long term trend was exacerbated in East Germany by the flight of many postwar German refugees to the west. As economic conditions remained bleak in the 1950s, East Germany's labor force was reduced further by the emigration of an additional 2.6 million citizens, a hemorrhage only stemmed in August, 1961, by a drastic remedy — the Berlin Wall.[17]

Many postwar phenomena affecting health care in the two Germanies are better understood in light of this labor shortage — for instance, West Germany's decision to admit millions of "guest workers" as long-term residents (but not naturalized citizens). In 1989 nearly 1.7 million foreign workers were obligatory members of West German sickness funds, making up 7.5 percent of those insured through the statutory health insurance system.[18] In East Germany, building up the labor pool became one of the communist regime's top priorities. It was reflected in the heavy emphasis placed on maternal and child health in the East German health system, a policy that became both the system's hallmark and its greatest success.

Incorporating Motherhood into the Workforce

The rights of women, for instance, were given great stress in the 1949 *Constitution of the German Democratic Republic*, and enlarged in Article 20 of the 1968 Constitution, which proclaimed that "Man and woman have equal rights and have the same legal status in all parts of social, national, and personal life. The promotion of women, especially in their work sphere, is a social and national task." If this was good Marxist doctrine, it was also and undeniably a practical necessity for the struggling new nation. It was vital for East German women to work, and work they did — or face social stigmatization. Seventy-nine percent of employable-age women were in the workforce in 1975, nearly half of all employed persons,[19] and the proportion approached 90 percent of working-age women in the late 1970s.[20] At the time of reunification, 73 percent of women had full-time jobs that kept them at work nearly nine hours a day.[21] Yet it was equally vital for women to bear children to replenish the nation's depleted stock of laborers — the more children the better. This double necessity led to an array of child-centered programs far surpassing anything the U.S. had achieved three and four decades later. They included

- an elaborate system of child-bearing financial incentives,
- liberal paid maternity leaves and infant day care programs at the worksite,
- maternal and child health initiatives with their own financial inducements to encourage participation,
- child-care accommodations for working mothers and their children encompassing more than half of children under three and 87 percent of children aged three to six in 1976,[22] and
- school health programs.

To induce people to have children, East German parents were offered an escalating schedule of monthly financial allowances for each child, interest-free housing loans, and a DM 1,000 cash bounty per infant. The **birth bounty** was paid in installments if the expectant mother kept her prenatal care appointments; 100

Figure 7.2

The Two Germanies' Shrinking Labor Pool*, 1939-70

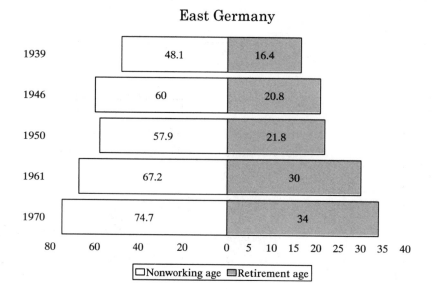

East Germany

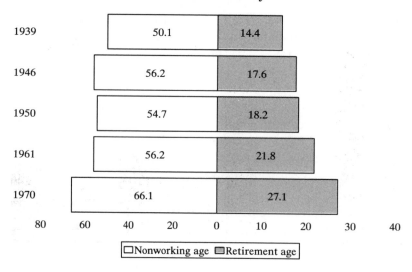

West Germany

*Number of persons of nonworking age (men under 15 and over 65, women under 15 and over 60) and of retirement age (men over 65, women over 60) per 100 persons of working age.

Source: H-J von Kondratowitz, Political Values and Health Care (1986), after K. Lungwitz (1974), Jahrbuch für Wirtschaftsgeschichte, Vol. I.

Figure 7.3

Official Infant Mortality Rates in Selected Years

(Deaths under 1 year of age per 1,000 live births.)

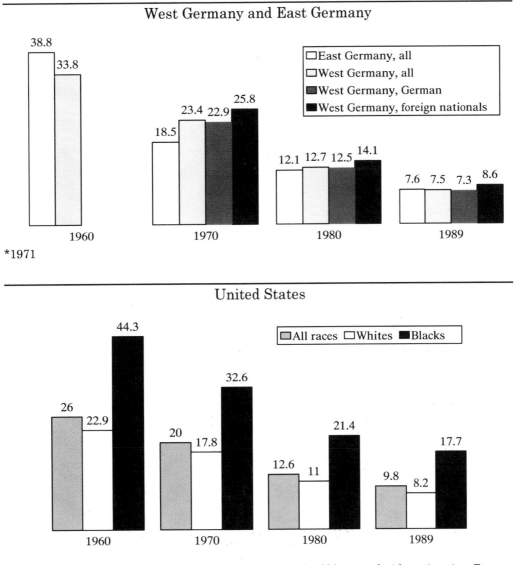

*1971

Note: Comparisons between East Germany and other nations should be treated with caution, since East Germany did not include infants who died soon after birth among "live-born infants, a definition which depresses rates of infant deaths per 1,000 live births. In 1973, the disparate definition accounted for about 2.5 points of the deaths/1,000 difference between West and East German rates. In later years, the definition accounted for proportionately samller degrees of difference between East Germany and other nations. The figures above are given to indicate trends and magnitudes of difference in infant mortality among the 3 nations.

Sources: Daten des Gesundheitswesens 1991, *Bundesministerium für Gesundheit;* Health United States 1991, *U.S. Department of Health and Human Services.*

marks was held back after the birth, to be paid in steps at each of four monthly postnatal care checkups.[23] These incentives were successful in increasing compliance with prenatal care guidelines beyond what the U.S. had achieved in 1989. In 1974, 84 percent of East German women began prenatal care in the first trimester of pregnancy.[24] Fifteen years later in the U.S., by contrast, the proportion of pregnancies with first-trimester care were 79 percent among white women, 60 percent of black women, 58 percent of American Indian women, and 59 percent of Hispanic women.[25] Only 1.1 percent of East German women began prenatal care during the eighth month or received no care prior to delivery in 1974,[26] compared to 7.9 percent of U.S. women in 1970 — and 6.4 percent as late as 1989.[27]

The extraordinary efforts invested in maternal and child health did not solve East Germany's labor shortage. In fact, birth rates dropped continuously throughout the 1960s and early 1970s,[28] though the pro-natalist campaign may have helped produce an upturn in the birth rate after 1975.[29] Thus, it is surprising that East Germany legalized abortions in 1972, which significantly depressed the birth rate.

Figure 7.4

Pregnancy-Related Maternal Mortality Trends 1956-89: Maternal deaths per 100,000 live births, East Germany, West Germany, U.S.

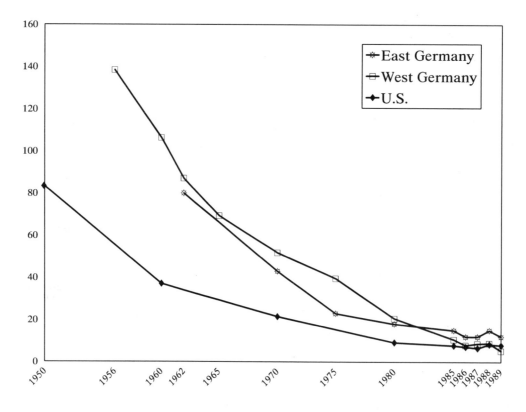

Sources: Daten des Gesundheitswesens 1991, *Bundesministerium für Gesundheit;* Health United States 1991, *U.S. Department of Health and Human Services; and Dr. Aloys Henning,* Political Values and Health Care *(1986).*

Due to East Germany's more liberal abortion laws, its rate of abortions per 1,000 live births was 2.5 to 4 times that of West Germany's by the late 1970s.[30] Legalizing abortion was partly an expression of women's rights and partly a successful attempt to reduce deaths of women undergoing unsafe illegal abortions.[31]

Infant Mortality Rates: Something To Brag About

East Germany's emphasis on pregnancy care did pay off in reductions of infant mortality and pregnancy-related maternal deaths, a record that stands up to comparison with much wealthier nations, including West Germany and the U.S. (Figures 7.3 and 7.4) Starting in 1960 with an infant mortality rate significantly higher than both of those nations, East Germany managed to reduce its rate to comparable or lower levels in the subsequent two decades.

One must interpret East German infant mortality rates with caution, since authorities there used a definition at variance with the World Health Organi-

Figure 7.5

Childhood Vaccination Rates: 1989

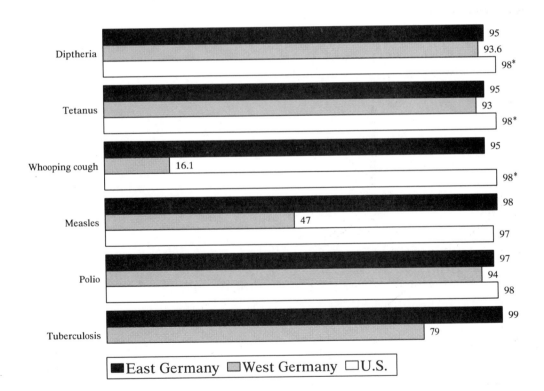

*In the U.S., a combined vaccine is administered for diptheria, tetanus and whooping cough.

Sources: Sachverständigenrat für die Konzertierte Aktion im Gesundheitswesen, 1991: and U.S. Center for Health Statistics, 1991.

zation standard. East Germany did not count deaths of infants soon after birth nor stillborn infants, which had the effect of making its infant mortality rates appear lower than other nations'. For instance, in 1973 the West German rate of 22.7 infant deaths per 1,000 live births would have been about 2.5 lower than that if West Germany had used the East German definition, according to one estimate.[32] As rates fell below that, the differential due to the disparate definition were presumably smaller. One former East German health planner acknowledges that officials there were very aware of the propaganda value of its infant mortality rate. "Infant mortality was a politically important measure, so we tried to emphasize it," says Berndt Schirmer, MD, former director of planning in the East German Ministry of Health.[33] Nevertheless, health statisticians consider East Germany's infant mortality successes to be genuine, and all the more impressive considering that society's low income levels. In addition, about 35 percent of all births in East Germany were illegitimate, since financial incentives to bear children did not require that mothers be married. Low income and illegitimacy are associated with higher infant mortality in most societies. As Hurst of the British Health Department put it, East Germany was able to "achieve good improvements in indicators such as infant mortality with relatively low expenditure and relatively poor facilities."[34] East Germany achieved higher childhood vaccination rates than West Germany. (Figure 7.5) Childhood preventive health programs could not avail against some hazards, however. High air pollution levels may have been responsible for 1988 respiratory death rates among children under five years old up to three times the West German rate, and 14 times the U.S. rate.[35]

The Downside of East German Priorities

East Germany's chronic labor shortage and its strategic decision to put its health care system at the service of national productivity had their dark side for older citizens. Discrimination in favor of the young and fit — and against the old and failing — was pervasive. For instance, in the delivery of medical and rehabilitation services, people who were temporarily incapacitated by illness or injury, and therefore could be returned to work, were "given priority over those permanently incapacitated by age or disability," report Peter Rosenberg, senior economist at the Federal Ministry of Labor and Social Affairs in Bonn, and Maria Elizabeth Ruban, senior researcher at the German Institute for Economic Research in Berlin.[36]

Keeping Elders At Work

More systematic was the nation's approach to occupational health among older workers. East Germany's birth rate was one of the world's lowest, and the population's average age one of the highest. It had one of the world's highest proportions of pensioners, and women pensioners outnumbered men by more than two to one, due to the decimating effects of World War II and a drastic decline in births during World War I.[37] Political leaders decided they had no choice but to keep older workers on the job as long as possible, according to von Kondratowitz of the German Center for Gerontology.[38]

Table 7.1

Suicide Rates Per 100,000 Inhabitants in East Germany, West Germany, U.S.: 1988

Age group in years	East Germany Male	East Germany Female	West Germany Male	West Germany Female	Age Group in years	U.S*. Male	U.S*. Female
0-15	1.5	.5	.5	.1	5-14	1.1	.4
15-20	9.9	3.1	11.0	3.3	15-14	23.4	4.6
20-40	33.1	8.3	22.2	7.3	25-34	25.7	6.1
40-60	56.4	20.4	31.1	9.3	35-44	24.1	7.4
					45-54	23.2	8.6
					55-64	27.0	7.9
60+	99.8	48.2	49.0	20.4	65-74	35.4	7.3
					75-84	61.5	7.4
					85+	65.8	5.3

*Whites only.

Source: Sachverständigenrat für die Konzertierte Aktion im Gesundheitswesen, 1991; and U.S. Department of Health and Human Services, 1991

The policy was explicit. For instance, in 1957, in the midst of East Germany's "second 5-year plan" for economic development, officials concluded that the labor supply was exhausted and the only alternative was to boost productivity. A nationwide system of factory-based health stations was set up to monitor the capabilities and limitations of older workers and, ostensibly, match them to the demands of particular jobs. The aim, according to the chief of one polyclinic, was "to preserve the capability to work for as long as possible beyond the pension age."[39] The emphasis on extending the working life of pensioners was even greater in the 1960s.[40] Despite a stated aim of finding suitable jobs, older workers often were treated as second-class citizens. They were placed in jobs that were unattractive to younger workers, and required to perform hard physical labor.[41] One study of three different kinds of factories found that more than half the aging workers were in a "markedly lowered" state of health.[42]

Yet most older workers could not afford to stop working, since pensions were miserably small — a deliberate policy to keep them in the workforce, according to von Kondratowitz. Pensioners who worked had twice the income of those who retired.[43] Rosenberg and Ruban reported in 1986 that

In 1980, when the average income was 1,030 marks per month, the average disability pension was 340 marks, the average old-age pension 321 marks, and the average old-age-plus-disability pension 302 marks. Retirement thus forces most workers and salaried employees to reduce their standard of living noticeably.[44]

In addition, East Germany's eligibility criteria for pensions were much tougher than in West Germany. Furthermore, elderly housing and nursing home beds were in short supply, according to interviews with East Germans and others. "Many elderly people couldn't get care, didn't have mobility, couldn't afford a telephone, didn't have social supports," says Hans-Konrad Selbmann of the University of Tübingen, who coauthored a 1991 report on health care reunification.[45] "Old people's lives in the German Democratic Republic were hard — *really* hard," adds Christian Reichmuth, a lawyer from former East Germany. "They had very low pensions, poor housing. Old people's homes often had six beds to a room, so they lost all their privacy and individuality."[46]

One disturbing index of despair was a suicide rate among middle-aged and elderly East Germans two to three times as high as West Germany's and five to ten times higher than those in the U.S. (Table 7.1) Diminished longevity among East Germans is another indicator of bleaker economic and health status. At age 65, remaining life expectancy for East German men was 1.5 to 2.3 years shorter than for West German or American men, and 2.5 to 3 years shorter for East German women. (Figure 7.6) These figures are probably the most reliable overall health indices, Selbmann points out, as they "cannot be manipulated easily."[47]

Failing the Chronically Ill

Mortality from leading chronic diseases was often (though not invariably) higher in East Germany than West Germany or the U.S. For instance, the reported age-adjusted mortality rate from heart and circulatory disease among East German males in 1988 was 40 percent higher than their West German counterparts, and among women it was more than 60 percent higher.[48,49] This is consistent with a 1992 study that reports higher prevalence of high blood pressure and hypercholesterolemia in East Germany before reunification. "Cardiovascular disease risk factor prevalence was in general higher in East Germany for all risk factors, with the exception of cigarette smoking for females only," report Uwe Helmert of the Bremen Institute for Prevention Research and Social Medicine and his colleagues.[50] In turn, West Germany's age-adjusted heart disease mortality in 1988 was 2.3 to 2.7 times higher than America's, which may reflect a strikingly higher number of West Germans with seriously elevated serum cholesterol levels.[51] Heart disease deaths declined significantly in both nations in recent decades. Age-adjusted cardiovascular mortality rates in West Germany fell between 1979 and 1989 by 19 percent among 25 to 74-year-old men and 21 percent during the same period for similarly aged women.[52] In the U.S. overall cardiovascular disease mortality for both sexes fell by 46 percent between 1971 and 1991.[53]

Age-adjusted cancer rates were reportedly 12 to 15 percent *higher* in West Germany than in East Germany, and death rates for specific types of cancer were ostensibly much higher in West Germany, including prostate cancer (68 percent higher) and female breast cancer (35 percent higher). Whether these discrepancies

Figure 7.6

**Life Expectancy in Years at Birth and Age 65 in 1988:
West Germany, East Germany, U.S.**

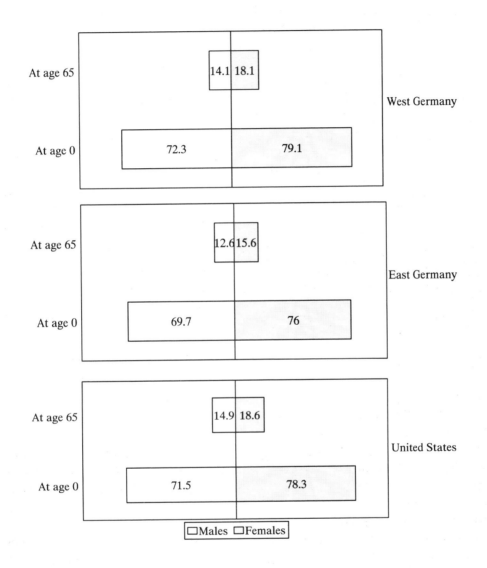

Differences in years (calculated from above)

	At birth		At age 65	
	male	female	male	female
West Germany/East Germany:	2.6	3.1	1.50	2.5
West Germany/United States:	0.8	0.8	-.08	-0.5
United States/East Germany:	1.8	2.3	2.30	3.0

*Sources: Health United States 1991, U.S. Department of Health and Human
Services.*

Table 7.2

Care of End-Stage Renal Disease in Germany: 1990

	New Federal* States	Old Federal** States
Number of dialysis treatment slots	800	8,000
Dialysis patients	2,500	24,000
Kidney transplants 1989	245	1,960
Dialysis patients/million residents	160	400
Kidney transplants/million residents	15	32

*Former East Germany.

**Former West Germany.

Sources: *Sachverständigenrat für die Konzertierte Aktion im Gesundheitswesen, 1991.*

represent systematic reporting error or actual differences in disease-specific mortality will probably take the Germans themselves a good deal of time and effort to sort out. However, it appears that cancer patients in East Germany are about three years younger than West Germany cancer patients when they die, a difference that may reflect more intensive anticancer therapy in the West.[54]

In their study of cardiovascular risk factors, Helmert and his coworkers found escalating risk associated with social class in both Germanies before reunification. "Although equity was a major political goal in East Germany," they write, "there have been health inequities comparable to those in Western Europe [sic] countries. But further investigations of these health inequalities in East Germany were hindered or even forbidden by state authorities, especially on important health indicators such as life expectancy started to fall behind the West German figures."[55]

Medical Care on the Front Lines: Scarcity and Scheming

After 1970, "the East German system became more run-down and rigid," notes sociologist Donald W. Light. "Morale dropped, coordination declined, and bureaucratic sclerosis set in."[56] Moreover, "the economic gap between the German Democratic Republic and the Federal Republic widened during the 1980s," notes Volker Wittke of the Social Research Institute of Göttingen.[57]

During East Germany's long decline toward eventual collapse in 1989, health care providers and their patients suffered myriad privations that became nearly intolerable in daily practice. As many explained in interviews, there was no alternative except to tolerate it and devise ingenious ways to cadge or reuse necessary supplies.

Supplying Charité

Administrators at the Charité, the venerable 260-year-old, 2,100-bed teaching hospital that was East Germany's flagship medical facility, tell of chronic shortages of such basic items as surgical gloves and drapes, intravenous tubing, and sterile syringes. In 1982, the Charité completed a sparkling new high-rise building, complete with East Germany's first total-body computerized tomography scanner and fully stocked supply cabinets. "We started proudly with disposable syringes and catheters imported from the West," recalls Tamara Benzet, an assistant to Charité's faculty dean. "We very soon realized there was no way to continue that and we again began to sterilize syringes and reuse gloves. There was no limit to staff, so rubber gloves were washed, sterilized, powdered, and sorted — all by hand. And gloves were only 1 of 101 supply problems."[58]

There were many instances, Benzet says, when surgeons would stand idle in the hospital's 26 operating suites while a driver was dispatched to the outskirts of East Berlin to the *Regierungskrankenhaus* — the hospital for high government officials — for rubber gloves or other supplies. "The *Regierungskrankenhaus* was very well-equipped," she explains. "If the situation here was very, very bad, in the last resort it was possible to send an ambulance there to fetch supplies. Only the Charité could do it. It was a privilege."

The anecdote is a glimpse of the inequality in East German health care that many commentators say was as pervasive as it was at odds with socialist ideals. Despite health care planning that blanketed the nation with a hierarchy of supposedly equal-access health care facilities rendering care from the preventive and primary to the tertiary (including organ transplants, open-heart surgery, and neonatal intensive care), some groups had special options. "It was mainly the political elite who had access to health care facilities with [the] West German standard," note Helmert and his colleagues.[59] Selbmann adds that East Germany "had several health care systems — for normal people, for the Army, for the *Stasi* [secret police], for Party officials, for athletes. They didn't know in their statistical yearbook how many doctors they really had. So when they started to make one system of health care, they found they had many doctors without employment — because they no longer needed a system for athletes, for state security, for Party members."[60]

High-Tech Care for Everyone...If Available

Every child in East Germany technically had equal access to high-tech care, according to Wolf-Rainer Cario, Dr.Sci.Med., a liver surgeon and, in 1991, director of the Second Pediatric Department at Berlin-Buch Hospital, a sprawling 4,000-bed institution in East Berlin that was the nation's biggest tertiary-care hospital. A child's chance of getting care at Berlin-Buch depended mainly "on the distance and whether the primary doctor would be interested and keen enough to get you to the next level," Cario says. "If you had a brain tumor you would have high priority. But if you develop a disorder of the brain, something not as acute, you might not have been referred."[61]

In a mirror of the problems with VIP care in affluent nations, high Party officials and their children did not always receive the best care at the *Regierungskrankenhaus* across the road from Berlin-Buch, according to Cario, who says he was not a Party member. "Doctors there [who treated the children of VIPs] only rarely saw severe diseases," he explains. "Often such children had to be transferred to us after being diagnosed over there — anonymously, so we wouldn't know who the parent was. There were very odd situations. In the government hospitals, doctors would feel incompetent to handle them, and they would transfer a child to me. I wouldn't have disposable syringes. They would be horrified and take the child back rather than give me the syringes."[62]

Elisabeth Saar, Berlin-Buch's chief of nursing, tells of how she and her staff sometimes manipulated Party officials into giving them sorely needed equipment:

> Until 1987, we had no infusion pumps [for delivering precisely calibrated doses of intravenous drugs]. We would have to hang up the IV drip and let it run. By a trick we were able to get six infusion pumps. For propaganda reasons, there was an interest in young doctors doing research. We had a team that got prizes at many levels. Before one visit from the deputy minister of health, I managed with difficulty to phone him in advance and ask if he wouldn't like to visit the children's tumor ward. The prizewinners diplomatically educated him about the dangers of wrong infusion techniques. He is a pharmacist of an age to have grandchildren, and he was moved. We got the six infusion pumps. But this technique didn't always work.

If East Germany's elite institutions had such shortages, the situation in ordinary doctors' offices was bleak during the declining years of the German Democratic Republic. "It was dearth, dearth, dearth," recalls Hartmut Reichwage, a 63-year-old family practitioner in the southern town of Geraberg, describing the availability of medical equipment, drugs, and supplies before the Wall fell on November 9, 1989. Reichwage, who earned a monthly salary of about $12,500 from the state, worked out of a one-physician office with medical technology straight out of the 1940s and light-years from the typical West German physician's office. He describes what he had to work with: "a stethoscope, a microscope for urinary sediment, a blood pressure cuff, an ear mirror — nothing else."

Liver Transplants or Tanks

Centralized health planning was a frustrating exercise in a nation with low and declining economic resources. Even though the German Democratic Republic had the strongest economy in the Eastern bloc, its industrial productivity was at least 30 percent below that of the Federal Republic of Germany, a structural problem "which creates a permanent demand for more labor and limits the expansion of social services," Aloys Henning notes.[63] In 1975, East Germany spent 15.4 percent of its budget on social services, including health care, compared to 29 percent in the West. Moreover, social spending in West Germany rose steadily (though not at the inflationary rates in the U.S.) while in the East it was static.[64] The situation did not improve in the 1980s, which saw annual budgetary increases for health care in the range of 3 to 4 percent, a rate that did not allow for inflation. "In the last years, in reality, we didn't have any real increase," says Berndt Schirmer, who was chief of planning in the East German Ministry of Health during this period.[65]

Despite its straitened circumstances, East Germany managed to acquire some modern medical technology and provide some advanced services while upgrading the general health of its population. For instance:

- East Berlin had three neonatal intensive care units which served the entire nation.[66]
- Open-heart surgery was available, but facilities were much scarcer than in West Germany, where nearly 70,000 cardiac operations were performed in 1992 in 57 centers.[67] East German figures are not available, but it was reportedly unusual for a patient to be referred for coronary artery bypass surgery.[68]
- Obstetricians at leading teaching hospitals acquired ultrasound machines, but not until 1984; as of 1988, only one East Berlin obstetrician had been certified in the use of obstetrical ultrasound.[69]
- Magnetic resonance imaging has been available since 1987 — but there was only one MRI scanner in East Berlin and one more at an Army hospital in Frankfurt-an-der-Oder, near the Polish border.[70]
- There were 31 computerized tomography (CT) scanners in East Germany by 1990, about 40 percent of West Germany's complement on a per-population basis.[71]
- By 1990 East Germany had acquired a half-dozen lithotripters for treating kidney stones.[72]
- East Germany's first liver transplant was performed in 1980, and the first pediatric liver transplant was in 1982.[73]

The Case of a Liver Failure in East Germany

The treatment of people with end-stage renal disease (kidney failure) offers a revealing glimpse of the capacities and shortcomings of high-tech care in East Germany — and of the way central health planning worked. Kidney dialysis and transplantation came into widespread use in most developed nations in the 1960s and early 1970s, and East Germany launched kidney transplant programs in 1968.[74] When the anti-rejection drug cyclosporin-A came into use in the 1980s, transplant surgeons in East Germany were able to obtain it for routine use by 1986, even though it cost more than 10 times more than previous, less effective immunosuppressive regimens, according to Peter Althaus, MD, the Mayo Clinic-trained chief of urology at the Charité Hospital.[75]

Kidney transplantation reportedly enjoyed a privileged status in East Germany because a prominent kidney transplant surgeon was a member of the Central Committee of the all-powerful *Sozialistische Einheitspartei Deutschlands* (*SED*). However, East Germany never was able to meet more than half the need for kidney transplants or 40 percent of the need for life-sustaining dialysis therapy. (Table 7.2) According to Berndt Schirmer, the former East German health planning chief, the behind-the-scenes debates over end-stage renal disease care represented just one of many decisions to forego more curative care.

> In 1987 we knew how many places for dialysis were available and rather well how many people we had with kidney diseases. We knew exactly how many people had which level of creatinine [a chemical in the blood, elevated levels of which indicate degrees of kidney failure]. We knew how much dialysis capacity we needed to do dialysis for various creatinine thresholds. We knew how much it cost and how much money we would have. We told the Planning Commission how many people would die if we didn't get more dialysis machines or drugs. We had a lot of arguments, a lot of polemics. But they said '3 percent and no more.' So we said, 'OK, in 1987, the level for us would be to do dialysis for everyone with a creatinine of 1,200 or over.' We knew that in Western Germany the criterion was a creatinine of 800, and we knew we couldn't reach that.[76]

Patients with kidney failure had a better chance than those with liver failure, however. Between 1982 and 1990, only six children received liver transplants; in the six months after the reunification treaty was signed, another half-dozen such operations were performed. Cario, who performed the first pediatric liver transplant in 1982, recounts how he watched success rates for the operation rise in the U.S. and West Germany and argued annually for an expansion of the program. The answer was always no. "The decision was because a Politburo member said it shouldn't be done," Cario says. "But for only one tank you could transplant 40 livers. So resource allocation was not part of those decisions."

Schirmer, who made a post-reunification metamorphosis from socialist planner to executive at Germany's leading private health insurer, says there was no explicit discussion, at least in recent years, about the tradeoffs between, for instance, more money for dialysis and more resources for premature infants. "We didn't evaluate it," he says. "We didn't want to know, I think." Schirmer adds that he and his colleagues at the top of the East German health bureaucracy used to congratulate themselves for their rational approach to planning. "We thought we had more regularity," he says. "We thought we had avoided the chaotic development of the West." But on further reflection, he thinks "planning" is a misnomer for the way health resources were allocated in East Germany. "We tried to plan, but the personnel and the methods were not very highly developed," he says. "We had theory and a big gap between that and practice....I thought we had some successes when I was responsible. Now I'm not so sure."[77]

Reunification: Back to the Future

The health care system West Germany inherited in 1990 posed a daunting challenge in physical terms alone. Not only was the state of medical technology far below West Germany's accustomed standards, but the crumbling infrastructure needed rescuing. The 539 hospitals in the East were more than 60 years old on average, compared to only nine years in the U.S. (A comparable statistic for

West German hospitals was not available.) Many had severe structural problems, including leaking roofs, inadequate sewage and sanitation facilities, damaged and dysfunctional heating systems, and dangerously outmoded electrical systems.[78] (Table 7.3) "It's incredible. We think every fifth hospital in the former German Democratic Republic should be closed and rebuilt," says Hans-Konrad Selbmann, coauthor of a federal status report on reunifying the German health care systems.[79] Between 1979 and 1988, East German hospitals' share of all spending for health and human services had declined by more than one-third.[80] Only 20 hospitals with a total of 15,000 beds had been built since 1970; at that rate, it would have taken East Germany another 200 years to renew its hospital system.[81]

The First Step

An inventory of available medical equipment revealed the need for an immediate infusion of DM 1.4 billion (about $700 million on a purchasing power parity basis) to bring East Germany's medical facilities up to standard. (Table 7.4) In 1990 the federal government launched an **immediate aid program** (*Soforthilfeprogramm*) of DM 520 million ($248 million) to begin the process of upgrading the East's failing health infrastructure. Among the most urgent needs:

Table 7.3

East Germany's Aging Hospitals*, 1988

	Number	Average age	Percent with severe structural defects
TOTAL	360	60.6	17.3%
General	294	56.3	13.8
Specialty total	66	76.7	28.0
Specialty psychiatric	38	81.2	30.2

*Community-level hospitals (not including teaching hospitals or other referral facilities).

Sources: Sachverständigenrat für die Konzertierte Aktion im Gesundheitswesen, Jahrestgutachten 1991.

- transportation for the disabled, including 240 specially equipped vehicles, 5,000 wheelchairs, and 1,300 hearing aids for children (cost: DM 55.6 million, or $26.6 million purchasing power parity or PPP);
- 85 ambulances (DM 10.5 million, or $5 million);
- 200 new dialysis machines and five prefabricated artificial kidney treatment centers (DM 23 million, or $11 million);
- beds, disposable supplies, and other equipment for nursing homes and retirement homes (DM 59, or $28.2 million);
- pharmaceuticals (DM 35.8 million, or $17.1 million);
- medical equipment for hospitals (DM 140 million, or $70 million); and
- immediate medical care for 1,305 eastern patients in western medical facilities (DM 25 million, or $12 million).[82]

The *Soforthilfeprogramm* was immediately followed by a more ambitious 1990-91 effort called "Soaring East" (*Aufschwung Ost*) of DM 5 billion ($2.4 billion in PPP) to restore and rebuild hospitals and facilities for the elderly and disabled. As of early 1993, the government planned a further **three-part financing program** for the decade beginning in 1995 that would funnel DM 700 million ($335 million) annually to eastern hospitals from the federal government, an equal yearly amount from each of the eastern state governments, and a third DM 700 million share from health, pension, and accident insurance funds in the form of an DM 8 per-bed annual subsidy.[83] By the end of 1992, DM 216 million in tax revenue ($103.3 million) had been allocated for hospital modernization.[84] *Aufschwung Ost* also included an **emergency drinking water program** of DM 120 million ($57.4 million).[85]

If these figures seem relatively modest compared with the need, they should be considered only down payments on the entire health care mortgage Germany has taken on. Selbmann estimated in 1991 that it would take DM 25 to 30 billion ($12 to $14.3 billion) over a decade to rebuild the hospital sector of the eastern states.[86] A 1992 estimate by the Federal Ministry of Health put the price tag at DM 20 billion ($9.6 billion). Hospital reconstruction will consume about 10 percent of the total amount that Germany figures it will spend on upgrading the entire infrastructure of the eastern states by the year 2000.

Deciding to shore up infrastructure was the easiest aspect of health care reunification. Far more complex and controversial was what organizational shape these financing and service-delivery systems should take. "The precise nature of the integration of the two health systems," notes Deborah Stone of Brandeis University, "was one of the most contentious issues in the debates leading up to unification."[87] The issues resolved into two big questions:

1. Should the new financing system duplicate the multiple sickness fund types in the West, or should there be a single-source payment mechanism?
2. Should medical care be delivered exclusively in the West German mode, by private ambulatory care physicians paid on a fee-for-service basis and salaried hospital-based doctors, or should alternative delivery modes be allowed, such as salaried group practices or American-style health maintenance organizations?

Choosing a System of Financing

For a brief period prior to reunification, there was some enthusiasm on both sides of the border for a departure from the complicated West German financing

Table 7.4

Medical Equipment in Germany's New Federal States: 1990 and 1995 goals

Type	Existing in 1990	Additional units needed by 1995 (est.)	Units needed to replace	Cost in millions	
Linear accelerators	23	78	18	116	55.5
Diagnostic x-ray units	2,200	1,800	1,200	600	287.0
Coronary catheter units	7	23	--	72	34.4
Digital subtraction angiography*	12	40	--	770	33.5
Conventional ultrasound (incl. Doppler ultrasound**)	14	50	--	--	--
Magnetic resonance imaging scanners	2	12	--	27.5	13.1
Gamma cameras	58	100	40	45.1	21.6
Lithotripters (kidney)	6	12	-	15	7.2
Laboratory autoanalyzers	200	350	40	34.2	16.4
Blood chemistry autoanalyzers	100	425	50	37.5	17.9
Blood gas autoanalyzers	190	400	15	9	4.3
Anesthesia machines/ ventilators	1,050	1,100	900	42.75	20.1
Kidney dialysis machines	630	1,435	300	44.2	21.1
TOTAL COST				**DM1,453.25**	**$695.3**

Sources: Sachverständigenrat für die Konzertierte Aktion im Gesundheitswesen, Das Gesundhietswesesen im vereinten Deutschland, Jahrestgutachten 1991.

model — perhaps something along the lines of the Swedish or Finnish systems, since these were seen by East Germans as embodying a high degree of social solidarity. In 1989 West Germany had just concluded a bruising political battle over health care reform in an attempt to rein in the system's spending, so transplanting the problems of that system to the "new states" gave many pause. East German officials had particular concerns about the inequities built into the West German system, such as the class-based distinctions between insurance coverage for blue-collar and white-collar workers (see Chapter Three). Their concerns were reinforced by the disenchantment they encountered among West Germans during the feverish negotiations of early 1990.

Schirmer, who led negotiations on health care provisions in the reunification treaty, remembers the first meeting with his counterpart in the West German Ministry of Labor. "At the first meeting, I knew nearly nothing about the West German system," he recalls. "I had read a lot, but you have to live here to understand. And he said, 'My first proposal is please don't build up a system of health insurance like West Germany's because it's such chaos and your decision to have a central payer is much better.'" The official, he adds, was not a member of the leftist Social Democratic Party, which has long favored a single-payer system, but a member of the conservative Christian Democratic Union Party. "He showed me what a wide range of opinions you found and will find in Western Germany."[88]

It became clear, however, that conditions were not as propitious for a dramatic experiment in health care financing as they initially appeared. The colossal failure of the Soviet-dominated states and the corset of Marxist-Leninist ideology that had kept the system upright for so long had tainted all forms of socialist organization, including democratic socialism. "No one thinks for a minute that the two systems are merging on an equal footing," Stone observed after a field trip to Germany in November 1990. "The starting assumption is that socialism has failed."[89] Those who wished to make more subtle arguments based on the distinction between socialist theory and socialist practice were at odds with both the new *Zeitgeist* and the vested interests of West German sickness funds, private insurers, and medical providers.

Second, practical realities intervened. The breakneck pace of reunification demanded fast decisions on how almost 16 million East Germans would have their medical bills paid after August, 1990. Once decided, the schedule allowed little time for implementing the new system. "We had only three months to prepare to start an *AOK* system in East Berlin," says one harried official of the *Allgemeine Ortskrankenkasse* or *AOK*, the "general local sickness fund" with primary responsibility to insure all comers.[90] Furthermore, the task had to be accomplished with thinly spread or untrained personnel and insufficient or nonexistent offices, computers, telephone lines, desks, and other mundane but vital necessities in the East. Somehow, in the six months following formal reunification, the Berlin *AOK* managed to enroll 350,000 new members in East Berlin at the rate of 8,000 to 10,000 a day, and at that point was expecting another 600,000.[91]

Another practical consideration was the elaborate, multivolume *Social Code of West Germany* that governs the whole structure of health insurance, health care providers, institutions, organizations, and federal-state relations in the realm of health care. "The complete transfer of the West Germany constitutional order made it difficult and even impossible to diverge from it in one particular area such as the health care system and look for other, different solutions," Schirmer concludes. "It is notably the legal system which influences more or less directly the emergence of specific structures in medical care."[92] At a minimum, it would have required heavy countervailing political pressure and lengthy debate to swim against this current.

Performing a Health Financing "Transplant"

In the end, the "new federal states" got an "articulated" (*gegliedert*) health insurance system identical to the West's — a highly segmented system of sickness funds differentiated by occupation, place of residence, income, and social class (to some degree) — despite the complexity, high administrative costs, and risk selection inherent in this model.[93] (The problem of risk selection among all Germany's sickness funds led to a major federal reform effort in late 1992 that is scheduled to set up a complicated risk-adjustment and cross-subsidization scheme among sickness funds during the 1990s.)

Only minor compromises were made in the financing structure installed in the "new states." For purposes of practical necessity, the *AOK* — which had hoped for an exclusive franchise for the new states — was given only a few months head start before other sickness funds were allowed in. In 1992, 13 *AOK* funds covered 61 percent of the eastern population, compared to their 42 percent market share in the western states, according to the Federal Ministry of Health. Private insurance companies were permitted to sell coverage in the East, over the objections of some who wanted to ban them altogether, but under the proviso that the 50 private insurers agree to offer only one product. It was argued that "*Ossies*" were so unfamiliar with the concept of private insurance that they would be easy prey for unscrupulous insurers. Private insurers, unsure of the market in the East for their product anyway, agreed to the restriction.

At the end of 1992, they had garnered only about 2 percent of the market in the "new states."[94] The most important accommodation needed to set up the new system was a complicated set of subsidies between sickness funds and government in the "old states" and the new eastern fledglings. The subsidies obviously put more pressure on "*Wessies*," mitigated only by the fact that health care providers are paid considerably less during a lengthy transition period.

Regardless of whether one considers the health care financing "transplant" operation to have been the right therapy, the patient did survive and is recuperating nicely. By June 1991, only 10 months after the *Treaty of Reunification* was signed, former East Germans were signing up at the rate of 284,000 a month and the "new states" already had 172 sickness funds covering three-quarters of the population. (Figure 7.7) By late 1992, there were 218 sickness funds in the East.[95]

At first, members and their employers had to pay a standard rate of 12.8 percent of each worker's income up to an income ceiling (shared equally between employer and employee). From 1992 onward, sickness funds were free to fix their own rates. None went up, according to the Federal Health Ministry, and the average contribution rate in 1992 was 12.7 percent compared to a national average of 12.6 percent. Strikingly, the eastern sickness funds had a collective *surplus* in 1991 of DM 2.7 billion ($1.3 billion). The principal reasons, according to federal health officials, were that Easterners

☐ have many fewer dependents — 24 dependents for every 100 primary sickness fund members compared to 46 per 100 in the West;

☐ use health care services at lower rates; and

☐ have a lower proportion of pensioners in their population, though this favorable ratio is changing due to emigration of younger workers to jobs in the West.[96]

The Fight Over Medical Turf

The fiercest and most fascinating struggle in the reunification of German health care was over nothing less than the collective soul of former East Germany's physicians. A dispirited bunch, some of the youngest and most ambitious voted with their feet. Out of the 40,143 active physicians who worked in East Germany when the Wall fell, the number who emigrated to the West is not known. Available data do not suggest the number was in the thousands, but neither was the phenomenon uncommon. In one medium-sized town in northeastern Germany, for instance, five doctors emigrated to the West as soon as the Wall fell, and four others tried to leave in the waning months of the communist regime but were caught and imprisoned.[97,98] The flight of doctors to the West was a problem considered serious enough that substantial monthly bonuses were offered to eastern doctors as an inducement to stay. These **not-to-flee bonuses**, as they were called, made up 15 percent of a typical generalist physician's income during the transition period.[99]

All but a tiny fraction of the doctors left behind were salaried by the state and most had known no other way. There were reportedly no more than 360 to

---

Figure 7.7

Growth of Sickness Funds in Germany's New Federal States: Mid–1991

Mo./Yr.	Total number	Of which ...						Substitute	
		Local	Company	Craft	Agricultural	Seamen	Miners	Blue-Collar	White-Collar
5/91	165	13	98	37	2	1	1	5	6
6/91	172	13	102	42	2	1	1	5	6

Source: Bundesministerium für Gesundheit, 1991.

Figure 7.7 continued

Share of Insured* by Type of Sickness Fund in Percent, June 1991

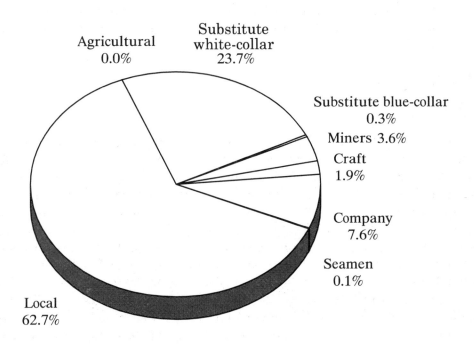

*Including pensioners but not family dependents.

Source: Bundesministerium für Gesundheit, 1991

Insurance Coverage in Germany's New Federal States: Mid–1991

(In thousands)

Mo/Yr	Obligatory members (w/o pensioners)			Pensioners			Voluntary members			Total insured		
	M	F	T*	M	F	T	M	F	T	M	F	T
5/91	3,905	3,912	7,187	961	2,186	3,147	354	230	474	5,219	6,219	11,438
6/91	4,037	4,047	8,084	924	2,197	3,121	384	131	515	5,345	6,357	11,722

*Indicates males, females, and total.

Source: Bundesministerium für Gesundheit, 1991.

400 private practitioners in East Germany at the time of the "turning point" (*Wende*), as it was known. A bare majority worked in hospitals (52 percent versus 49 percent in the West), and 40 percent worked in polyclinics or other ambulatory settings, mostly in groups that employed nonphysician personnel — a very different practice setting than the individualistic, entrepreneurial mode of ambulatory-care doctors in West Germany. Only 5 percent or 2,139 practiced alone (though their practices belonged to the state). Despite East Germany's 40-year emphasis on preventive services, a majority of physicians were specialists, just as in the West.[100] The density of physicians (doctors per 100,000 residents) was 23 percent lower than West Germany's in 1989, though it was 8 percent higher than the U.S. ratio.[101,102] (Table 7.5)

A New Face for the Eastern Doctors

The debate over how these eastern doctors should work — in what settings, under what economic arrangements, whether solo or in groups, and in what

---

Table 7.5

Physician Practice Settings, Population Ratio, Specialty Status, and Gender; East Germany, West Germany, U.S. 1989

	East Germany	West Germany	U.S.
Total practicing MDs	40,143	188,225	577,200
MDs/100,000 population	244	315	255
Ambulatory practice	40%	39%	63%*
Hospital-based practice	52%	49%	25%*
Administration, govt. research & other	8%	12%	8%*
Unclassified/Unknown	N.A.	N.A.	3%*
Specialists	55%	46%	65%
Female	>50%	30%	15.2%*

*1986 figures

Bundesministerium für Gesundheit 1991; Sachverständigenrat für die Konzertierte Aktion im Gesundheitswesen, 1992; U.S. Physician Payment Review Commission 1992, American Medical Association 1987.

---

relationship to hospitals and other health professionals — was substantively different from the argument over total system financing. It was obvious that some new financing scheme was necessary for the system *in toto*, since the state was effectively the payer in East Germany and the East German state was no more. (This is true even though technically most of the population was covered through the Free German Trade Union, with an estimated 33 percent subsidy from the government.) But it was not so obvious that the doctors of former East Germany had to be transformed *en masse* from salaried group practitioners to entrepreneurial solo practitioners. It was open to possibility, in a way that total system financing was not, that there could be a mixture of physician practice settings and payment arrangements in the new eastern states. Many on both sides of the border argued that the situation presented a unique opportunity to reinvigorate medical care in all of Germany by introducing new practice models. "At first I thought this is really a chance to get some new ideas into our system," said J. Matthias Graf von der Schulenburg, director of the Institute for Insurance Studies at the University of Hannover in western Germany.[103] The issue of what to preserve from the East German system — if anything — was and is "a very ideological question," observes Schirmer, the former East German health planning chief. "Some people said all things connected with former Socialism we have to sweep away. And you also had people who said there are a lot of interesting things and we should preserve them. For example, polyclinics, prevention, programs, special clinics in the workplace, child care, maybe other things."[104]

As Deborah Stone of Brandeis points out, the context of the debate was a turf battle — specifically, who would own the franchise for ambulatory medical care. "The nice word for this monopoly in German is the *Sicherstellungsauftrag*, which means 'the task of assuring the supply of services,'" explains Wulf-Dietrich Leber, the Berlin representative of the Federal Association of Local Sickness Funds.[105] "Of course, nobody explicitly talked in terms of a monopoly franchise," Stone writes. "Instead, everyone talked politely about assuring an adequate supply of services in East Germany."[106]

The debate had deep historical roots. In a struggle that stretched back to the 19th century, German physicians had won — and West German physicians had assiduously preserved — the exclusive statutory right to provide ambulatory care as solo practicing entrepreneurs. To execute that right, independent practitioners were organized into professionally autonomous regional groups called *kassenärztliche Vereinigungen*, a phrase which means "associations of doctors authorized to treat sickness fund patients." Physicians in the territory of former West Germany have strong feelings about this hard-won franchise. It symbolizes their professional and economic independence. From a policy standpoint, it has had benefits as well: It is the main reason West Germany has been able to count on the cooperation of organized medicine in cost control efforts during the 1970s and 1980s (see Chapter Four). The question was whether it was time to move away from this exclusive model of ambulatory care delivery.

Death of a Model

The focus of controversy was the fate of **polyclinics**, multispecialty groups of salaried physicians working in conjunction with public health workers, social workers, physical therapists, psychologists, and other personnel. In 1989 there were 626 polyclinics in East Germany employing the great majority of doctors in the ambulatory care sector.[107] At the time of reunification, polls showed that polyclinics had the support of nearly 90 percent of physicians as well as most of the public.[108] Patients liked the convenience. "Everything is under one roof," said Claudia Himmelreich, 30, a Berlin office assistant. "Why have separate machines in every doctor's office? Why destroy the polyclinics? It's pointless." Polyclinics also provided services which sickness funds do not cover or are barred from covering, such as family counselling, social service, and special preventive and rehabilitative services for the chronically ill.[109] According to one account, only a small fraction of the services provided by an East German pediatrician would be considered billable under West German fee-for-service rules.[110]

Many doctors argued that polyclinics should be preserved as an alternate practice mode because of their administrative efficiencies as well as the medical benefits of interdisciplinary groups. For a brief period in 1989 and 1990 a group of eastern doctors and other health workers sprang up to defend polyclinics. It called itself the Rudolf Virchow Association (*Rudolf-Virchow-Bund*), a name that not only honored the 19th century German pioneer of public health but quixotically echoed that of the powerful *Hartmannbund*, which represents the economic interests of fee-for-service practitioners in the West. "We had the idea that the doctor as a single actor is outdated," explains Harald Mau, dean of the faculty of medicine at Humboldt University in Berlin, who was a leader of the short-lived group. Noting that the first polyclinic was established in 1806 at the Charité Hospital in Berlin, Mau adds that

> the term "polyclinic" has been spoiled by overuse in the socialist system. It has nothing to do with socialism whatsoever. Polyclinics are the ideal way of working for specialists because it enhances medical and economic efficiency. Polyclinics, however you want to term them, will be the future form of provision of medical care.[111]

Polyclinics' critics countered that polyclinics were thoroughly discredited, not only by their association with a Communist regime but because they were simply inefficient and contained insufficient incentives for doctors to work hard. One critic, voicing a common opinion in the national weekly newspaper *Frankfurter Allgemeine Zeitung*, accused polyclinics' defenders of "wishful thinking" and socialist-style "perfectionist thinking." In reality, this correspondent wrote in 1991, polyclinics delivered impersonal, bureaucratic care and were rife with featherbedding.

> According to work instructions, a general internist was supposed to be available 33 hours a week for patient care. This proved to be an illusion. There was a drop-out of some 30 percent of the total work time due to illness, holidays, postgraduate training, or "work for the society." Since only 60 percent of the remaining time was used for consultations, only an average of four hours per day were left for patient care.[112]

Defenders acknowledged that polyclinics often had low productivity and were frequently overstaffed, but said the problems were inherent in the East German situation rather than the idea of multispecialty salaried group practice. For instance, 65 to 70 percent of polyclinic doctors were women, and women in East Germany enjoyed much more liberal maternity leave and other benefits than women in the West, where thousands of female doctors simply drop out of the profession during child-rearing years. In addition, polyclinics often had their own staff carpenters, electricians, plumbers, and even gardeners because they found they could not otherwise obtain these support services. "The lack of dedication to work is not intrinsic to polyclinics. It's intrinsic to a guaranteed employment system," comments Harald Möhlmann, assistant director of the Local Sickness Fund (*Allgemeine Ortskrankenkasse* or *AOK*) of Berlin. "That's why I don't like the Berlin model, in which the state owns the polyclinics. You have to be able to fire the doctor."[113]

Polyclinic proponents criticize the incentives of fee-for-service medicine to perform unnecessary services. "In the interest of maximizing profits, every doctor must be afraid of referring patients to another doctor," says Möhlmann. In a salaried practice, "a doctor doesn't have an interest in gaining or losing patients, though perhaps he has an incentive to minimize his work."[114] The average West Berlin patient who visits his physician for a particular problem "is summoned back for four to seven follow up visits," Stone notes. "His East Berlin counterpart receives care in an outpatient department or ambulatory care clinic, where the physicians are salaried, and he is summoned back for only one to two follow up visits. East Germany doesn't have to worry about those perverse incentives of fee-for-service in the first place."[115]

The debate might have gone on for years, but it was cut short by a swift decision of the Kohl government in 1990. The West German system of physician payment and organization would be duplicated in the East. Chancellor Helmut Kohl had been heavily lobbied by West German physician groups, who feared that polyclinics would be the end of their monopoly over ambulatory care services. Organized medicine in West Germany opposed any role for polyclinics not only because of their salaried nature and the payment they permit for psychologists, social workers, and other nonphysicians, but also because polyclinic physicians have hospital privileges. In Germany, the wall between ambulatory and hospital care proved more durable than the Wall separating East from West, although a federal reform law passed in December 1992 makes an earnest assault on the barrier between hospital and outpatient care.

Under the August 1990 *Treaty of Reunification*, polyclinics were allowed a five-year grace period, during which they can receive sickness fund reimbursement. After that a special commission with representatives from the polyclinics and the *kassenärztliche Vereinigungen* would decide if salaried group practices are still "necessary to assure the supply of medical services." In reality, the "grace period" was a death warrant, according to many observers, because in order to be competitive the polyclinics would need to persuade banks to loan them capital to upgrade their facilities and buy new technology. "We call the polyclinics a dying model," Leber said in early 1991. "No one will want to invest in a venture that is likely to go out of business in five years."[116]

The Social Transformation of East German Medicine

The decision to grant the *Sicherstellungsauftrag* for ambulatory care to fee-for-service doctors touched off a mad scramble among East German doctors to set up office practices lest they be left out in the cold. By all accounts it was a harrowing time, particularly for older doctors (more than a third of all polyclinic doctors were over age 50) and for women physicians (about 70 percent of polyclinic doctors). Older doctors worried that they would not be able to pay back the bank loans they would need to set up shop. For East German doctors accustomed to making perhaps DM 21,600 a year ($10,334 in PPP) the necessary amounts seemed astronomical. Women physicians were concerned about juggling the demands of running their own business and caring for their children at the same time.[117]

The Stampede to Private Practice

In many polyclinics, paychecks suddenly stopped. "There was a stampede to take control of the polyclinic buildings and to set up private practices," Leber recalls.[118] West German physician groups set up workshops all over the East in a sort of "sister city" arrangement to teach eastern doctors how to set up a practice, what equipment they would need, how to work the complicated billing system, how to duplicate the multilayered system of physician organizations, how many patients they would need to see to amortize their debt, and other matters. The federal government launched a parallel effort to indoctrinate eastern health personnel on the proper West German procedures. The government also made special allowances for older doctors, allowing them to work beyond the new mandatory retirement age of 68 (a measure to combat Germany's growing surplus of physicians) so they could convince banks that loans would be repaid.

East German medicine was transformed in the space of two years from an almost entirely salaried, state-run enterprise to an entirely private and overwhelmingly fee-for-service model. In 1989, only about 340 physicians and 450 dentists in East Germany owned their own practices, according to the Federal Health Ministry. By late 1990, a few months after formal reunification, 10 percent of the 17,000 ambulatory care doctors had "settled down" into private practice, as the German phrase goes (niedergelassen). The proportion rose to 30 percent in January, 1991, and 91 percent by late May, 1992.[119] The number of polyclinics dwindled to a few dozen at most, staffed mainly by older doctors and women physicians who did not want to launch private practices. In Berlin, 13 polyclinics have been preserved as city-operated health centers, but others have been converted to private doctors' offices with, as one patient describes it, "spacious hallways and waiting rooms, tasteful colors, comfortable furniture, soft carpeting instead of shappy linoleum, and pretty receptionists behind hotel-like counters attending to patients instead of constantly busy nurses peeping out of the consultation room every half-hour at the most to collect appointment cards."[120]

Learning the Western Way

The adaptation of eastern doctors to the unfamiliar new situation seems astonishingly rapid. "When the first doctors began to work in office-based situations, very quickly they saw that their situation was much better," says Schirmer. "They were their own boss, they had a lot more money to build up their office, and there was much more money to earn. And because doctors are rather intelligent people, rather quick to understand the situation, after one year they changed their minds."[121] Asked in 1992 what complaints she had, one doctor replied: "One major problem is drugs. Before we only could prescribe about 2,000 drugs. Now there are about 24,000. There are days when I have six or seven pharmaceutical representatives in my office. I go mad if I have to talk to all of them." Yet, she added, she appreciates all the free samples. "I pass them on to my patients and ask them later if it helped them or not."[122]

Eastern patients learned quickly too. Their expectations are higher now. "They want new drugs from the West. They want a very thorough physical exam. They claim a checkup once a year. They would like to have an electrocardiogram once every three months. They would like to have ultrasound," says Sieglinde Böhme, MD, who launched a solo practice in 1992 in the medium-sized town of Stendal, about 100 kilometers west of Berlin. Asked if she tries to persuade patients they may not always need these services, she replies: "No. I'm afraid I might overlook something. And if they want it, why not?"[123]

Yet all has not been smooth sailing for eastern physicians. Many spontaneously discuss the shock they felt upon plunging into the capitalist ways of fee-for-service medicine. As one doctor told the national newsmagazine *Der Spiegel*, "We didn't realize how brutally important money is."[124] Most distressing to many was the way the new era set colleague against colleague. "Collegiality declined drastically," says Böhme. "There is a lot of competition for patients. For example, if I refer someone to a specialist, they try to keep hold of a patient to make sure they bring the next *Krankenschein* to them and not somebody else." (A *Krankenschein*, or sickness certificate, is a quarterly voucher issued to all Germans insured through statutory sickness funds. Presented to the ambulatory physician of their choice, it is the patient's ticket to receive outpatient care and the physician's ticket to get paid for it.)

The Elusive Perfect Balance

Hartmut Reichwage, the general practitioner from tiny Geraberg, probably mirrors the mixed feelings of most of his eastern colleagues in the wake of the profession's "turning point." In the spring of 1990, the 61-year-old physician was depressed and anxious about the future. Two younger female colleagues in his district had attempted to take over his 30-year family practice. "They tried to sway people against me," Reichwage said at that time. "I had to make a fast decision. I jump now into the cold water and try to make the best of it." He sorely regretted "that now we must look for money all the time."[125]

Reichwage's 93-year-old mother, Dr. Annemarie Reichwage, was also shaken by the dog-eat-dog atmosphere that had suddenly come over her profession. The daughter and granddaughter of Prussian physicians — a medical lineage stretching back to Bismarck's time — the *Frau Doktor* said she was happy Germany was one nation again. "But I am not always happy with what has happened in the last year. Before the change there was a perfect feeling of collegiality. Now it's very, very depressing because colleagues fight against each other."[126]

By the end of 1992, Hartmut Reichwage was more cheerful with his "new beginning," as he put it in a letter. With the 850 to 1,000 patients he sees every quarter and the new fee-for-service billing system, he makes up to DM 120,000 a year ($57,416 PPP) — a far cry from the DM 21,600 ($10,335) he was earning in 1990. Moreover, he sees fewer patients than before the "change," so has more time for each one. He has a brand-new Siemens 12-lead electrocardiograph machine. He has been able to hire a professional nurse, and his wife does the billing and bookkeeping — a new task for them that he reports takes "roughly an hour" every day. The 1993 German health care reform aimed at reducing physicians' drug prescribing and other unnecessary utilization "will hit me little, as far as I can see." Reichwage still has mixed feelings about the changes that have overtaken health care in eastern Germany. But he does not yearn for the old days and former ways. He writes:

> We former GDR inhabitants have experienced that the determination to accomplish something *[Leistungswille]* wearies with salaried payment. There must be a financial incentive for good performance. How this could be better done than with the current system I don't know. Currently I see the danger that physicians provide unnecessary services, and that they charge more for their work than justified. An ideal solution does not exist.

References and Notes

1. Light, DW (1993). Comparative Models of "Health Care" Systems with Application to Germany. Unpublished paper, p. 22.

2. Hurst, JW (1991). Reform of Health Care in Germany. *Health Care Financing Review*. Vol. 12, No. 3, p. 84.

3. Schirmer, B (1992). "Reorganization of the Health Care Systems in Eastern Europe: How to Use Our Experiences of a New Start in Eastern Germany after German Reunification." Address at the Harvard School of Public Health, October 16, 1992.

4. Kirchberger, S (1986). Public Health Policy in Germany, 1945-1949: Continuity and a New Beginning. *Political Values and Health Care: The German Experience*. ed. Light, DW and A Schuller. Cambridge: MIT Press, p. 215.

5. Kirchberger, S (1986), p. 196.

6. Ibid, p. 215.

7. Ibid, p. 195.

8. Henning, A (1986). Mother and Child Care. *Political Values and Health Care: The German Experience*. Ed. DW Light and A Schuller. Cambridge: MIT Press, p. 471.

9. Kirchberger, S (1986), p. 216.

10. Rosenberg, P and Ruban, ME (1986). Social Security and Health-Care Systems. *Political Values in Health Care: The German Experience*. Cambridge: MIT Press, p. 265.

11. Light, DW (1993), p. 21.

12. Henning, A (1986), p. 471.

13. Rosenberg, P and Ruban, ME (1986), p. 265.

14. Stone, DA (1991). German Unification: East Meets West in the Doctor's Office. *Journal of Health Politics, Policy and Law*. Vol. 16, No. 2, p. 404.

15. Ibid.

16. von Kondratowitz, H-J (1986). Occupational Health and the Older Worker. *Political Values and Health Care: The German Experience.* Ed. DW Light and A Schuller. Cambridge: MIT Press, p. 499.

17. Ibid.

18. Sachverständigenrat für die Konzertierte Aktion im Gesundheitswesen (1992). *Ausbau in Deutschland und Aufbruch nach Europa.* Baden-Baden: Nomos Verlagsgesellschaft, p. 143.

19. Henning, A (1986), p. 472.

20. Rosenberg, P and Ruban, ME (1986), p. 279.

21. Rothmaler, S (1992). The Impact on Child Care in Germany and Gender: The Effects of Unification on German Women in the East and the West. *German Politics and Society.* Vol. 24 & 25, Winter 1991-1992, p. 107.

22. Ibid.

23. Henning, A (1986), p. 472-475.

24. Ibid.

25. U.S. Department of Health and Human Services (1991). *Health United States.* Washington: U.S. Department of Health and Human Services, p. 56.

26. Henning, A (1986), p. 475.

27. U.S. Department of Health and Human Services (1991), p. 130.

28. Henning, A (1986), p. 480.

29. Keiner, G (1986). The Question of Induced Abortions. *Political Values and Health Care: The German Experience.* Cambridge: MIT Press, p. 446.

30. Ibid.

31. Henning, A (1986), p. 474.

32. Müller, CKE (1977). Die Säuglingssterblichkeit in der Bundesrepublik Deutschland und in der Deutschen Demokratischen Republik. Dissertation, Universität Bonn, quoted by Henning, A (1986), p. 484.

33. Schirmer, B (1992). Personal interview, December 17, 1992.

34. Hurst, JW (1991), p. 84.

35. Sachverständigenrat für die Konzertierte Aktion im Gesundheitswesen 1991, p. 194; and U.S. Center for Health Statistics, May, 1991, personal communication.

36. Rosenberg, P and Ruban, ME (1986), p. 284.

37. von Kondratowitz, H-J (1986), p. 515.

38. Ibid, p. 501.

39. Ibid, p. 505.

40. Ibid, p. 515.

41. Ibid, pp. 515, 518.

42. Ibid, p. 517.

43. Ibid.

44. Rosenberg, P and Ruban, ME (1986), p. 278.

45. Selbmann, H-K (1991).

46. Reichmuth, C (1991), personal interview.

47. Selbmann, H-K (1992). "The German Health Care System: A Model for the United States?" Presentation at a Goethe Institute symposium on German health care, October 15, 1992.

48. Sachverständigenrat für die Konzertierte Aktion im Gesundheitswesen (1991), p. 206.

49. Selbmann, H-K (1992).

50. Helmert, U; Mielck, A; and Classen, E (1992). Social Inequities in Cardiovascular Disease Risk Factors in East and West Germany. *Social Science Medicine*, Vol. 35, No. 10, pp. 1283-1292.

51. Kohlmeier, L and Hoffmeister, H (1990). Consequences of Current Lipid Guidelines for the Federal Republic of Germany. *Klinische Wochenschrifft*, Vol. 68, pp. 454-459.

52. Selbmann, H-K (1992).

53. National Heart, Lung and Blood Institute (1992). *NHLBI Fiscal Year 1992 Fact Book*. Bethesda: National Heart, Lung and Blood Institute, p. 41.

54. Selbmann, H-K (1992).

55. Helmert, U, et.al. (1992), p. 1,290.

56. Light, DW (1993), p. 22.

57. Wittke, V (1991). "The Economics of German Unification." Presentation at a conference on The Economic Impact of German Unification at the Harvard Center for European Studies, April 6, 1991.

58. Benzet, T (1991), personal interview, March 6, 1991.

59. Helmert, U, et.al. (1992), p. 1,290.

60. Selbmann, H-K (1991).

61. Cario, W-R (1991), personal interview, March 6, 1991.

62. Ibid.

63. Henning, A (1986), p. 485.

64. Ibid.

65. Schirmer, B (1992), personal interview.

66. Cario, W-R (1991).

67. Deutsche Presseagentur (DPA newswire), February 24, 1993.

68. Böhme, S (1992), personal interview, December 16, 1992.

69. Benzet, T (1991).

70. Ibid.

71. Sachverständigenrat für die Konzertierte Aktion im Gesundheitswesen (1991), p. 238.

72. Ibid.

73. Cario, W-R (1991).

74. Ibid.

75. Althaus, P (1991), personal interview, March 6, 1991.

76. Schirmer, B (1992), personal interview.

77. Ibid.

78. Sachverständigenrat für die Konzertierte Aktion im Gesundheitswesen (1991). *Das Gesundheitswesen im vereinten Deutschland*. Baden-Baden: Nomos Verlagsgesellchaft, p. 236.

79. Selbmann, H-K (1991).

80. Sachverständigenrat für die Konzertierte Aktion im Gesundheitswesen (1991), p. 239.

81. Ibid, p. 237.

82. Bundesministerium für Gesundheit (1992). *Bilanz: Entwicklung des Gesundheitswesens in den neuen Bundeslandern*. Bonn: Bundesministerium für Gesundheit, pp. 10-11.

83. Meier, M (1992), personal communication.

84. Bunsdeministerium für Gesundheit (1992), p. 14.

85. Ibid, p. 15.

86. Selbmann, H-K (1991), personal interview.

87. Stone, DA (1991), p. 403.

88. Schirmer, B (1992), personal interview.

89. Stone, DA (1991), p. 402.

90. Möhlmann, H (1991), personal interview with Harald Möhlmann, assistant to the managing director, *AOK/Berlin*, March 5, 1991.

91. Ibid.

92. Schirmer, B (1992), Harvard presentation.

93. Stone, DA (1991), p. 408-409.

94. Schirmer, B (1992), personal interview.

95. Schmeinck, W (1992). "Statutory Health Insurance: Its Role, Structure, and Functioning." Presentation at a Goethe Institute conference on German health care, Boston, October 16, 1992.

96. Bundesministerium für Gesundheit (1992), p. 24.

97. Böhme, S (1992). Personal interview with Dr. Sieglinde Böhme, December 6, 1992.

98. There were also rumors that hundreds of West German physicians were applying for licensure in the East in 1990 so they could open practices there, but Deborah Stone of Brandeis University could not substantiate these rumors (Stone, 1991, p. 406).

99. Reichwage, H (1991), personal interview with Hartmut Reichwage, MD, March 5, 1991.

100. The specialist-to-generalist ratio in East Germany in 1989 was 55:45, according to 1991 figures of the Federal Health Ministry. This counts as generalists those who were certified as specialists in "general medicine." (Bundesministerium für Gesundheit, *Daten des Gesundheitswesens 1991*, p. 327)

101. Bundesministerium für Gesundheit (1991). *Daten des Gesundheitswesens*. Baden-Baden: Nomos-Verlagsgesellschaft, pp. 325-327.

102. Some commentators consider the effective ratio of physicians per 100,000 population in the East to be equivalent to the West under the conditions extant before 1990, because a high proportion of physicians were women who were entitled to generous maternity benefits. According to Selbmann, women physicians in the German Democratic Republic worked 70 percent of the hours put in by their male colleagues. (Personal interview, 1991)

103. von Schulenburg, J-M (1991). Personal interview, March 10, 1991.

104. Schirmer, B (1992), personal interview.

105. Leber, W-D (1991). Personal interview with Wulf-Dietrich Leber, March 5, 1991.

106. Stone, DA (1991), p. 403.

107. Bundesministerium für Gesundheit (1991). *Daten des Gesundheitswesens 1991*, pp. 327, 332.

108. Schirmer, B (1992), personal interview.

109. Bundesministerium für Gesundheit (1992), pp. 27-28.

110. Stone (1991), p. 408.

111. Mau, H (1992). Personal interview with Dr. Harald Mau, December 6, 1992.

112. Flöhl, R (1991). Impersonal Relationship to Patients: Bureaucracy Hampered Function of Polyclinics in the former GDR. *Frankfurter Allgemeine Zeitung*, No. 73, March 27, 1991.

113. Möhlmann, H (1991).

114. Ibid.

115. Stone, DA (1991), p. 403.

116. Leber, W-D (1991).

117. Stone, DA (1991), p. 408.

118. Leber, W-D (1991), personal interview.

119. Bundesministerium für Gesundheit (1992), p. 27-28.

120. Himmelreich, C (1993), personal communication.

121. Schirmer, B (1992), personal interview.

122. _____ (1992), personal interview with general practitioner in eastern Germany in December, 1992, name withheld on request.

123. Böhme, S (1992), personal interview, December 6, 1992.

124. Halter, H (1990), *Der Spiegel* 46: pp. 273-280, quoted by Stone, DA (1990), p. 412.

125. Reichwage, H (1991). Personal interview.

126. Reichwage, A (1991). Personal interview, March 4, 1991.

CHAPTER 8

The Opportunity
To Do Better:
Lessons Old and New

I f a cryo-preserved social policy analyst from the early part of this century were thawed out in 1993, he would be thunderstruck by our current interest in "what the U.S. might learn from Germany" about the financing and delivery of health care. The question was already a matter of considerable debate on this side of the Atlantic between the 1890s and 1930s. In fact, the American seed of what might have become a European-style social insurance mechanism was planted as long ago as 1798, when the U.S. government established the U.S. Marine Hospital Service, deducting 20 cents a month from each merchant seaman's wages to prepay his care. But unlike similar initiatives abroad, the program did not flourish into health coverage for the population at large (although it did grow into the U.S. Public Health Service).[1]

A century later, Chancellor Bismarck's health insurance system for German workers began to attract the notice of U.S. reformers concerned about the failings of charitable health care in a rapidly urbanizing America. In 1911, the U.S. Commissioner of Labor published a report on European workers' insurance plans.[2] President Theodore Roosevelt made national health insurance a plank in his Progressive Party platform in the election of 1912. "Legislation to study and plan for national unemployment, old age, and sickness insurance was introduced in Congress in 1916 and 1917 by its only Socialist member," notes a 1993 report by the National Institute of Medicine.[3]

Support was not limited to a few ragtag socialists. The American Medical Association established a Committee on Social Insurance in 1916 to work with a similar group of the **American Association for Labor Legislation**, whose members included such distinguished Americans as Jane Addams, Louis Brandeis, and Woodrow Wilson.[4] The panel came up with a set of criteria that was strongly influenced by Germany's model. (Figure 8.1) The AMA committee, which concluded that voluntary health insurance was unworkable and called for state legislation, was chaired by Teddy Roosevelt's personal physician, Alexander Lambert, and staffed by a Socialist physician, I.M. Rubinow, author of a 1916

Figure 8.1

Proposed U.S. Standards for Model State Health Insurance Legislation*, 1914

Coverage

- ☐ Compulsory participation by workers
- ☐ Voluntary participation for the self-employed
- ☐ Emphasis on illness prevention when possible

Organization and operation

- ☐ Financing through contributions from employer, employee, and the public
- ☐ Administration by employers and employees under public supervision
- ☐ Separate program of disability insurance to replace lost income

*Adopted by the American Association for Labor Legislation

Source: National Institute of Medicine, 1993, after Anderson, 1968.

book on the topic. In the same year, the AMA elected the U.S. Surgeon General, Rupert Blue, MD, as its president, who called for adequate health insurance in his inaugural address. An AMA trustees' report argued that it was wiser for organized medicine to "initiate the necessary changes than have them forced on us."[5] The AMA House of Delegates actually approved the trustees' report in June 1917, though it did not reflect sentiment in many state medical societies.[6]

From German Model to "Prussian Menace"

Interest was stirring in some states. Legislation proposing health insurance (and other varieties of social insurance) was debated in New York, California, Illinois, Michigan, and Wisconsin — which actually enacted a social insurance law in the 1920s. In Massachusetts, a contingent of progressive AMA members apparently persuaded Governor Samuel McCall, who served three one-year terms beginning in 1916, that the German model was the way to go. According to a 1935 history of Massachusetts politics,

In his Second Inaugural Address, Governor McCall dwelt at length on the benefits and desirability of health insurance and asked that the Legislature give the subject serious consideration. "I am strongly of the opinion that there is no form of social insurance that is more humane, sounder in principle, and that would confer a greater benefit upon large groups of our population and upon the Commonwealth as a whole, than health insurance," he told members of the Legislature. He recommended the establishment of a compulsory system with considerable benefit during the period of sickness, and that the system be made to include members of the family as is done in many of the German funds.[7]

When the Massachusetts Legislature did not spring to action, McCall brought it up again, "at considerable length," in his Third Inaugural. "The Legislature took the ground that the advent of the European War made it inadvisable to act, and the governor agreed with them," the historian reports circumspectly. In fact, the anti-German feeling of the day swamped all discussion of following Germany's lead. Paul Starr, PhD, of Princeton University reports in *The Social Transformation of American Medicine* that

the entry of America into the war in April [1917] proved a major turning point in the insurance movement. Many physicians went into the service; the A.M.A. closed down its committee on social insurance....In Massachusetts, debate was suspended on a bill that had the support of prominent Boston physicians and progressive social and political leaders. Anti-German feeling rose to a fever, the government's propaganda bureau commissioned articles denouncing German social insurance, and opponents of health insurance now assailed it as a Prussian menace inconsistent with American values.[8]

Another Attempt, Another War

The administration of Franklin Delano Roosevelt presented another opportunity to enact national health insurance legislation. Many social reformers pushed for it, and concern was mounting over the insupportable costs of medical care for the Depression-ravaged population. The principal draftsman of the Old Age and Survivors Insurance provisions in Roosevelt's landmark *Social Security Act* of 1935, B.N. Armstrong, had published a "lessons-from-abroad" book on social insurance (including health coverage) in 1932.[9] But the Social Security Act was silent on health care. "Led by organized medicine, the opposition to inclusion of such benefits was formidable, and the cabinet Committee [on Economic Security] and its staff were concerned that the inclusion of health insurance would jeopardize enactment of the entire measure," writes Rashi Fein, PhD, professor of the economics of medicine at Harvard Medical School.[10]

Another world war intervened, and although Presidents Harry S. Truman and Richard M. Nixon would later propose forms of national health insurance, they were careful not to associate the idea with such "alien" ideas as European social insurance. Meanwhile, America had gone in a different direction — voluntary employment-based health insurance. The movement was born during the Depression with the establishment of regional hospital sponsored prepayment programs that became Blue Cross plans and the subsequent physician prepayment programs called Blue Shield. A wartime wage freeze gave a big boost to employment-based health insurance in the 1940s, attracting commercial companies into the market, because labor unions could trade medical benefits for foregone wage raises. Health insurance became a major agenda item in contract negotiations — as it is today, but in a rear guard, negative sense.

The Rise of Voluntary Health Insurance

The voluntary health insurance movement took the steam out of Truman's 1948 push for a national system. Fein notes that by 1949, 61 million Americans already had protection against medical costs through Blue Cross, commercial insurers, and other plans, and enrollment was galloping ahead at rates of up to 17 percent a year. "There was little middle-class pressure for a compulsory health insurance system," Fein writes.[11] The steady expansion of voluntary employment-based insurance, which had reached 157.7 million Americans or 72 percent of the nonelderly population by 1992,[12] spawned an American conviction that eventually everyone would be covered in one way or another without enacting European-style compulsory programs. The mistaken assumption that voluntary workplace-based health insurance would eventually cover all employed Americans is what permitted U.S. policymakers to believe that Medicare (for the aged and disabled) and Medicaid (for the unemployed poor) would be enough to plug the coverage gaps.[13] That faith would hold until the 1990s, when middle-class Americans realized in sizable numbers that their coverage was neither affordable nor secure. (Figure 8.2)

The growth in public discontent about the ragged state of U.S. health coverage represents a sea change in long-standing attitudes about voluntary job-based health insurance. Previously there was a stigma attached to being medically uninsured, an attitude linked to 19th century notions of poverty as an individual failing rather than a social responsibility. In the early 1990s, many Americans came to realize that most of the uninsured *are* employed, and that it's not their fault if their jobs do not provide health insurance. Given the escalating cost of even a minor illness, many people also understand that it is not just the "deserving poor" who need social support against this contingency. The long *laissez-faire* policy of the federal government toward health insurance for most Americans had reached a dead end. And so it is that the U.S. is looking again across the Atlantic to see if it can glean some fresh ideas from tested European health systems.

Lesson One:
Get a Structure

Addressing the question "What can Americans learn from Europeans," Bengt Jönsson of the department of health and society at Sweden's Linköping University observes that "compared with Europe, the U.S. federal government seems to have less control over the totality of the system, at the same time that it is more directly involved in detailed regulation of efficacy, safety, and price setting."[14]

Jönsson's observation is telling. Control over "the totality of the system" is precisely what the U.S. lacks, and why many policy analysts of varying ideological stripes are convinced that tinkering with halfway measures, such as private insurance industry reform, will not suffice. Since the collapse of President Jimmy Carter's cost-control initiatives in the late 1970s, federal policy

Figure 8.2

Americans' Health Insurance Anxieties

Percent of Americans who say they worry "a great deal" or "quite a lot" that . . .

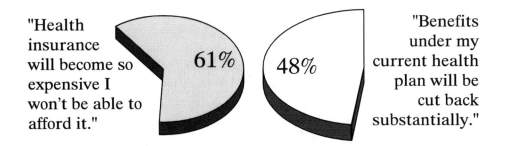

"Health insurance will become so expensive I won't be able to afford it." 61%

48% "Benefits under my current health plan will be cut back substantially."

Source: Robert J. Blendon et al., data from Kaiser Foundation/Commonwealth Fund/Louis J. Harris Associates national opinion survey of April, 1992.

Why Americans Worry About Their Health Coverage

☐ 1 in 4 lose insurance during any 2-year period[1]

☐ Nearly half of employed Americans have had benefits cut during the last 2 years[2]

☐ 1 in 4 households has someone locked into a job for health insurance reasons[3]

☐ 1 in 4 see high out-of-pocket costs as their most serious problem[4]

☐ 1 in 20 have been denied coverage for preexisting medical conditions[5]

[1]CBS News Poll, June 1992; [2]ABC News/Washington Post Poll, December 1991; [3]ABC News/Washington Post Poll, December 1991; [4]Louis Harris Associates, 1991; [5]Kaiser Family Foundation/Commonwealth Fund/Louis Harris Poll of April 1992

Source: Robert J. Blendon et al., January 1993.

toward health care has taken the narrow view that constraining government outlays was the only thing that really mattered. The government set an official example of shifting costs to more vulnerable payers, a policy which fragmented the payment system even further and contributed to the unravelling of the private health insurance system. New structures that organize the U.S. health financing and delivery system *into a totality* with some hope of coordinated response to government priorities and signals are what is necessary, and what Germany, more than other possible models for a U.S. reform, seems to have devised.

The Next Question: Comparability

Referring to the long, if sporadic, history of American interest in the German model, William A. Glaser, PhD, professor of health services management at the New School for Social Research, says it is time for the U.S. debate over health financing reform to "rediscover its original road."[15] A number of other respected analysts agree. But there is still a contingent which argues that Germany's health care system (or indeed any other nation's) is alien to American values and fraught with cultural and demographic differences that invalidate it as a useful model — an attitude Victor G. Rodwin of New York University calls "American exceptionalism." This outlook is not unique to Americans. "Nations throughout the world rely on [an] 'assumption of uniqueness' to reject ideas from abroad," Rodwin says. The problem is that this attitude "tends to make us conservative; and, therefore, it supports the *status quo* in the United States."[16]

America's "Greater Burden"

Skeptics advance a number of arguments about why the U.S. is unique. While these arguments do not strike at the heart of the matter — the United States' 15 percent rate of uninsured citizens and its lack of control over health cost increases — they deserve to be taken seriously. One of the most frequently heard claims, especially from physicians, is that a major reason the U.S. health system is so expensive is that it is burdened with social problems unique in scale, from urban poverty and crack babies to AIDS and drug-resistant tuberculosis. "If Canada, Germany or Sweden had our social problems, a comparable poor population and behavioral risk factors, their sickness and death rates surely would be much worse and their health care costs would be much higher," argue Leroy L. Schwartz, MD, and Mark W. Stanton of Health Policy International, a New Jersey consulting firm.[17]

One possible counter-argument is that societies with such formidable social risk factors have an even greater need for health care that is effective, efficient, and universally available. Leaving that argument aside, claims that U.S. health costs are heavily influenced by social "pathology" are inherently difficult to quantify, and apparently there has been no systematic attempt to do so. It seems likely that social problems account for some fraction of the difference in health care costs between the U.S. and Germany. However, the picture is not a simple one.

The U.S. clearly has more residents living in poverty. Although truly comparable figures are not obtainable, one rough set of indicators is that about 6 percent of Germany's population was receiving welfare payments in 1990 (a proxy for "poverty"), while 13.5 percent of U.S. residents were classified as having incomes below the federal poverty standard — a difference of more than two-fold.[18,19,] However, unemployment rates in Germany were consistently higher than America's during the 1980s, averaging 7.9 percent in Germany between 1980 and 1991 versus about 6.2 percent in the U.S.[20,21,] Furthermore, the U.S. is a richer nation than Germany, even though the gap between rich and poor is greater and more obvious in the U.S. In 1990, America's per capita gross domestic product was $20,774 — 30 percent higher than Germany's $15,943 (on a purchasing power parity basis).[22]

Less Difference Than Many Suppose

Acquired Immune Deficiency Syndrome is obviously a large burden for the U.S., which logged 43,352 new cases of AIDS in 1991[23] compared to Germany's 6,936 new cases.[24] However, when population size is accounted for, AIDS incidence in the U.S. is not 2 or 3 times higher but only 56 percent higher — 17.2 cases per 100,000 in the U.S. in 1990 versus 11 per 100,000 in Germany. Other infectious disease indices yield similarly counterintuitive results. For instance, the incidence of active tuberculosis, a disease classically linked to poverty and poor living conditions, is actually twice as high in Germany — 20.2 cases per 100,000 versus 10.3 in the U.S. — perhaps because the rate among the 4.5 million foreigners living in Germany was 63 per 100,000 in 1989.[25,26] The incidence of hepatitis B, a viral infection often associated with intravenous drug use and promiscuous sexual activity, is also higher in Germany.

Illicit drug use is an especially vexatious phenomenon to compare internationally, for intrinsic reasons and because nations do not measure this risk factor in the same way. For instance, the U.S. Center for Health Statistics periodically surveys households and asks whether individual members used various illicit substances in the previous month, a measure of current use. Germany collects statistics on the number of young people who say they have used a given illicit substance "at least once." One would expect the latter method to yield a higher figure than current use. Granting that the U.S. undoubtedly has a bigger drug problem, the available data do indicate that drug use in Germany is prevalent. (Figure 8.3) About 8 percent of German youths between the ages of 12 and 24 say they have tried cocaine, and nearly half have used marijuana at least once.[27] Data on habitual alcohol use are more comparable, and they show that alcohol use is twice as high among U.S. teenagers and young adults.[28,29] (Figure 8.4) Comparative figures on alcohol abuse are more difficult to come by.

Germany's low rate of infant mortality, one of the cardinal indices of public health, probably does reflect, in part, a lower-risk population of childbearing-age women than in the U.S. For instance, only 1 in 166 German mothers (in both the East and West) is under age 16,[30] compared to 1 in 21 American mothers.[31] However, it is reasonable to assume that Germany's low infant mortality rate — 25 percent below the U.S. rate — is at least partly due to the fact that virtually every pregnant woman is insured. Not only that, but over decades Germany has built up an elaborate system of benefits and services for pregnant women. The system encompasses generous paid maternity leave, both before and after delivery, as well as a highly organized system of prenatal medical care. Every pregnant woman gets a *Mutterpass* ("mother's pass"), a checklist on which to record the results of each checkup. Women are legally entitled to time off work to attend prenatal care appointments. Family planning and genetic counseling services are well-organized and widely available.[32] Out-of-pockets costs are never an issue.

Figure 8.3

Illicit Drug Use Among U.S. Teens and Young Adults, 1990

Those who say they have used . . . in the past month

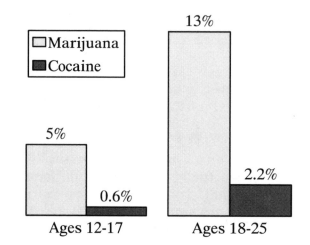

Source: National Institute on Drug Abuse, 1991.

Illicit Drug Use Among German Teens and Young Adults, 1986-87

Those who say they have tried . . . at last once, former West Germany

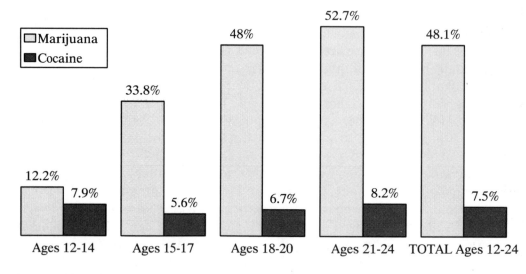

Source: Bundesministerium für Gesundheit, 1991.

Figure 8.4

Alcohol Use* Among U.S. and German Teens and Young Adults, 1990

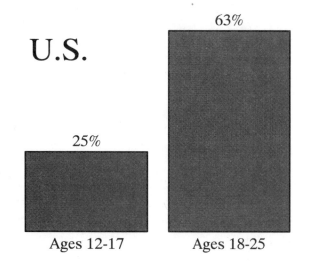

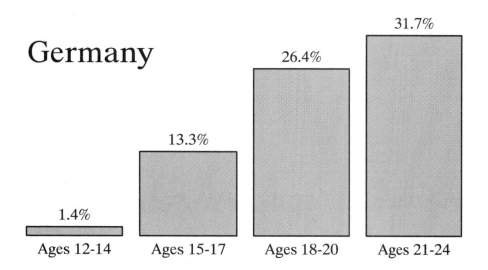

*U.S.: "In the past month." Germany: "Habitually," former West Germany only

Sources: National Institute on Drug Abuse 1991, Bundesministerium für Gesundheit, 1991.

Another suggestion that nationally organized systems of care actually do affect pregnancy outcome and infant survival lies in Germany's success in reducing its perinatal mortality rate. This index, a measure of death among late-stage fetuses and infants in the first seven days of life, reflects both the adequacy of prenatal care and the quality of obstetrical services. In the early 1970s, Germany's perinatal mortality rate was higher than America's. Recognizing the problem, German authorities launched a national perinatal surveillance system, beginning in Bavaria in 1975. Between 1974 and 1984, the perinatal mortality rate in Bavaria dropped from 26.3 per 1,000 to 7.1 per 1,000.[33] By 1991, the system embraced about 90 percent of all deliveries. It provides hospitals with statistical feedback of their performance relative to other institutions. The system is credited with reducing Germany's perinatal mortality rate below any other European nation's, and one-third below the U.S. rate.[34] (Figure 8.5)

Germany's Clear Disadvantages

Under the heading of "behavioral risk factors," Germany has population-wide problems that offset its advantages over the U.S. in other areas. Blood

---

Figure 8.5

Perinatal Mortality Rates: West Germany and U.S.

Number of late fetal deaths plus infant deaths within seven days of birth per 1,000 live births plus late fetal deaths.

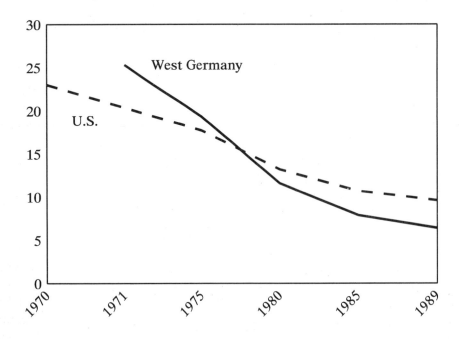

Sources: Daten des Gesunheitswesens 1991, *Bundesministerium für Gesundheit;* Health United States 1991, *U.S. Department of Health and Human Services.*

---

cholesterol levels are substantially higher in Germany and the disparity is growing. Forty percent of all German adults have borderline-high cholesterol levels versus 30 percent in America; 33 percent of Germans have cholesterol levels considered dangerously high versus 27 percent in the U.S. These numbers somewhat understate the differences, because Germany defines seriously high cholesterol as over 250 milligrams per deciliter while U.S. health officials define it as over 240 milligrams. The prevalence of high blood pressure, another major cardiovascular risk factor, is lower among Germans. But obesity is much higher in Germany — almost three times more frequent among men and nearly twice as high among women. (Figure 8.6) Moreover, Germans are still smoking at higher rates than Americans, especially German men. (Figure 8.7)

Germany's most serious disadvantage is demographic. Although much attention is focused on the contribution of America's elderly to health spending, the proportion of over-65 residents is actually 25 percent higher in Germany. The portion of all residents who are over 80 years old is 37 percent larger in Germany. (Figure 8.8) The Germans have more reason to worry about the future impact of aging on their pay-as-you-go sickness funds than Americans do about the soundness of Medicare trust funds. The indications point to a society that will inexorably shrink and age in the next decades because:

- the proportion of (West) German children under age six in 1988 was only 75 percent of what it was in 1950;[35]
- the number of marriages has declined steadily since 1960, and the fertility rate in western Germany has dropped 50 percent since 1950;[36]
- between 1971 and 1989 there was an excess of deaths over births;[37] and
- the number of working-age adults is projected to decline by 13.3 million between 1990 and 2030, while the number of those over age 60 is expected to increase by 4.6 million.[38]

The absorption of East Germany may not offset these trends. Although a somehow higher proportion of the population in the "new federal states" are young children, the share of over-65 citizens (13.3 percent in 1989) is even higher than in the West.[39] Furthermore, reunification was accompanied by a 50 percent drop in the number of live births among women in the East. Hans-Konrad Selbmann of the University of Tübingen calls this "the largest impact of unification in the health area,"[40] although of course it may represent only a temporary phenomenon due to the uncertainty young Easterners feel about their future.

All in This Thing Together

Clearly, it is difficult to say whether either Germany or the U.S. is better or worse off than the other in the burdens each nation's health care system must bear. The larger point is that both societies must cope with an array of strikingly similar problems. In addition to those mentioned above, both have troublesome problems with their respective physician supplies, in terms of number and specialty mix. Both must grapple with the relentlessly rising price of technological success — a factor to which economist Joseph P. Newhouse, PhD, professor of health policy and management at Harvard University, ascribes more weight than the combined effects of aging, generous insurance benefits, income growth, and oversupply of physicians.[41]

Rather than argue about how much weight to give this or that explanation for why U.S. health expenditures are 73 percent higher per capita, it is more profitable to ask what the U.S. can learn from Germany. As Theodore Marmor,

Figure 8.6

Blood Cholesterol Levels Among U.S. and German Adults

U.S. (1976–80)		Borderline High** 200–240 milligrams/dl	Severely High** >240 milligrams/dl
All adults		30.3%	26.8%
Men	35-44 yrs old	33	27.9
	45-54	35.2	36.9
	55.64	37.3	36.8
	65-74	34.8	31.7
Women	35-44 yrs old	31.7%	20.75
	45-54	34.2	40.5
	55.64	34	52.9
	65-74	32.5	51.6

Germany* (1985)		Borderline High* 200–250 milligrams/dl	Severely High* >250 milligrams/dl
All adults		40.3%	33.2%
Men	30-39 yrs old	40.1	24.5
	40-49	44.4	36.8
	50-59	44.5	39
	60-69	39.2	42.8
Women	30-39 yrs old	41.2%	17.8%
	40-49	49.1	24.1
	50-59	35.9	57.1
	60-69	27.6	65.7

*Former West Germany only
**In Milligrams Total Cholesterol Per Deciliter of Blood

Sources: U.S. Department of Health and Human Services, Health United States 1991; *Bundesministerium für Gesundheit,* Daten des Gesundheitswesens 1991.

Figure 8.6 continued

High Blood Pressure* in U.S. and German Adults

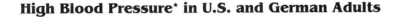
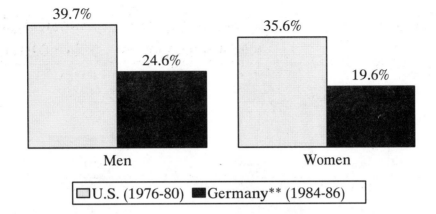

*Blood pressure >140 mmHg systolic or >90 mmHG diastolic
**Former West Germany only

Sources: U.S. Department of Health and Human Services, Health United
States 1991; *Hans-Konrad Selbmann, University of Tübingen, 1992.*

Obesity* in the U.S. and Germany**

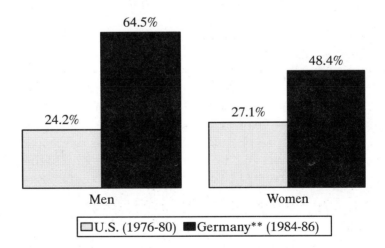

*U.S. defined as body mass index > 27.8 kg/m³ for men, 27.3 kg/m³ for women;
Germany defined as body mass index > 25 kg/m³
**Former West Germany only

Sources: U.S. Department of Health and Human Services, Health United
States 1991; *Hans-Konrad Selbmann, University of Tübingen, 1992.*

Figure 8.7

Smoking Rates Among Men and Women Age 25 and Over in the U.S. and Germany*, 1988

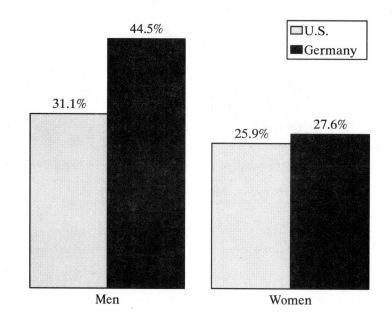

*West Germany only

Sources: U.S. Department of Health and Human Services, Health United States 1991; *and Bundesministerium für Gesundheit,* Daten des Gesundheitswesens 1991.

professor of public policy and management at Yale University, puts it: "Perhaps the only advantage of being the last industrial democracy without universal health insurance is that we can learn from the experiences of others."[42] The learning does not have to be one-way. "Most countries, irrespective of their particular health system, face common problems with regard to the efficient and equitable allocation of scarce health care resources," Rodwin notes. The aim, he adds, should be "how the best features of each system might be combined."[43]

A large caveat is necessary, of course. American culture already owes a substantial debt to Germany — not only in terms of music, art, religion, philosophy, literature, and other aspects of "high" culture, but also for innumerable contributions to American society made by German immigrants and their descendants. Nevertheless, Americans are certainly not Germans, nor vice versa. It would be as big a mistake to assume that German ways could simply be transplanted to the U.S. and function in the same fashion as it would to dismiss Germany's health care experience as simply irrelevant.

However, a thoughtful adaptation of certain features of German health care is certainly possible. Clearly, German policymakers are receptive to

Figure 8.8

The Aged in Germany* and U.S., 1988

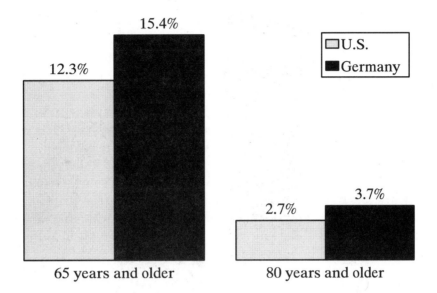

*West Germany only

Sources: Organization for Economic Cooperation and Development Health Data File, 1992.

learning from some aspects of U.S. health care. Two emerging realms for cross-fertilization follow.

Diagnosis-linked hospital reimbursement. Germany is planning its own kind of diagnosis-specific hospital payment mechanisms for the 1990s, adapted to their circumstances, to replace the problematic per-diem method that has predominated there. They can learn from the workings of the diagnosis-related group (DRG) method used by Medicare since the early 1980s. And U.S. reimbursement experts might well learn something useful from the way German DRG hospital payments evolve.

Risk-adjustment among health insurance plans. Beginning in 1996, Germany plans to calculate risk profiles of each sickness fund's enrollees and adjust each fund's revenues accordingly by transferring money from those with lower-risk populations to those with higher-risk enrollees. The aim is to permit free competition among sickness funds on grounds other than risk selection — the Germans are quite mindful of the disastrous American experience in this regard. Many U.S. analysts believe America must build risk adjustment into any health reform if it to achieve the "right" kind of competition among health plans. Therefore, it will profit both nations to learn from the other's experience in this relatively uncharted territory. Risk adjustment is an undeveloped science. The standard variables of age, sex, and family composition only a tiny fraction of the total variation in annual variation in health spending on individuals. Newhouse found that only about 15 percent of cost variation is explained by all identifiable patient characteristics.[44]

What Germany Can Teach Us

Americans interested in the lessons to be gleaned from Germany's health care system should view the scene through two different lenses. One focuses on Germany itself, isolating the main elements within a German frame of reference. The other lens views German health care with explicit reference to the evolving debate over the future of America's health care system. The point, after all, is pragmatic: to focus on those German experiences most relevant to American needs. This is a speculative exercise. No one can know what paths U.S. health care reform will take from 1993 onward, even if some of the outlines of possibility are (perhaps) emerging from the fog. In fact, the firmest prediction one can make is that both U.S. and German reform will take unexpected twists and turns, enter some cul-de-sacs, and take shape over a period of years if not decades.

Lessons Tried and True

Looking through our first lens, Germany offers both "old lessons" and "new lessons" that the U.S. would do well to heed as it attempts to reform its health care system. The "old" lessons, derived from more than a century's experience and revisions, include the following general principles:

1. **An explicit national policy.** The starting point must be a unified national health care policy, with clearly spelled out values, goals, and roles (of public and private participants).
2. **Sharing the burden.** The central value should be an acknowledgement that equitable access to a standard set of health benefits requires the economically advantaged to subsidize the less-advantaged, the young to contribute to the care of the old, and those without children to subsidize families with children. A system without such cross-subsidization does not work, as the unravelling U.S. health insurance system demonstrates. The Germans call this principle **social solidarity**, but a more American term might be **fairness-based financing**.
3. **Virtual universality.** Nearly everyone in the society must be covered, not only as a value in itself but as a crucial element in making the system work. This means that participation in the system must be compulsory for the great bulk of the population.
4. **Guarding the boundaries.** The rules governing who is allowed to opt out of the compulsory system must ensure that these people are not permitted, by their numbers or the advantages they can buy, to undermine the integrity or stability of the compulsory system.
5. **Structured financing.** There must be a national system of mechanisms to translate national health care goals into a health care financ-

ing and delivery system that is coherent at the federal, regional, and local levels. Although there may be regional variation within federally set criteria, this crucial link should not be left to vague incentives and theories about how the health care market should work.

6. **All play the same game.** It is vital that all payers and all providers be bound by the same rules, whether those rules pertain to uniform health care benefits, reimbursement, or relationships among payers and providers. This does not mean there cannot be a multiplicity of payers or providers, who compete for subscribers, patients, and resources on the circumscribed playing field.

7. **Inclusive policy setting.** All stakeholders, including payers, health care providers, and consumers (in Germany normally represented through labor unions), must be involved in negotiating the rules, the operational details, and the allocation of money and resources. Participants must be carefully counterbalanced. This process must be made publicly accountable through government-sponsored mechanisms as well as by government oversight.

8. **Government as referee.** Government involvement should be limited to rule-setting, convening, backstopping (mechanisms for decision-making when negotiations deadlock), oversight, and occasional course correction. The temptation to micromanage the system, either by government initiative or at the behest of stakeholders, should be strongly resisted. However, government must intervene promptly when the system departs from the stated goals, and when the system of countervailing private interests becomes imbalanced. Problems should never be left to fester and worsen.

Those with intimate knowledge of the German health care system (and perhaps a quotient of European cynicism) will rightly point out that Germany does not always adhere to these principles. To take one timely example, the health care reform laws of 1989 and 1993 raise the interesting and important question of whether the German federal government is departing from its traditional "subsidiary" role into a more interventionist one. Nevertheless, it is fair to say that these principles do characterize the German system's main features as they have evolved between 1883 and 1993.

Lessons Necessary and New

The "new" lessons Germany has to teach span a time period of approximately 1972 to the present day. Concerned more with operational strategies than with fundamental principles, these elements are nonetheless important for U.S. policymakers who need to understand what has worked in a universal, all-payer health system — and what has needed retooling under the pressures of escalating costs. These include (but are not limited to) the following.

1. **Societal affordability**. Money spent for health care should be pegged to the revenues raised for that purpose — not the other way around. These "contributions" from workers, employers, and tax funds should be kept stable and allowed to rise only for explicitly recognized reasons. Germans call this a **revenue-oriented expenditure policy**.[45]

2. **Budgets, budgets, and budgets**. Health care spending can only be contained by budgets. There should be a global budget for the entire

system and separate budgets encompassing different provider sectors. These budgets should be set through negotiating processes, and backstopped by mechanisms to set spending levels if negotiations deadlock. Under Principle 5 above, there are mechanisms to apply national budget limits to the regional and ultimately to the individual provider level (hospital, physician, pharmacy, etc.).

3. **Attending to the supply side**. Restrictions on the supply of medical services are an inescapable component of cost-containment policy. These restrictions (as Germany is learning) must embrace both physical assets, such as facilities and technology, and service personnel, especially physicians.

4. **Controlling volume**. Price-setting mechanisms are a necessary but not sufficient instrument of cost containment. They must be coupled with controls on the volume of service. These controls — sets of financial incentives and disincentives — must operate as directly as possible on front-line providers, and there should be prompt feedback on the provider's performance in order to influence behavior concurrently. Controls targeted to individual providers should be mixed with collective controls for maximum effectiveness.

5. **Involving the regulated**. Volume controls work best when the affected providers have a meaningful hand in their formulation and implementation, with appropriate checks and balances, and with clear consequences for failing to meet expenditure targets or caps.

Although the main lessons from Germany tend to fall into these two types — principles and strategies — the overall point to bear in mind is that they are interrelated. The strategies cannot easily be implemented (if at all) in the absence of a system that is universal in coverage and coherent in operating principles. But the principles by themselves will not, as Germany has painfully discovered, ensure an efficient and affordable health care system.

Each of the above points is illustrated by descriptions, examples, and historical background in earlier chapters of this book. There are, in addition, innumerable lessons to be learned from close comparisons of the inner workings of German and American health care. For instance, what Germans sacrifice, if anything, from their lower capacity for open-heart surgery — 1.1 open-heart units per million residents in western Germany[46] versus 3.5 per million in the U.S.[47] What are the indications and health outcomes of a German prescription drug utilization rate three times the U.S. rate? (See Chapter Six.) What is the case mix and treatment intensity in German hospitals compared to U.S. institutions? Such studies have not yet been done, but experts in international health believe they could yield important insights into both systems of care.[48]

"Managed Competition" vs a German Model

Enthusiasm over "managed competition" in the Clinton Administration has raised questions in many observers' minds about the relevance of any foreign health care system to the direction the U.S. may take. Although President Clinton has made occasional admiring references to the German system, Administration officials were avoiding mention of foreign models and ideas in early 1993. "They have decided against encouraging any overseas analogies," says Robert J. Blendon, ScD, chairman of health policy and management at Harvard School of Public Health, who has consulted for the Clinton Administration on public attitudes toward health care reform. "They have decided that an American plan with no foreign analogies will sell better. They want to highlight the fact that managed competition is strictly an American idea."[49]

As America's early 20th-century experience has shown, it may be tactically smart to stress the home-grown nature of managed competition-based reform. But it is also misleading. In fact, there is a striking convergence between many aspects of German health care and current notions of **managed competition** — even as managed competition has recently been articulated by its inventors. One of the major problems in this area is that "managed competition" is such a complex and shifting set of concepts that it means many different things to different people. For better or worse, this state of affairs is likely to persist. There are political advantages in it, and in fact the content and emphasis of "managed competition" is very likely to evolve during debate and implementation.

The belief that managed competition and a German-style approach to health care are inimical is based on a false understanding of both. It assumes that:

☐ Managed competition must rely solely on market forces — not global budgeting — to set prices and control total spending, albeit within a framework that maximizes the incentives of purchasers, payers, and providers to pick economical health plans, pay wisely for provider services, and practice economically; and that

☐ Germany's system relies on top-down budgeting to control total spending and bargaining to set prices within this global budget.

Each of these characterizations is a caricature of the respective models. Some leading exponents of managed competition say their model can and must accommodate national-level global budgeting along with managed regional competition among health plans and bargained payment rates. Germany has always had a good deal of "play" in the application of federally set budgets — which are not really budgets, in any case, but expenditure targets. Additionally, Germany has regional bargaining among provider groups and a confined group of payers. And the German Parliament in late 1992 adopted a reform plan that requires much more "managed competition" among sickness funds than ever before by 1996.

Managed Competition: The Original Version

As originally proposed and proselytized by Alain C. Enthoven of Stanford University and others, managed competition is a restructuring of the market for health insurance and health care delivery on a regional basis. "Its goal is to divide providers in each community into competing economic units and to use market forces to motivate them to develop efficient delivery systems," Enthoven explains.[50] It has two key structural elements:

1. **Sponsors of health coverage.** These can be either large employers or newly organized regional entities, often termed **Health Insurance Purchasing Cooperatives** or **Health Alliances**. These organizations would be "gatekeepers" to all or most of the health insurance market in a region, empowered to purchase health insurance on behalf of everyone not sponsored by a large firm.

2. **Organized systems of care.** Hospitals, doctors, and other health care providers in each region of the nation would be organized into a rigorously defined and limited universe of groups. All would be required to provide a uniform nationally determined set of benefits for a capitated amount negotiated between the provider groups and the sponsors.

In operation, the lowest-priced plan in each region would set the standard for what employers and enrollees were obligated to pay, or what government was obligated to purchase or subsidize on behalf of the poor, the unemployed, and low wage earners. Those who opted for more expensive plans would have to pay the difference out of their own pockets (with taxable income, according to the strong preference of Enthoven and other proponents). The basic premiums would be community rated, implicitly requiring the healthy to subsidize the sick, the young to pay for the not-so-young, small families to pay more than large families, large employment groups to bear some of the burden for small groups, and so on. Furthermore, HIPCs would have the responsibility to risk-adjust capitation payments to provider groups to eliminate or minimize any incentive to compete on the basis of enrolling lower-risk customers. Through these and other reengineering measures, proponents assert, the health care marketplace could offer universal and cost-effective care without intrusive government price-setting, rate-regulation, and centrally imposed budgets.

The debate over managed competition revolves around its untested potential to contain societal health spending. Advocates can point to instances in which large managed care systems have provided care more efficiently. However, managed care providers in the real world have had a mixed record. Robert D. Reischauer, director of the Congressional Budget Office, urges policymakers to scale down their expectations of managed competition's cost-controlling ability. "Most Americans do not consider [staff and group-model] HMOs an attractive option, and many of the proposals for reform rely on looser forms of managed care," Reischauer told the U.S. House Ways and Means health subcommittee on March 3, 1993, adding that

> If everyone could be cajoled into enrolling in a staff or group model HMO, national health expenditures could drop by as much as 10 percent, and insurable personal health care spending could drop more than 10 percent. Although substantial, that amount represents roughly one year's increase in health care spending. Thus, although managed care could lower the level of current health expenditures, it probably would not affect the long term growth of those costs.[51]

Managed competition proponents can also cite subsets of Americans, such as groups of federal and state employees, who have purchased care with relative efficiency through arrangements that resemble HIPCs. But it has been impossible to show, in the fragmented and risk-based U.S. private health insurance system, that some of the apparent efficiencies and lower costs in these "managed" systems were not derived from the selection of lower risks and the shifting of cost to other payers. Enthoven acknowledges this uncertainty. "Managed competition offers the most powerful force for reducing national health expenditures," he writes. "However, as is the case with any other policy, there is no guarantee that managed competition will automatically hold spending growth to acceptable levels, even if implemented optimally."[52]

Managed Competition: The Compromise

Enthoven and other members of the Jackson Hole Group, a nucleus of managed competition proponents founded by Paul Ellwood, MD, dislike **top-down global budgets** and have often insisted that the two approaches are incompatible. However, another recent school of thought contradicts that position. It holds that federally set limits on overall health spending not only can but must be married with managed competition to ensure that costs are contained — an economic and political necessity if all Americans are to be brought into the system.

Sociologist Paul Starr articulated this view in a 1992 book, *The Logic of Health Care Reform.* In a March 1993 essay, Starr and Walter A. Zelman, PhD, a deputy insurance commissioner in California, further assert that posing managed competition and global budgeting as irreconcilable alternatives is "a misleading polarization" motivated by pro-market ideologues who simply dislike government intervention. "With new rules and institutions in the market, we can — and almost certainly will — have both," they assert, calling this model "managed competition with a cap." In fact, they add, since managed competition emphasizes payment of health plans on a capitation basis, "managed competition provides a better platform for global budgeting than exists in the current system."[53]

Uwe E. Reinhardt, professor of political economy at Princeton University and a long-time exponent the German system as a model for U.S. health care reform, is one of managed competition's most vocal critics. Nevertheless, he has recently accepted Starr's view. Reinhardt argues in a 1993 paper that managed competition "is merely a cost-control mechanism that could be coupled with any scheme of funnelling money into the health system's insurance fund or funds."[54] He sketches the following scenario:

> The reforms now being contemplated by the Clinton Administration and Congress are likely to give managed competition the chance to demonstrate its ability (a) to please patients and (b) to control the cost of health care, without imposing top-down budgeting onto the entire American health system. If managed competition should fail to control total national health spending visibly and soon, the health system is likely to be put under a top-down global budget for all Americans except those in the top 10 to 15 percent of the income distribution....And herein lies a small irony apparently overlooked by the proponents of managed competition: While staunchly opposing top-down global budgeting and marketing their concept as an alternative, they are actually developing the ideal infrastructure for its imposition....Managed competition based on *capitated* managed-care plans furnishes the ideal platform for the imposition of top-down budgets.[55]

Blendon agrees that the U.S. may evolve toward a globally budgeted system to control spending. "Managed competition will be difficult to manage and control," he predicts. "If you have trouble with that, what else can you do but put in a globally budgeted, all-payer system. But you can only make that work if everyone sits down and negotiates."[56]

The forthcoming U.S. scenario may have other wrinkles that will require explicit budgetary limit-setting. Many areas of the U.S. do not lend themselves to the managed competition framework advocated as the standard model. For instance, one out of three Americans lives in an area with fewer than 360,000 residents — the minimum considered necessary by leading managed competition advocates to support three health maintenance organizations and thus ensure meaningful competition.[57] Moreover, some jurisdictions may elect not to adopt the managed competition approach. Thus, other models are likely to be tried concurrently with "pure" managed competition, and some of those models may well resemble Germany's methods of controlling costs in a fee-for-service universe. In such regions, Starr notes,

> ...the principle health plan or the HIPC itself would most likely negotiate global budgets with hospitals. Elsewhere, depending on state policy, global hospital budgets might be set in negotiations under the auspices of the HIPC involving all plans in a region [a concept very much like the "concerted" budget-setting negotiations between groups of sickness funds and hospitals in Germany]. As in the German system, the total compensation pool for physicians outside managed-care plans would also be fixed annually. Physicians would be paid fee-for-service, but the value of fees would depend on the volume and mix of services and the size of the compensation pool.[58]

Even Enthoven has left the door ajar to a compromise between managed competition and "top-down global budgets." Although he warns that federal health care budgeting "would focus the whole health services industry on political efforts to raise or maintain the ceiling as a percentage of gross national product," Enthoven sketches out how a hybrid model could work.

> Government could define as the "global budget" the lowest capitation rate in each HIPC, multiplied by the number of people residing in each HIPC area, added up over all HIPCs. These would be market-determined global budgets and would encompass all publicly supported and tax-subsidized national health expenditures. Government could then decide on a public policy that sets a target for this global budget relative to GNP. If the global budget grows faster than the target, the president and Congress should direct the National Health Board to develop and implement a set of targeted interventions designed to reduce health spending based on solid and current data....In other words, government should examine the causes of excess spending and apply specific remedies, rather than trying to sweep the problems under the carpet of a national global budget.[59]

Putting It All Together

Under any of the above scenarios, it would appear that the U.S. will have much to learn in the years ahead from another national health care system based on
- compulsory job-based coverage for the working population,
- government-subsidized coverage for the unemployed and poor,
- federally negotiated expenditure targets,
- structured health insurance choices,
- a nationally uniform benefit package with limited cost-sharing,
- community rating of insurance premiums,
- risk adjustments among insurers based on enrollees, and
- negotiations between payers and providers over payment rates.

Moreover, this other system — Germany's, of course — is characterized, like America's, by heavy emphasis on curative care and advanced medical technology, a demanding population, and a keen interest in controlling costs.

There are aspects of German health care that the U.S. would *not* want to emulate. The rigid separation between inpatient and ambulatory care is a major and well-recognized flaw that seriously hinders Germany's efforts to coordinate care, reduce expensive duplication, and shift some kinds of care to cheaper settings. Certainly no one suggests duplicating Germany's excess supply of hospital beds, its 17-day hospital stays, its oversupply of physicians, or its weak system of care for chronically ill elders. For its part, Germany will find it difficult, if not impossible, to copy managed care. Organized medicine there is too fiercely opposed to anything that smacks of salaried outpatient practice, as illustrated by its recent success in squelching experiments with polyclinics following reunification (see Chapter Seven). The rescinding of Germans' freedom to choose doctors is unlikely. "Closed panels and lock-ins are no longer legally possible," Glaser flatly states.[60] It will presumably be even more difficult to encourage alternatives to fee-for-service care while Germany has a large and still-growing surplus of doctors, since managed care reduces the need for physicians.

When it comes to global budgeting, Starr and Zelman warn against confusion between "true" global budgets, which they define as "an overall budget limit on health care services, regardless of where the funds originate," and spending limits set separately for each provider sector (hospitals, doctors, pharmaceuticals, etc.). The latter type of budgeting tends to lock in existing spending patterns rather than permit more economical redistribution of funds. "Fee-for-service global budgeting seems a fine recipe for blocking structural reform, heightening conflict, and discrediting the concept of a budget," they write.[61]

Yet Germany, which has a totally fee-for-service health care universe, has both types of budgeting. Its national Council for Concerted Action in Health Care sets a recommended limit for increases in the revenues raised for health care in the coming year, and also recommended sector-by-sector spending limits. These serve as guidelines for negotiations between sickness funds and groups of providers, and the guidelines seem surprisingly effective. This, apparently, is partly due to everybody's knowledge that if negotiations deadlock, the budget will be set by a neutral arbitrator, who will almost certainly rely on the recommended federal guidelines. Rainer Hess, JD, chief legal council for Germany's Federal Chamber of Physicians (*Bundesärztekammer*), says in his 20 years with the organization he can recall only once instance in which regional negotiations were kicked into arbitration.[62] Setting budgets by provider sectors may, as Starr and Zelman warn, hamper Germany's ability to reallocate health resources more rationally from hospitals to other settings. But the German experience also suggests that budget-setting at both global and sectoral levels can work and has positive features.

A Question of Values

Ultimately the most important lessons to be learned from Germany concern values. This is not to say that the U.S. should or could adopt another culture's value system. But there is abundant evidence that the root of America's long-standing stalemate over health care reform, in the face of severe, painful, and worsening problems, is a confusion of values. "We lack an adequate understanding of why the moral ideal of 'health care as a human right' is not a part of our public policy," notes Richard J. Botelho, MD, of the Jacob W. Holler Family Medical Center in Rochester, NY. "Most importantly, we pay inadequate attention to the value system that underpins our actual health care policies and practices."[63] Until the U.S. identifies, clarifies, and reorders the values that have blocked comprehensive reform for most of the past century, the nation seems doomed to either timid, incremental remedies or continued social policy paralysis.

A close look at Germany's health system, with all its resemblances and differences, throws America's confusion into sharp relief. Americans seem unable to choose which values should govern a reformed health care system — whether, for instance:

- □ universal access to care should take precedence over preserving the undoubted high quality and technological prowess instantly available to America's well-insured;
- □ America's unique commitment to doing everything possible for the individual patient should give way to an acknowledgement of reasonable limits and a more rational distribution of resources; or
- □ the autonomy of health care providers (doctors and hospitals in particular), which has been a predominant value in U.S. health care since the Flexner Report (1910), should be allowed to block reforms that would reorganize the way care is delivered and resources allocated.

Germany is hardly free of value conflicts in health policy. In fact, debate there has, if anything, a stronger ideological cast due to its multiparty parliamentary system. German politics features a wide spectrum of carefully delineated philosophies (left, left-center, right-center, right) within parties as well as across them. Yet Germans of every ideological stripe seem to have a clearer idea of what they expect a health system to do. To an American observer inured to confusion and ideological dissonance over health care, the remarkable thing is the solid and durable social consensus on the fundamental values that undergird the German health care system. Almost no one questions that

- □ all residents of Germany, including all ethnic groups as well as noncitizens, should have access to health care;
- □ everyone has access to the same generous set of benefits;
- □ financing should be fair, and based on enrollees' income as much as possible;
- □ out-of-pocket medical expenses should be kept at nominal levels for most medical goods and services;
- □ professional autonomy, while if anything more sacrosanct than in the U.S., must sometimes give way to preserve the integrity of the total system.

Consensus on these central values, summed up in the frequently used term **social solidarity** (*Solidarität*), largely explains another remarkable feature of German health politics well worth copying: the vigilance and responsiveness of the political system in identifying and correcting problems, flaws, and imbalances. It is no accident that the (West) German *Bundestag* has passed no fewer than 12 major federal health reform acts since 1972[64] — an average of one every 20 months. Some of the explanation is due to Germany's parliamentary government structure, which features a highly stable and professional bureaucracy within the ministries that keep watch over health care. These civil servants (assisted by expert advisers from academia) identify emerging problems, fashion solutions, and help line up corrective action. But the continuous cycle of reform would not have been possible without a strong underlying value structure by which to judge when things were going awry and what sorts of remediable measures were justified.

A Comparison of Health Care Values

Reinhard Priester of the University of Minnesota's Center for Biomedical Ethics has dissected the values that currently underlie the U.S. health care enterprise, and, with colleagues in the Center's "New Ethic" project, has laid out a proposed new value system.[65] Using the Minnesota matrix, one can assay the major differences between U.S. and German values affecting health care. (Figure 8.9) In some cases, these differences are considerable. Americans are radically individualistic, the Germans believe in social solidarity. Americans distrust government, while Germans respect authority. It has only very recently begun to dawn on Americans that there may be limits to their accustomed horizons of improving prosperity or their ability to indulge in death-defying technology. Germans, having suffered terrible privation and disastrous wartime defeats within living memory — not to mention centuries of cultural preoccupation about insufficient *Lebensraum*, or "living space" — are deeply conscious of limits.

In other respects, the German-U.S. values differential is more a matter of degree. For example, technology is a national fetish for both cultures, although Germans try to balance technological fixes with a belief in "natural" healing to a degree that would strike most Americans as downright odd. Physician autonomy is high in both societies, to a dysfunctional degree, but in Germany the medical profession has retained a degree of clout not seen by U.S. organized medicine since the 1960s. This may derive from a strong German tendency to respect authority, which affects not only professional autonomy but also the autonomy of the German patient, who is less insistent on his rights than the typical American.

Seen through this prism, it is easier to understand the underpinnings of the German health system and the failure of the U.S. to enact anything remotely similar. For instance, Botelho argues that American society's traditionally strong belief in individual liberty over social equity, coupled with "the myth of unlimited resources," has allowed the U.S. to place a higher value on a "negative right" — the right not to be interfered with by society or government — than on the positive right to health care for all.[66] Germans, with their bedrock belief in fairness, find this attitude reprehensible.

Deemphasizing Dysfunctional Values

These very real and fundamental differences should not be taken to mean that the U.S. has nothing to learn from German experience. First, as argued earlier in this book, there are also striking similarities between both systems, as well as convergences in the pressures operating on both. Second, value systems may be slow to change, but they are not immutable. Neither should political leaders and concerned citizens view themselves as helpless to alter the *status quo* in health care-related values.

Figure 8.9

Values Underlying the U.S. and German Health Systems

U.S. Values	German Values

Fundamental outlook

Faith in individualism	Faith in social supports
Distrust of government	Respect for authority
Preference for private solutions to social problems	Belief in social solidarity as solution to social problems
Belief in power of technology	Belief in technology balanced by belief in natural forces
Standard of abundance as normal state of affairs	Current abundance as something to be guarded and preserved

Principal health care values

Professional autonomy	Professional autonomy, buttressed by high respect for authority
Patient autonomy	Patient autonomy tempered by deference to authority
Consumer sovereignty (freedom to choose both health plan and physician)	Limited consumer sovereignty (limited freedom to choose health plan, freedom to choose physician)
Patient's interests first	Patient interest primary, but societal interests a factor
Access of individual presenting patient to highest quality care	Universal access to high quality of care

Source: Adapted from Reinhard Priester, "A Values System for Health Care Reform," Health Affairs, Vol. 11, No. 1.

This is not a theoretical argument. Recent examples are at hand illustrating how health care values are being reordered in both societies. In both instances, they involve changes in the political and professional dominance of physicians — a value that has been determinative for decades in health policy setting.

The German example is the cataclysmic defeat suffered by organized medicine in its 1992 attempt to fend off some of the most far-reaching limits on doctors' professional autonomy in the history of the German system. The *Health Care Structural Reform Act* that took effect on January 1, 1993, puts German physicians on stringent budgets when prescribing medication. It also clamps down on the number of physicians permitted to enter ambulatory care practice (see Chapter Four). Two more dramatic incursions on German physicians' traditional prerogatives can scarcely be imagined, and the profession fought fiercely against them. This was barely a year after the West German medical establishment preempted any inclination of reformers to seize reunification as an opportunity to experiment with alternatives to fee-for-service practice. Whether or not doctors regain their former clout, the abrupt turnabout indicates how determined Germans are to protect their health care system from financial destabilization. And it shows how deeply ingrained values can change when circumstances require.

The U.S. example is less dramatic, but perhaps no less fundamental. As recently as the 1970s, the American Medical Association held near-absolute veto power over federal health legislation as well as who might or might not be appointed to high federal health posts. The AMA's price for not blocking enactment of Medicare in 1965 was President Johnson's agreement not to let the new program interfere with the practice of medicine and to require it to pay doctors' "usual and customary" fees. But the AMA and state medical societies have long since lost their ability to fend off salaried group practice. Complain as they do about the "hassle factor," U.S. physician groups also seem impotent to stave off a slew of recent intrusive innovations in medical practice and physician payment. And during the deliberations of Hillary Rodham Clinton's health reform task force in early 1993, Clinton Administration officials minced no words when telling AMA Executive Vice President James S. Todd that his organization was merely one special interest voice among many that would not be allowed a seat at the task force's table.

More Changes on the Way

Germany's 1993 reform was apparently the beginning of a new cycle of health care changes that promises to challenge other long-held German values. Opening up all sickness funds to German-style "managed competition" is intended to wipe away structural barriers that predate Bismarck's health program in order to preserve the more important values of systemwide equity and efficiency. More startling, there is considerable discussion among German policymakers about limiting the system's generous benefit package and requiring more cost-sharing by beneficiaries. This is no easy thing to do in a society that harbors "a strong sense of entitlement that grows from one hundred years of ever-expanding insurance," as political scientist Deborah Stone of Brandeis University puts it.[67]

An earlier reform in 1989 featured bruising battles over the government's successful attempt to impose sharp limits on sickness funds' payments for taxi trips to doctors' appointments, and on curtailment of *Sterbegeld*, or funeral benefits. The latter, said one high-ranking health ministry official, was said to spell "the end of Western funeral culture as we know it."[68] As Stone explains it: "Aunt Hildegard paid into the system all her life, why should she have to pay five Marks a day for hospital care? Her grandmother and great grandmother paid their premiums and got their care. Why shouldn't she?"[69] But from the additional cost-sharing in the 1993 reform act, it appears that the ice has been broken and German policymakers intend more thorough examinations and challenges of the prevailing benefits and their underlying values. As novel as it seems from an American vantage point, they are trying to anticipate future pressures on the system from a rapidly aging society, which brings a pressing need for long term care insurance as well as other demands. "We must decide whether certain benefits cannot be left up to the insured persons themselves," says Gerhard Schulte, the third-ranking official in the Federal Health Ministry. "The wealth of the past decades has made us far too accustomed to classifying everything conceivable as solidarity."[70] Schulte offered some examples:

> If we want to continue to be in a position in the future to pay for a hip operation or a kidney transplant for a 75-year-old, within the framework of the statutory health insurance system, then our citizens must be prepared to pay at least the cost of their food in the hospital. It is also questionable whether we will be continue to be able to afford to send all insured persons for a four- to six-week course of treatment at a health spa at three-year intervals in the future.[71]

Schulte's American counterparts can only wish for such problems!

Achieving Value Change

If modification of long-held values is *sine qua non* of meaningful health care reform, it is also a tall order. Germany's example suggests that it helps to start with a clear articulation of the important values, something the U.S. has never managed. "Explicit values can help us reach agreement on what we should reasonably get out of the system, make clear the trade-offs we face, and force us to have more realistic expectations," Priester says.[72] It is up to leaders of all types, starting with the President and encompassing reformers at all levels of professional and civic life, to achieve consensus on a clear and concise set of health care values that should govern the new system. Then it is their responsibility to articulate and sell these core values, a task far more important than explaining all the complicated and necessary details.

In articulating this new value system, the overriding lesson from Germany is that fair access to a reasonable set of health care benefits should head the list. The long dominance of provider autonomy (which has come to encompass hospitals, insurers, health plans and other strong provider interests as well as physicians) should be made subordinate to fair and universal access as *the* guiding principle of the U.S. health care system. Cost control, in this schema, would not be a fundamental or isolated value as it has been, without success, throughout the 1980s. Important as it is, controlling costs should be seen as necessary only in order to achieve and maintain fair and universal access to a decent standard of care.

Though the Germans call this idea solidarity, Americans will need to find their own language for the new operative ideal of fairness. Call it what you will, this is the controlling idea of humane and effective health care policy. It is the take-home message for any American who would learn the secret of Germany's long success in health care.

References and Notes

1. Field, MJ and Shapiro, HT, editors (1993). *Employment and Health Benefits: A Connection at Risk*. Washington: National Academy Press, p. 57.

2. Glaser, WA (1993). Unpublished manuscript.

3. Field, MJ and Shapiro, HT (1993), p. 58.

4. Ibid.

5. Field, MJ and Shapiro, HT (1993), p. 59.

6. Starr, P (1982). *The Social Transformation of American Medicine*. New York: Basic Books, p. 252.

7. Hennessey, ME (1935). *Four Decades of Massachusetts Politics: 1890-1935*. Norwood, MA.: Norwood Press, p. 244.

8. Starr, P (1982), p. 253, quoting from Ronald L. Numbers (1978). *Almost Persuaded: American Physicians and Compulsory Health Insurance*. Baltimore: Johns Hopkins University Press, pp. 75-77.

9. Glaser, WA (1993).

10. Fein, R (1986). *Medical Care, Medical Costs: The Search for a Health Insurance Policy*. Cambridge, MA: Harvard University Press, p. 42.

11. Fein, R (1986), p. 49.

12. Employee Benefit Research Institute (1993). *Sources of Health Insurance and Characteristics of the Uninsured*. Washington: EBRI, p. 5.

13. Glaser, WA (1993).

14. Jönsson, B (1989). What Can Americans Learn from Europeans? *Health Care Financing Review*, Annual Supplement 1989, p. 92.

15. Glaser, WA (1993).

16. Rodwin, VG (1987). American Exceptionalism in the Health Sector: The Advantages of "Backwardness" in Learning from Abroad. *Medical Care Review*, Vol. 44, No. 1, pp. 119-152.

17. Schwartz, LL and Stanton, MW (1992). Social Problems That Escalate America's Health Care Costs. *The Internist*, July-August, 1992, p. 16.

18. Statistische Bundesamt (1992). *Statistische Jahresbuch 1992*. Bonn: Statistische Bundesamt, p. 504.

19. U.S. Department of Health and Human Services (1991). *Health United States 1991*. *Washington: HHS, p. 122.*

20. Statistische Bundeasamt (1992), p. 127.

21. *Statistical Abstract of the U.S.* (1992), p. 383.

22. Wicks, EK (1992). *German Health Care: Financing, Administration, and Coverage.* Washington: Health Insurance Association of America, p. 16.

23. U.S. Centers for Disease Control, personal communication, April, 1993.

24. Bundesministerium für Gesundheit (1991), p. 114

25. Ibid, p. 75.

26. U.S. Department of Health and Human Services (1991), p. 187.

27. Bundesministerium für Gesundheit (1991), p. 54.

28. U.S. Department of Health and Human Services (1991), p. 209.

29. Bundesministerium für Gesundheit (1991), p. 46.

30. Selbmann, H-K (1992). The German Health Care System: A Model for the United States? Presentation at a Goethe Institute symposium on German health care, October 16-17, 1992.

31. U.S. Department of Health and Human Services (1991), p. 132.

32. Henning, A (1986). Maternal and Child Care. *Political Values and Health Care: The German Experience.* Cambridge, MA: MIT Press, pp. 477-480.

33. Jost, TS (1990). *Assuring the Quality of Medical Practice: An International Comparative Study.* London: King Edward's Hospital Fund, p. 61.

34. Selbmann, H-K (1992).

35. Bundesministerium für Gesundheit (1991), p. 18.

36. Ibid, p. 19.

37. Ibid.

38. Wicks, EK (1992), p. 16.

39. Bundesministerium für Gesundheit (1991), p. 299.

40. Selbmann, H-K (1992).

41. Newhouse, JP (1992). Medical Care Costs: How Much Welfare Loss? *Journal of Economic Perspectives*, Vol. 6, No. 3, pp. 3-21.

42. Marmor, TR (1991). Misleading Notions: Social, Political and Economic Myths Prevent Us from Learning from Other Countries' Experiences in Financing Health Care. *Health Management Quarterly*, Vol. 13, No. 4, p. 18.

43. Rodwin, VG (1987), pp. 120, 136.

44. Newhouse, JE (1986). Rate Adjusters for Medical under Capitation. *Health Care Financing Review*, 1986 annual supplement, pp. 45-46.

45. Henke, K-D (1991). Fiscal Problems of German Unity: The Case of Health Care. *Staatswissenschaften und Staatspraxis*, Vol. 2, No. 2, p. 174.

46. Selbmann, H-K (1992), personal interview.

47. American Hospital Association (1992-93). *Hospital Statistics: A Comprehensive Survey of U.S. Hospitals*. Chicago: AHA, p. 208.

48. Lohr, KN, et.al. (1992). Health Care Systems: Lessons from International Comparisons. *Health Affairs*, Vol. 11, No. 4, pp. 239-241.

49. Blendon, RJ (1993). Personal interview, April 8, 1993.

50. Enthoven, AC (1993). The History and Principles of Managed Competition. *Health Affairs*, Vol. 12, special supplement, p. 29.

51. Reischauer, RD (1993). Written testimony before the Subcommittee on Health, Committee on Ways and Means, U.S. House of Representatives, March 2, 1993, p. 15.

52. Enthoven, AC (1993), p. 42.

53. Starr, P and Zelman, WA (1993). A Bridge to Compromise: Competition Under a Budget. *Health Affairs*, Vol. 12, special supplement, p. 8.

54. Reinhardt, UE (1993). The Jackson Hole Initiatives for a 21st Century American Care Health Care System: A Comment. *Health Economics*, forthcoming.

55. Ibid.

56. Blendon, RJ (1993).

57. Chupp, N et.al. (1993). Managed Competition: An Analysis of Consumer Concerns. Working paper, January, 1993, p. 3.

58. Starr, P (1992). *The Logic of Health Care Reform: Transforming American Medicine for the Better*. Knoxville, Tenn.: Grand Rounds Press, p. 71.

59. Ethoven, AC (1993), pp. 43-44.

60. Glaser, WA (1993). The Competition Vogue and Its Outcomes. *The Lancet*, Vol. 341, p. 810

61. Starr, P and Zelman, WA (1993), p. 18.

62. Hess, R (1992). Presentation at a Goethe Institute conference on German Health in Boston, October 16, 1992.

63. Botelho, RJ (1991). Overcoming the Prejudice Against Establishing a National Health Care System. *Caring for the Uninsured and Underinsured*. Chicago: American Medical Association, p. 146.

64. Schneider, M (1991). Health care cost containment in the Federal Republic of Germany. *Health Care Financing Review*, Vol. 12, No. 3, pp. 90-91; and other sources.

65. Priester, R (1992). A Values Framework for Health System Reform. *Health Affairs*, Vol. 11, No. 1, pp. 88-107.

66. Botelho, RJ (1991), p. 150.

67. Stone, D (1991). German Unification: East Meets West in the Doctor's Office. *Journal of Health Politics, Policy and Law*. Vol. 16, No. 2, p. 410.

68. Vielhaber, T (1991). Personal interview, March 8, 1991.

69. Stone, D (1991), p. 410.

70. Schulte, G (1992). Problems of Health Care in the Conflict Area between Market Economy and Governmental Economic Control. Presentation at a Goethe Institute conference on German health care in Boston, October 16, 1992.

71. Ibid.

72. Priester, R (1992), p. 85.

GLOSSARY

Allgemeine Ortskrankenkassen — Local sickness funds, called *AOK* for short. (*Allgemeine* means "general" and *Ort* means "place" or "locality"). *AOK*s must insure all applicants within their service areas. They cover 37 percent of the population, more than any of the other seven sickness fund types.

Allgemeine Patienten Verband — Patients' Defense Union, one of two national patient advocacy groups.

ambulatories — Primary care centers in East Germany. Part of a network of health care established by Soviet decree in 1947 that included ambulatories and polyclinics.

AOK — *Allgemeine Ortskrankenkassen*, local sickness funds.

Ärztekammer — State "physicians' chamber," a government- chartered organ of physician self-government. Each state's *Ärztekammer* is essentially a physician licensure agency. Membership is compulsory for all practicing physicians. The chamber promulgates and enforces a detailed code of ethics and medical practice regulations which has the force of law. It also certifies specialists and handles matters of professional discipline. At the federal level there is a Federal Physicians' Chamber, or *Bundesärztekammer*, which represents physicians in professional matters in federal-level negotiations, but is not a "body of public law" as state chambers are.

Associations of Sickness Fund Physicians — Called *kassenärztliche Vereinigungen* or *KV*s, they function as the intermediary between sickness funds and individual doctors in ambulatory practice. They collect capitated funds from sickness funds for the outpatient care of subscribers in their region, and distribute payments to member doctors based on the fee-for-service bills submitted by physicians. In order to receive sickness fund reimbursement for ambulatory care, a doctor must belong to the local *KV*.

Aufschwung Ost — "Soaring East," a 1990-91 aid effort, mounted by the federal German government, to restore and rebuild hospitals and facilities for the elderly and disabled in eastern Germany. It was estimated to cost $2.4 billion in PPP terms.

Bavarian Contract — An experiment launched in 1979 in the German state of Bavaria that relieved doctors from a ceiling on physician spending if they could demonstrate savings in other sectors subject to their control.

Bedarfsplan — Hospital "need plan" (plural: *Bedarfspläne*), developed by each German state to govern major capital expenditures by hospitals.

Beitragssatz — "Contribution rate" or premium charged by sickness funds for coverage. The *Beitragssatz* is split evenly between employers and employees.

Beratung — Physician consultation.

Betriebskrankenkassen — Sickness funds based in medium-sized to large firms, similar to self-insurance plans in the U.S. (*Betrieb* means "business enterprise" or "factory.") *Betriebskrankenkassen* are the most numerous type of sickness fund, but they cover only about 11 percent of the German population.

birth bounty — DM 1,000 paid in cash to pregnant East German women in installments after each prenatal care appointment and after four postnatal care checkups.

Bundesärztekammer — German Medical Association, a federal-level organization that represents physicians on professional matters (see *Ärztekammer*).

Bundesrat—The upper chamber of the German parliament made up of representatives from state governments.

Bundesverband der Pharmazeutischen Industrie e.V. (BPI) — German Pharmaceutical Industry Association.

Christian Democratic Union — Center-right German political party with leading role in governing coalition since 1987. Closely allied with the Christian Democratic Union (*CUD*), a conservative party based in Bavaria.

Central Health Administration — Set up in East Germany in 1946, it was the first central authority in German history responsible for the entire health system.

Charité Hospital — A 260-year-old, 2,100-bed teaching hospital in the formerly communist sector of Berlin. It is one of the oldest hospitals in the nation.

Concerted Action in Health Care — *Konzertierte Aktion im Gesundheitswesen*, an advisory panel created by the German Parliament in 1977 to help "steer" the system. Chaired by the Minister of Health, it is made up of more than five dozen representatives of payers, labor unions, physicians, hospitals, pharmaceutical companies, medical equipment manufacturers, and other interested parties.

comfort services — Refers to private rooms and more immediate attention from staff in hospitals, services available to those who are privately insured.

Committee on Social Insurance — A group established by the American Medical Association in 1916 to examine reform of the U.S. health system on a model similar to the German system.

corporatism — The organization of society into formal interest groups which, by custom or by law, are authorized to represent their members in the operation of a social function. In German health care, nongovernmental groups of consumers (usually represented by labor unions), employers, payers (sickness funds), and providers (physicians, hospitals, and others) negotiate the terms of their relationships and carry out the daily operation of the system with the oversight of federal and state governments. The governing principle is that socially undesirable concentrations of power in one or another vested interest can be prevented by giving these organizations powers over one another.

DÄV—*Deutsche Ärztevereinsbund*

detailers—A term applied to drug salespeople who visit doctors to provide scientific "information" and patient samples.

Der Spiegel — A leading national newsmagazine in Germany.

Deutsche Ärztevereinsbund — Umbrella group of medical associations in late 19th and early 20th centuries whose goal was to promote a national medical code. The national government ruled this was the province of the states, and the *DÄV* was superseded by state *Ärztekammer* and the *Hartmannbund*.

diagnosis-related group (DRG) — A U.S. payment system, used by the Medicare program and a growing number of private insurers, which reimburses hospitals a fixed amount for each of about 480 diagnoses, regardless of length of stay or utilization of specific services.

Ersatzkassen — "Substitute funds," sickness funds for salaried white-collar workers and certain blue-collar workers. *Ersatzkassen* are part of Germany's statutory health insurance system (*Gesetzliche Krankenversicherung* or *GKV*), but for historical reasons are not part of the original group of statutory funds, called *Reichsversicherungsordnung* (*RVO*) funds. *Ersatzkassen* insures about 31 percent of the German population, making them next in size to the *AOK* funds (see above). They pay physicians somewhat higher rates and their governance is by members exclusively rather than by members and their employers.

Fallpauschalen — Lump sum payments to cover costs of particular treatments and procedures related to certain diagnoses.

Federal Health Agency — The German equivalent of the U.S. Food and Drug Administration.

Federal Republic of Germany (FRG) — Founded in 1949 after the defeat of the Third Reich in World War II, the FRG until 1990 was known as West Germany. It now encompasses the former German Democratic Republic (GDR). The FRG consists of 16 states and city-states with a population of 80.3 million in 1992.

Festbetrage — Fixed price or "reference price" for certain classes of pharmaceuticals, an innovation contained in a 1989 federal reform law intended to reduce health care cost inflation. (Plural: *Festbeträge*.)

Finanzausgleich — A risk equalization scheme among sickness funds contained in a 1993 federal health care reform law. It is intended to adjust for varying risk profiles among sickness funds, taking into account members' income levels, age, sex, and number of dependents. In combination with open enrollment among sickness funds, officials hope *Finanzausgleich* will lead to greater competition among sickness funds on the basis of their quality of service and efficiency.

Frankfurter Allgemeine Zeitung — A leading German newspaper, based in Frankfurt.

Free Democratic Party — The junior member of the ruling coalition in Germany. It has an economically conservative philosophy and is often thought to represent businessmen and professionals.

führer — Director, manager, or chief (of an enterprise or department).

Free German Trade Union — Provided health and other social insurance for 89 percent of the citizens of communist East Germany. The rest were covered by the state.

GDP — Gross domestic product, the total value of all goods and services produced within the borders of a nation.

gegliedert — "Articulated," in reference to the German health system, a segmented system of sickness funds whose members are differentiated by occupation, residence, income, and social class.

German Democratic Republic — Formal name for former East Germany.

Gesetzliche Krankenversicherung (GKV) — Statutory Sickness Insurance. Germany's system of compulsory health insurance for all citizens whose earnings fall below a certain ceiling. It includes eight different types of sickness funds.

Gesundheitsreform Gesetz (GRG) — Health Reform Law passed in 1989, designed to control rising costs, especially of pharmaceuticals.

Gesundheitsstruktur Gesetz (GSG) — Health Care Structural Reform Law passed in December, 1992, and effective on January 1, 1993.

global budget — A fixed expenditure limit, applied either to total health care spending or to spending by a particular provider sector, such as physicians or hospitals.

guilds — Organizations of tradesmen founded in the Middle Ages which defined the qualifications needed to practice a trade or craft and limited entry into the field. Guild sickness funds provided the original self-help model upon which Germany's statutory sickness funds were based in 1883.

Hartmannbund — A national organization of office-based doctors, founded in 1900 as the *Leipziger Vorband* and named after its original leader, Herman Hartmann, MD. Its full name is Union of German Physicians for the Defense of Their Economic Interests.

HICCA — *Health Insurance Cost Containment Act.*

Health Care Structural Reform Act — *Gesundheitsstruktur Gesetz.* Passed in December, 1992, a comprehensive health cost containment law.

Health Insurance Act of 1883 — Law introduced by Chancellor Otto von Bismark that founded the German system of compulsory employment-based health insurance.

Health Insurance Cost Containment Act — A 1977 law which launched a series of cost containment efforts that persists into the 1990s. Among its provisions was one that established a national council called Concerted Action in Health Care.

HIPC — Health Insurance Purchasing Cooperative (see "managed competition").

Hospital Financing Act — Passed in 1972, this legislation set up the German hospital planning apparatus linking "need plan" compliance with capital funding and the guarantee of full operating cost reimbursement.

Hospital Cost Containment Acts of 1981 and 1982 — Laws which brought hospitals into the Concerted Action mechanism and removed their exemption from cost controls.

HMO — health maintenance organization.

Imperial Insurance Decree — Also called *Reichsversicherungsordnung* or *RVO*, a 1911 set of regulations which codified the German health insurance system.

Innungskrankenkassen — Craft-based sickness funds (*Innung* means "guild").

IPA — Independent practice association, a U.S. form of health financing and delivery in which independent fee-for-service physicians agree to provide care for reduced rates and with utilization controls in order to gain access to IPA members, who typically pay a fixed monthly premium for comprehensive benefits with limited out-of-pocket expenses.

Krankenversicherung der Rentner — "Sickness Insurance for Pensioners," or the system of health insurance for German retirees, which provides for a system of cross-subsidization among sickness funds depending on their respective proportions of pensioners.

kassenärztliche Vereinigungen (KVs) — Regional associations of sickness fund physicians which serve as intermediaries between office-based doctors and sickness funds (see Associations of Sickness Fund Physicians).

Kassenlöwen —"Fund lions" or utilization reviewers employed by *KV*s to monitor physician billing activity and look for statistical outliers.

Kellertreppeneffekt — "Cellar stairs effect," a term used by German hospital officials to describe how cost-cutting in one year results in lower per diem rates the following year, punishing hospitals that are more economical.

Knappschaftskassen — Miners' sickness funds (*Knappschaft* means "body of miners").

Konzertierte Aktion im Gesundheitswesen — Concerted Action in Health Care panel.

Kopfpauschale — "Lump sum per head" or capitation rate for each sickness fund member.

Krankenschein — Sickness certificates presented to physicians by sickness fund members for treatment. Physicians list procedures performed for each patient on the *Krankenschein* and submit the certificates to the regional *kassenärztliche Vereinigung* on a quarterly basis. The *KV* tallies the amount owed, pays the doctors, and monitors its members for excessive utilization.

Kurkliniks — Resort spas which offer mineral baths and other restorative treatments, physical therapy, exercise regimens, and rehabilitation.

Kurkrankenhäuser — Spa hospitals, specializing in rehabilitation.

KV — *kassenärztliche Vereinigungen*, Associations of Sickness Fund Physicians.

Länder — German states (singular: *das Land*).

Lebensraum — "Living space."

Leipziger Vorband — Physicians' economic lobbying group founded in 1900 in Leipzig with 21 original members. Became known as the *Hartmannbund* after its founding leader, Herman Hartmann, MD.

Leistungswille — The determination to accomplish something.

managed competition — A proposed U.S. system of health care delivery featuring regionally organized groups of health care purchasers who negotiate over the price of a standard comprehensive benefit package with organized groups of care providers.

Marburgerbund — Trade union of hospital-based salaried doctors and salaried health officials.

Medicaid — Publicly funded insurance coverage for low income individuals in the U.S.

Medical Service Organization (MSO) — German utilization review agencies created by a 1989 reform law. Similar in concept to American Professional Review Organizations (PROs), their purpose is to ensure that medical care is appropriate, high-quality, and efficient.

Medicare — U.S. system of health care insurance for those over 65 years old and for the disabled, funded by payroll taxes and general revenues.

Mutterpass — "Mother's pass," a German checklist on which doctors record the results of pregnant women's checkups, designed to encourage early and regular prenatal care.

negative list — A German "blacklist" of drugs shown to have no value or to be useful only for minor ailments, such as coughs and colds. Introduced in a 1989 reform law, the statute forbade sickness fund payments for drugs on the list.

New Hospital Regulation Law — German federal statute implemented in 1985 which put responsibility for hospital capital investment solely on state governments, ending a 13- year era of joint federal-state responsibility.

Neue Bundesländer — Five new states of reunified Germany that once made up East Germany.

niedergelassen Arzt — "Settled-down doctor" or office-based physician.

OECD — Organization for Economic Cooperation and Development.

Ossies — Slang term for former East Germans.

orientation parameter — Term for a voluntary global budget used in reference to a drug-expenditure ceiling included in *HICCA* to alter physician prescribing patterns.

outliers — Values which lie outside a statistical norm.

panel doctors — Doctors admitted to sickness fund practice. In the early 1900s, sickness funds recruited physicians to their panels who were willing to work for low wages, often because they had not passed their board exams.

Pflegesatz — Per diem rates paid by sickness funds to hospitals for the care of fund members.

Physician Chambers — Regional organizations that, by law, German physicians must belong to. They have authority over licensing, specialty certification, and physician discipline.

PMA — Pharmaceutical Manufacturer's Association (U.S.)

polyclinics — Multispecialty group clinics in eastern Germany. Part of a network of health care established by Soviet decree in 1947. Their staffs included salaried physicians, social workers, physical therapists, psychologists, and other personnel.

PPO — Preferred provider organization, a U.S. form of health care financing which offers subscribers comprehensive coverage and relatively low out-of-pocket costs if they go to "preferred providers" — doctors, hospitals, pharmacists and others who give the insurer a discount. If subscribers choose to go to other than preferred providers, they must pay an additional cost.

PPP — Purchasing power parities.

Preisvergleichsliste — A comparative list of single-agent drugs and their prices.

Price Office — State agencies in Germany which had ultimate rate-setting powers over hospital charges between 1981 and 1985. They retain approval power over arbitrated prices set by state hospital associations and state associations of statutory sickness funds.

Professional Medical Code — A detailed body of regulations, which carry the force of law, developed and occasionally revised by the German Medical Association (*Bundesärztekammer*).

purchasing power parities — PPPs are an international monetary conversion formula based upon comparisons of a price-weighted "market basket" of goods and services. PPPs have advantages over monetary exchange rates because they are more stable and may more accurately reflect the purchasing power of a given unit of currency. PPPs are used in this text wherever possible.

reference pricing system — A system of allowable reimbursement levels for drugs. Any amount over the reference price must be paid by the patient.

Regierungskrankenhaus — Hospital for high government or communist party officials in former East Germany.

Regresspflicht — Liability for monetary restitution.

Reichstag — The German Parliament prior to the establishment of the Federal Republic of Germany in 1949.

Reichsversicherungsordnung (RVO) — A 1911 set of regulations which codified the German health insurance system.

Richtgrössen — Prescription volume controls that put individual doctors at direct financial risk for the volume of drugs they were prescribing.

Rudolf-Virchow-Bund — A short-lived group of public health-oriented doctors and other health workers created after reunification in 1990 to defend the East German polyclinic system of health care delivery.

RVO **funds** — Sickness funds regulated by the *Reichsversicherungsordnung*, which include all but the two types of *Ersatzkassen*.

Selbstkostendeckungs-Prinzip — "Self cost-reimbursement principle," a guarantee that hospitals would be reimbursed for their full costs.

Selbstverwartung — Principle of "self-regulation" under which the countervailing powers of workers, employers, and health care providers are supposed to produce a compromise that works for all parties with a minimum of government interference.

Sicherstellungsauftrag — "Task of assuring the supply of services." Some consider this a polite description of "monopoly franchise."

sickness funds — Nonprofit health insurers in Germany. Based on self-help medieval organizations in which members paid fixed amounts in exchange for cash benefits in times of sickness, injury, or death.

Social Code of West Germany — Multivolume set of laws and regulations governing the whole structure of health insurance, health care providers, institutions, organizations, and federal-state relations in the realm of health care.

Soforthilfeprogramm — "Immediate aid program," a federal initiative which provided $248 million in 1990 to begin the process of rebuilding eastern Germany's failing health care infrastructure.

Solidarität — Social "solidarity," a value system that is the cornerstone of the German health care system. It involves a social consensus that the risks and costs of health care must be shared.

Sonderentgelte — "Special payments," a system of flat-rate payments for particular specialized hospital services, outside the usual per-diem system of hospital reimbursement.

Sozialistische Einheitspartie Deutschlands (SED) — The communist party of East Germany.

Stasi — East Germany's secret police agency.

Sterbegeld — "Death money," funeral benefits traditionally paid by sickness funds, curtailed by a 1989 reform law.

substitute funds — *Ersatzkassen*. A category of nationally based sickness funds, seven in number, open primarily to white-collar workers. They provide almost identical benefits as the primary sickness funds (*RVO* funds) but carry a degree of social cachet because membership is a sign of higher employment status. Substitute funds pay doctors twice as much as *RVO* funds, which reportedly buy their members better physician service.

tariffs — Private health insurance premiums in Germany.

thalidomide — A drug used by women in some European countries in the 1960s to prevent morning sickness until it was determined that the drug was causing extensive birth defects in their babies. Thalidomide was never approved for use in the U.S.

transparency list — A government pharmaceutical list detailing the price of a drug along with its pharmacokinetic data, active-agent content, identity, purity, and stability. Doctors are technically required to consider these attributes when prescribing pharmaceuticals.

Treaty of Reunification — Treaty reuniting East and West Germany, signed August 31, 1990.

VAT — Value-added tax, a tax added at each stage in the production of a product.

verboten — "Forbidden."

Weimar Settlement — A 1931 agreement between sickness funds and physician groups which more than doubled the number of doctors that funds were obliged to admit into their panels, and which established associations of sickness fund doctors to negotiate collectively with the funds over reimbursement.

Weltanschauung — "World-view," "philosophy," or "ideology."

Wende — "Turning point," "new epoch," the colloquial reference to reunification.

Wessies — Slang term for West Germans.

Zeitgeist — "Spirit of the times."

Zentrum **Party** — "Center Party," a conservative political party allied with the Roman Catholic Church influential in Germany until the 1890s. It was philosophically opposed to government intervention in social affairs as contrary to "natural law," which requires individuals to be dependent only on God.

INDEX